Modules in Applied Mathematics: Volume 4

Edited by William F. Lucas

Modules in Applied Mathematics

Volume 1
Differential Equation Models
Martin Braun, Courtney S. Coleman, and Donald A. Drew, *Editors*

Volume 2
Political and Related Models
Steven J. Brams, William F. Lucas, and Philip D. Straffin, Jr., *Editors*

Volume 3
Discrete and System Models
William F. Lucas, Fred S. Roberts, and Robert M. Thrall, *Editors*

Volume 4
Life Science Models
Helen Marcus-Roberts and Maynard Thompson, *Editors*

Life Science Models

Edited by
Helen Marcus-Roberts
and Maynard Thompson

With 80 Illustrations

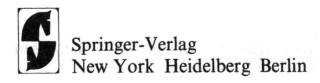

Springer-Verlag
New York Heidelberg Berlin

Helen Marcus-Roberts

Department of Mathematics and Computer Science
Montclair State College
Upper Montclair, NJ 07043
USA

Maynard Thompson

Department of Mathematics
Indiana University
Bloomington, IN 47405
USA

AMS Subject Classifications: 00A69; 92A01, 02, 07, 10, 15, 17

Library of Congress Cataloging in Publication Data

Modules in applied mathematics.
  Includes bibliographies.
  Contents: —v. 2. Political and related models / edited by Steven J. Brams, William F. Lucas, and Philip D. Straffin, Jr.—   —v. 4. Life science models / edited by Helen Marcus-Roberts and Maynard Thompson.
  1. Mathematics—1961– .   2. Mathematical models. I. Lucas, William F., 1933– .
QA37.2.M6 1982 510 82-10439

This book was prepared with the support of NSF grants Nos. SED77-07482, SED75-00713, and SED72-07370. However, any opinions, findings, conclusions, and/or recommendations herein are those of the authors and do not necessarily reflect the views of NSF.

Softcover reprint of the hardcover 1st edition 1983

Typeset by Asco Trade Typesetting Ltd., Hong Kong.

9 8 7 6 5 4 3 2 1

ISBN-13: 978-1-4612-5461-4   e-ISBN-13: 978-1-4612-5459-1
DOI: 10.1007/978-1-4612-5459-1

Preface

The purpose of this four volume series is to make available for college teachers and students samples of important and realistic applications of mathematics which can be covered in undergraduate programs. The goal is to provide illustrations of how modern mathematics is actually employed to solve relevant contemporary problems. Although these independent chapters were prepared primarily for teachers in the general mathematical sciences, they should prove valuable to students, teachers, and research scientists in many of the fields of application as well. Prerequisites for each chapter and suggestions for the teacher are provided. Several of these chapters have been tested in a variety of classroom settings, and all have undergone extensive peer review and revision. Illustrations and exercises are included in most chapters. Some units can be covered in one class, whereas others provide sufficient material for a few weeks of class time.

Volume 1 contains 23 chapters and deals with differential equations and, in the last four chapters, problems leading to partial differential equations. Applications are taken from medicine, biology, traffic systems and several other fields. The 14 chapters in Volume 2 are devoted mostly to problems arising in political science, but they also address questions appearing in sociology and ecology. Topics covered include voting systems, weighted voting, proportional representation, coalitional values, and committees. The 14 chapters in Volume 3 emphasize discrete mathematical methods such as those which arise in graph theory, combinatorics, and networks. These techniques are used to study problems in economics, traffic theory, operations research, decision theory, and other fields. Volume 4 has 12 chapters concerned with mathematical models in the life sciences. These include aspects of population growth and behavior, biomedicine (epidemics, genetics and bio-engineering), and ecology.

These four volumes are the result of two educational projects sponsored by The Mathematical Association of America (MAA) and supported in part by the National Science Foundation (NSF). The objective was to produce needed material for the undergraduate curriculum. The first project was undertaken by the MAA's Committee on the Undergraduate Program in Mathematics (CUPM). It was entitled Case Studies and Resource Materials for the Teaching of Applied Mathematics at the Advanced Undergraduate Level, and it received financial support from NSF grant SED72-07370 between September 1, 1972 and May 31, 1977. This project was completed under the direction of Donald Bushaw. Bushaw and William Lucas served as chairmen of CUPM during this effort, and George Pedrick was involved as the executive director of CUPM. The resulting report, which appeared in late 1976, was entitled *Case Studies in Applied Mathematics*, and it was edited by Maynard Thompson. It contained nine chapters by eleven authors, plus an introductory chapter and a report on classroom trials of the material.

The second project was initiated by the MAA's Committee on Institutes and Workshops (CIW). It was a summer workshop of four weeks duration entitled Modules in Applied Mathematics which was held at Cornell University in 1976. It was funded in part by NSF grant SED75-00713 and a small supplemental grant SED77-07482 between May 1, 1975 and September 30, 1978. William F. Lucas served as chairman of CIW at the time of the workshop and as director of this project. This activity lead to the production of 60 educational modules by 37 authors.

These four volumes contain revised versions of 9 of the 11 chapters from the report *Case Studies in Applied Mathematics*, 52 of the 60 modules from the workshop Modules in Applied Mathematics, plus two contributions which were added later (Volume 2, Chapters 7 and 14), for a total of 63 chapters. A preliminary version of the chapter by Steven Brams (Volume 2, Chapter 3), entitled "One Man, N Votes," was written in connection with the 1976 MAA Workshop. The expanded version presented here was prepared in conjunction with the American Political Science Association's project Innovation in Instructional Materials which was supported by NSF grant SED77-18486 under the direction of Sheilah K. Mann. The unit was published originally as a monograph entitled *Comparison Voting*, and was distributed to teachers and students for classroom field tests. This chapter was copyrighted by the APSA in 1978 and has been reproduced here with its permission.

An ad hoc committee of the MAA consisting of Edwin Beckenbach, Leonard Gillman, William Lucas, David Roselle, and Alfred Willcox was responsible for supervising the arrangements for publication and some of the extensive efforts that were necessary to obtain NSF approval of publication in this format. The significant contribution of Dr. Willcox throughout should be noted. George Springer also intervened in a crucial way at one point. It should be stressed, however, that any opinions or recommendations are those of the particular authors, and do not necessarily reflect the views of NSF, MAA, the editors, or any others involved in these project activities.

There are many other individuals who contributed in some way to the realization of these four volumes, and it is impossible to acknowledge all of them here. However, there are two individuals in addition to the authors, editors and people named above who should receive substantial credit for the ultimate appearance of this publication. Katherine B. Magann, who had provided many years of dedicated service to CUPM prior to the closing of the CUPM office, accomplished the production of the report *Case Studies in Applied Mathematics*. Carolyn D. Lucas assisted in the running of the 1976 MAA Workshop, supervised the production of the resulting sixty modules, and served as managing editor for the publication of these four volumes. Without her efforts and perseverance the final product of this major project might not have been realized.

July 1982   W. F. LUCAS

Preface for Volume 4

Most of the ongoing work in formulating and developing mathematical models in the life sciences is in one or more of these fields: populations, epidemics, genetics, ecology, pharmacokinetics and physiology. Each of these fields has several major subfields, and to adequately represent them all would require several volumes this size. The chapters included here do, however, provide a selection from some of the more important and highly developed areas. In addition, a variety of mathematical levels and techniques is illustrated.

Part I of this volume is concerned with population models. In addition to their importance in the biological sciences, population models also contribute to our understanding of problems in actuarial science, economics, political science and sociology. It is customary to classify population models according to the biological systems to which they apply, single species or multi-species; and also according to their mathematical character, deterministic or stochastic, discrete or continuous, analytic or simulation, etc. The first three chapters are concerned with the time evolution of a single species population. In the first, Hoppensteadt surveys both discrete and continuous models, and in the second Fennell gives a more detailed development of a discrete model. The third, by Marcus-Roberts, explores some of the relations between two important classes of population models: deterministic and stochastic. The fourth chapter of Part I by van der Vaart, provides a systematic introduction to multi-species models, and especially to the use of such models in ecosystem analysis. Each of the first four chapters is concerned with the time evolution of populations. In contrast, Chapter 12 by Solomon is another example of a population model, but one which is concerned with questions of spatial rather than temporal distribution.

The five chapters of Part II of this volume are devoted to biomedical models. Modern work in mathematical biomedicine is concerned, among other things, with the spread of epidemics, with inheritance, with bio-engineering, and with physiology. The study of the spread of communicable diseases was stimulated by the efforts of Kermack and McKendrick beginning in the 1920's. More recently, the 1957 book *The Mathematical Theory of Epidemics* by N. T. J. Bailey (revised as *The Mathematical Theory of Infectious Diseases and Its Applications*, 1976) served as a starting point for many developments. Chapter 5 on malaria, by Marcus-Roberts and Roberts, presents several models for the population dynamics of the malaria parasite, the causative organism of an historically important tropical disease. Another tropical disease, schistosomiasis, is the topic of the review of Mac-Donald's work by Ludwig and Haytock. Schistosomiasis and other helminth infections are considered by the World Health Organization to have major impacts on many tropical populations. The last chapter on epidemics is by Braun and is concerned with a model for the spread of gonorrhea over long time periods.

The mathematical study of genetics goes back to the pioneering work of Gregor Mendel, and has given much insight into the mechanisms of inheritance, both in individuals and in populations. In fact, the theoretical and practical advances in genetics resulting from the use of mathematical ideas has been a major stimulus to the search for other ways to use mathematical ideas in the life sciences. Here we present a single example of the application of mathematics in the study of problems of inheritance, specifically to the diversity of inherited traits. This is in Chapter 8 by Marcus-Roberts.

Much of mathematical biomedicine has been influenced by the mathematics of engineering. Chapter 9, by Drew, contains an example of a bio-engineering model. The chapter focuses on one aspect of the important medical problem of cigarette smoking, and specifically on the effect of a filter on a cigarette.

The three chapters in Part III of this volume are devoted to models of the behavior of biological populations. The first two chapters in this final part consider problems of energy use in food acquisition. Chapter 10 by Roberts shows how optimization questions arise in biological settings through a study of food acquisition by humans. Here the mathematical techniques of linear programming are illustrated. These techniques expand the set of mathematical tools (calculus, differential equations, combinatorics and probability) used in this volume. The second of the two chapters on energy use in obtaining food, by Roberts and Marcus-Roberts, is a parallel study of animal populations, making use of techniques of calculus, simulation, and probability. It is concerned with optimal foraging strategies of an energy efficient predator. The last chapter, by Solomon, studies the spatial distribution of cabbage butterfly eggs. It relates to the previous chapter in which the spatial distribution of food supply is studied. Both of these chapters use probabilistic methods to study spatial distributions. This final chapter makes the important point that even though a model may lead to good predictions, it does not necessarily follow that the model describes the actual biological mechanisms.

The biological models described in this volume represent a broad but certainly incomplete sample of the many ways in which mathematics relates to the life sciences. A particularly conspicuous omission is the use of mathematical models and computer simulations to study such physiological processes as circulation, digestion, and respiration, and such diseases as heart disease, cancer, and nervous disorders. Such methods have also been used profitably as an alternative to analytic models in the study of communicable diseases.

In some of the instances studied in this volume, e.g., genetics, the use of mathematics has led to significantly better understanding of the biology of the situations. In other instances, e.g., human demography, predictions based on mathematical models have had major social and economic implications. Although not all mathematical models in the life sciences are as useful as those applied in genetics and demography, there are expectations that as the models are refined with new mathematics and computing capability, and the basic processes are more completely understood, there will be significant contributions in other fields as well.

July, 1982   HELEN MARCUS-ROBERTS
                                                                            MAYNARD THOMPSON

Contents

Part I. Population Models

Chapter 1. Population Mathematics   1
Frank C. Hoppensteadt

  1. Introduction   1
  2. Formulation of a Model   2
  3. A Stable Age Distribution   5
  4. Population Waves   9
References   17

Chapter 2. Population Growth: An Age Structure Model   18
Robert E. Fennell

  1. Introduction   18
  2. An Example   18
  3. Powers of a Nonnegative Matrix   21
  4. Prediction and Implementation   24
  5. Conclusion   26
Appendix   28
Solutions to the Exercises   29
References   30
Notes for the Instructor   31

Chapter 3. A Comparison of Some Deterministic and Stochastic
Models of Population Growth   32
Helen Marcus-Roberts

  1. Introduction   32
  2. Basic Philosophy of Model Building   33

3. Probability Generating Functions (pgf's)   37
4. Derivation of the General System of Differential Equations for the Pure
   Birth Process   43
5. Models of Population Growth   46
References   77
Notes for the Instructor   77

Chapter 4. Some Examples of Mathematical Models for the
Dynamics of Several-Species Ecosystems   78
H. R. van der Vaart

Preface   78
1. Introduction   79
2. Predator-Prey   92
3. Mutualism and Competition   108
4. Some Remarks on *N*-Species Systems   111
Appendix A   114
Appendix B: Bibliography   148
References   149
Appendix C: Suggestions and Solutions   154

Part II. Biomedicine: Epidemics, Genetics, and Bioengineering

Chapter 5. Malaria: Models of the Population Dynamics of the
Malaria Parasite   161
Helen Marcus-Roberts and Fred S. Roberts

 1. Introduction   161
 2. Malaria   162
 3. The First Model   162
 4. The Second Model: Survival Proportions   163
 5. A Look at Data   166
 6. The Third Model: Varying Survival Proportions   167
 7. The Fourth Model: Varying Reproduction Numbers   169
 8. First Probabilistic Model   170
 9. Second Probabilistic Model: Survival Probabilities   172
10. Third Probabilistic Model: Varying Survival Probabilities 173
11. Fourth Probabilistic Model: Varying Reproduction Probabilities 173
12. Discussion   174
Exercises   175
References   177
Notes for the Instructor   177

Chapter 6. MacDonald's Work on Helminth Infections   178
Donald Ludwig and Benjamin D. Haytock

1. Introduction   178
2. The Schistosomiasis Model   179

3. The Poisson Probability Distribution   180
4. Calculation of $P(m)$ 182
5. Analysis of Equation (6)   184
Appendix: An Alternate Model   186
Appendix: Reprint of MacDonald's Article   189
References   207

Chapter 7. A Model for the Spread of Gonorrhea   208
Martin Braun

Exercises   216
Notes for the Instructor   217

Chapter 8. DNA, RNA, and Random Mating: Simple Applications
of the Multiplication Rule   218
Helen Marcus-Roberts

1. Introduction   218
2. Multiplication Rule   218
3. DNA and RNA   223
4. Random Mating   229
Exercises   235
References   236
Notes for the Instructor   237

Chapter 9. Cigarette Filtration   238
Donald A. Drew

Exercises   246
Appendix: Discussion of Density and Flow Rate   246
Reference   248
Notes for the Instructor   249

Part III. Ecology

Chapter 10. Efficiency of Energy Use in Obtaining Food, I: Humans   250
Fred S. Roberts

1. Introduction   250
2. Energy and Food: Some Biological and Physical Background   252
3. Efficiency and Optimally Efficient Behavior   253
4. Human Energy Use for Food   266
References   283
Notes for the Instructor   285

Chapter 11. Efficiency of Energy Use in Obtaining Food, II: Animals   286
Fred S. Roberts and Helen Marcus-Roberts

1. Introduction: The Problem   286
2. The Allometric Law   287
3. Predators as Efficient Users of Energy   294
4. Pure Pursuers   297
5. Pure Searchers   331
6. Discussion   346
References   346
Notes for the Instructor   348

Chapter 12. The Spatial Distribution of Cabbage Butterfly Eggs   350
Daniel L. Solomon

1. Purpose   350
2. The Biology   350
3. Biological Assumptions I   352
4. Biological Assumptions II   354
5. Biological Assumptions III   356
6. Suggestions for Further Study   357
Appendix: Probability Generating Functions   358
Solutions to the Exercises   362
References   365
Notes for the Instructor   365

Contents of the Companion Volumes

VOLUME 1. DIFFERENTIAL EQUATION MODELS

Part I. Differential Equations, Models, and What To Do with Them

1 Setting Up First-Order Differential Equations from Word Problems
   Beverly Henderson West

2 Qualitative Solution Sketching for First-Order Differential Equations
   Beverly Henderson West

3 Difference and Differential Equation Population Growth Models
   James C. Frauenthal

Part II. Growth and Decay Models: First-Order Differential Equations

4 The van Meegeren Art Forgeries   *Martin Braun*

5 Single Species Population Models   *Martin Braun*

6 The Spread of Technological Innovations   *Martin Braun*

Part III. Higher Order Linear Models

7 A Model for the Detection of Diabetes   *Martin Braun*

8   Combat Models   *Courtney S. Coleman*

9   Modeling Linear Systems by Frequency Response Methods
    William F. Powers

Part IV. Traffic Models

10   How Long Should a Traffic Light Remain Amber?   *Donald A. Drew*

11   Queue Length at a Traffic Light via Flow Theory   *Donald A. Drew*

12   Car-Following Models   *Robert L. Baker, Jr.*

13   Equilibrium Speed Distributions   *Donald A. Drew*

14   Traffic Flow Theory   *Donald A. Drew*

Part V. Interacting Species: Steady States of Nonlinear Systems

15   Why the Percentage of Sharks Caught in the Mediterranean Sea Rose
     Dramatically during World War I   *Martin Braun*

16   Quadratic Population Models: Almost Never Any Cycles
     Courtney S. Coleman

17   The Principle of Competitive Exclusion in Population Biology
     Martin Braun

18   Biological Cycles and the Fivefold Way   *Courtney S. Coleman*

19   Hilbert's 16th Problem: How Many Cycles?   *Courtney S. Coleman*

Part VI. Models Leading to Partial Differential Equations

20   Surge Tank Analysis   *Donald A. Drew*

21   Shaking a Piece of String to Rest   *Robert L. Borrelli*

22   Heat Transfer in Frozen Soil   *Gunter H. Meyer*

23   Network Analysis of Steam Generator Flow   *T. A. Porsching*

VOLUME 2. POLITICIAL AND RELATED MODELS

1 The Process of Applied Mathematics   *Maynard Thompson*

2 Proportional Representation   *Edward Bolger*

3 Comparison Voting   *Steven J. Brams*

4 Modeling Coalitional Values   *William F. Lucas and Louis J. Billera*

5 Urban Wastewater Management Planning   *James P. Heaney*

6 An Everyday Approach to Matrix Operations   *Robert M. Thrall and E. L. Perry*

7 Sources of Applications of Mathematics in Ecological and Environmental Subject Areas, Suitable for Classroom Use   *Homer T. Hayslett, Jr.*

8 How To Ask Sensitive Questions without Getting Punched in the Nose   *John C. Maceli*

9 Measuring Power in Weighted Voting Systems   *William F. Lucas*

10 To the (Minimal Winning) Victors Go the (Equally Divided) Spoils: A New Power Index for Simple *n*-Person Games   *John Deegan, Jr. and Edward W. Packel*

11 Power Indices in Politics   *Philip D. Straffin, Jr.*

12 Committee Decision Making   *Peter Rice*

13 Stochastic Difference Equations with Sociological Applications   *Loren Cobb*

14 The Apportionment Problem   *William F. Lucas*

VOLUME 3. DISCRETE AND SYSTEM MODELS

1 Foresight—Insight—Hindsight   *James C. Frauenthal and Thomas L. Saaty*

2 Five Natutical Models   *Roberts L. Baker, Jr.*

3   An Optimal Inventory Policy Model   *Oswaldo Marrero*

4   An Arithmetic Model of Gravity   *Donald Greenspan*

5   Four-Way Stop or Traffic Lights? An Illustration of the Modeling
    Process   *Edward W. Packel*

6   A Model for Municipal Street Sweeping Operations   *A. C. Tucker and
    L. Bodin*

7   Finite Covering Problems   *Ronald E. Prather*

8   A Pulse Process Model of Athletic Financing   *E. L. Perry*

9   Traffic Equilibria on a Roadway Network   *Elmor L. Peterson*

10 An Optimal Mix Problem: Capacity Expansion in a Power Field
    Jacob Zahavi

11 Hierarchies, Reciprocal Matrices, and Ratio Scales   *Thomas L. Saaty*

12 Multiple Choice Testing   *Robert J. Weber*

13 Computing Fixed Points, with Applications to Economic Equilibrium
    Models   *Michael J. Todd*

14 Production Costing and Reliability Assessment of Electrical Power
    Generation Systems under Supply and Demand Uncertainty
    Jacob Zahavi

PART I

POPULATION MODELS

CHAPTER 1

Population Mathematics

Frank C. Hoppensteadt*

1. Introduction

The estimation of the size and age composition of various biological populations is a significant concern to many decisionmakers. For example, such
information is needed in planning the use of renewable natural resources
such as fish and waterfowl and the long-range educational and economic
policies for human populations. Although the ideas and techniques introduced in this unit have obvious relevance for a whole set of biological
populations, we will use the terminology of human population growth just
to have a specific example at hand.

Attempts to use mathematics to describe the growth of human populations
go back at least as far as the late 18th century, and one of the most familiar
elementary models was proposed by the English economist and demog-
rapher, T. R. Malthus (1766–1834). The Malthus model is based on the
assumption that the instantaneous rate of growth of a population is proportional to the size of the population. Here and in the future the size of a
population is assumed to be measured in convenient, continuously divisible
units (biomass or a similar quantity), so using differential equations presents
no inherent difficulty. Malthus' model leads to the prediction of unlimited
population sizes; a conclusion that leads one to view the underlying assumptions with some skepticism. Various modifications of the Malthus
model have been proposed that remove the objectionable conclusion. For
example, a model proposed by a 19th century Belgian sociologist, P. F.
Verhulst, and subsequently rediscovered by others leads to predicted population sizes that tend asymptotically to a constant value as time increases.

* Department of Mathematics, University of Utah, Salt Lake City, UT 84112.

However, the Verhulst model and many more recent ones, some of which lead to differential-delay equations or functional-differential equations of considerable mathematical interest, do not consider directly the influence of the age composition of a population on its development. This will be the primary concern of this module.

We have a number of decisions to make. First of all, shall we view the situation as a deterministic or a stochastic one? Obviously, the biological–social situation we are modeling induces random events. However, if we are concerned with large populations, then we have some confidence that a deterministic model will provide a good first approximation. Also, the mathematical techniques required for an analysis of the deterministic model proposed here are less sophisticated than those needed for the analysis of a stochastic model of similar generality. The choice of model is ultimately a decision of the investigator, and we choose a deterministic model.

Our second decision is whether or not to consider the spatial as well as the temporal variation of the population. For various reasons, among these a lack of adequate data for spatially distributed populations, we shall restrict our attention to the changes in the size and age composition of the population through time.

Our last decision is whether time should be considered as a continuous or discrete variable. Here we will compromise and introduce two models, one in the module proper and another in a project. Most of the module is devoted to a discussion of a continuous-time model first introduced by A. J. Lotka and subsequently refined by many researchers. The Lotka model has served as the taking off point for much of the research in population dynamics. The topic of one of the projects is a discrete-time model due to P. H. Leslie. Both models are discussed in N. Keyfitz's book *Introduction to the Mathematics of Population* [5]. This book, the article [6], and especially the book [7] contain data and applications of conclusions based on the model to problems in economics, education, social services, etc. In addition, [7] contains computer programs for many of the calculations. A few references are provided at the end of the module. The items [2] and [6] contain other references to the vast literature on the subject.

2. Formulation of a Model

In this section we will formulate a continuous-time model for the dynamics of the female population. The dynamics of the entire population can be determined from a knowledge of the dynamics of the females, assumptions relating the number of male and female births, and assumptions regarding male survivorship. We begin with some definitions and notation.

Let $B(t)$ denote the rate of additions to the female population, the birth rate, at time t. Our first goal will be to relate B to three quantities that can be determined from available data. Specifically, we suppose that the *age distribution of the initial population*, the age specific *mortality rate*, and the age specific *fertility rate* are known quantities. Suppose that we identify $t = 0$ as the time at which our analysis of the population begins, and let $u_0(a)$ denote the density of the initial age distribution. That is, we assume that the number of individuals with ages between a_1 and a_2 at $t = 0$ is given by $\int_{a_1}^{a_2} u_0(a)\, da$. The mortality rate will be defined indirectly by a function $l(a)$ that gives the proportion of births that survive to age a. The function l is usually given as a *life table*, a listing of age a and survivor ratio $l(a)$, which is obtained from census data for the population. A sample life table is given in Table 1.

The fertility rate is obtained from a table of the number of female births produced by females of various ages. In particular, suppose that $\bar{b}(a)$ is the rate at which female offspring are produced by 100,000 females of age a. Then we define $b(a)$, the fertility rate, by $b(a) = 10^{-5}\bar{b}(a)$. That is, the fertility rate is the average rate at which females of age a bear female offspring. We assume that $b(a) = 0$ for large age a, say $b(a) = 0$ for $a \geq A$. In human populations it is customary to assume $b(a) = 0$ for $a \leq 15$ and $a \leq 55$. Notice that we are assuming that the fertility and mortality rates,

Table 1. A Sample Life Table

a Age	$l(a)$ Proportion of Births Surviving to Age a
0	1.0
5	0.76
10	0.72
15	0.69
20	0.65
25	0.61
30	0.56
35	0.52
40	0.48
45	0.44
50	0.40
55	0.36
60	0.32
65	0.27
70	0.20
75	0.12
80	0.07
85	0.03
90	0.00

though age dependent, are independent of time t. That is, l and b depend only on a, not on t.

Next we turn to the derivation of an expression for the birth rate $B(t)$ at time t. These births can (potentially) arise from two sources. First, they can be births to females in the initial population; second, they can be births to females born since $t = 0$. In the first case the density of females surviving from the initial population to attain age a at time t, $a \geq t$, is

$$[l(a)/l(a - t)]u_0(a - t).$$

Indeed, $l(a)/l(a - t)$ is the proportion of the initial population which will survive from age $a - t$ to age a, and $u_0(a - t)$ is the density of females in the initial population which, if they survived, could be of age a at time t. Each of these females will bear female offspring at the rate $b(a)$. Therefore,

$$b(a)[l(a)/l(a - t)]u_0(a - t)$$

is the density function for the rate at which female offspring will be produced by the survivors of the initial population who have reached age a at time t. The contribution of individuals at all ages can be obtained by integrating. Consequently, the total birth rate at time t due to the initial population is

$$\int_t^\infty b(a)[l(a)/l(a - t)]u_0(a - t)\,da.$$

Since $b(a) = 0$ for $a \geq A$, this integral is equal to

$$\begin{cases} \int_t^A b(a)[l(a)/l(a - t)]u_0(a - t)\,da, & \text{if } t < A \\ 0, & \text{if } t \geq A. \end{cases}$$

The second source of new females in the population is births to those born after $t = 0$. At time t consider the females of age a. These females were born at the rate $B(t - a)$ at time $t - a$ and the proportion $l(a)$ of them survived to age a. Therefore, the number of females of age a to $a + da$ at time t is $l(a)B(t - a)\,da$. Since each of them will bear children at the rate $b(a)$, the rate of additions to the population at time t due to new females is

$$\int_0^t b(a)l(a)B(t - a)\,da.$$

Combining these results we obtain an equation for B where $t < A$

$$B(t) = \int_t^\infty b(a)[l(a)/l(a - t)]u_0(a - t)\,da + \int_0^t b(a)l(a)B(t - a)\,da,$$

and for $t > A$

$$B(t) = \int_0^t b(a)l(a)B(t - a)\,da.$$

which we write as

$$B(t) = h(t) + \int_0^t b(a)l(a)B(t - a)\,da. \tag{1}$$

This integral equation for the birth rate B is called the *renewal equation,* since it describes the way the population reproduces itself.

If we could solve equation (1) for the function B, then we could predict the size and age structure of the population; in fact, if $f(a, t)$ denotes the age density of females of age a at time t so that the number of females of age a_1 to a_2 at time t is given by $\int_{a_1}^{a_2} f(a, t)\,da$, then

$$f(a, t) = \begin{cases} l(a)B(t - a), & a < t \\ [l(a)/l(a - t)]u_0(a - t), & t < a. \end{cases}$$

3. A Stable Age Distribution

Unfortunately, the renewal equation (1) is not an easy equation to solve. Using the method of successive approximations it is fairly straightforward to show that, under quite general conditions on the functions h, b, and l in (1), the renewal equation has a unique solution on $(0, \infty)$ (see, for example, [1, p. 217]). However, we are interested in certain properties of the solution, in particular its asymptotic behavior, which are more difficult to obtain. Most of the facts of interest to us, which we will use without proof, can be deduced with the use of Laplace transform methods (see [1, p. 231 ff.]).

First, we know that the solution B has the form

$$B(t) = B_\infty e^{pt} + R(t) \tag{2}$$

where B_∞ and p are constants and the remainder R is a complicated function that satisfies

$$\lim_{t \to \infty} e^{-pt} R(t) = 0.$$

Consequently, R is negligible compared to the first term on the right-hand side of (2) for large values of t.

What the value of p must be is easy to determine. From (1) we have

$$e^{-pt}B(t) = e^{-pt}h(t) + \int_0^t b(a)l(a)e^{-pa}e^{-p(t-a)}B(t - a)\,da.$$

Taking the limit $t \to \infty$, we have

$$B_\infty = B_\infty \int_0^\infty b(a)l(a)e^{-pa}\,da + \lim_{t \to \infty}\int_0^A b(a)l(a)e^{-pa}e^{-p(t-a)}R(t - a)\,da$$

$$= B_\infty \int_0^\infty b(a)l(a)e^{-pa}\,da.$$

Therefore, p must satisfy the *characteristic equation*

$$1 = \int_0^\infty b(a)l(a)e^{-pa}\,da. \tag{3}$$

This equation was first derived by Lotka in 1922 [9, p. 340]. It has a unique real solution for p, say p^*. The constant p^* is called the *intrinsic rate of natural growth* or the *biotic potential* of the population. This constant is analogous to the growth rate in the ordinary exponential or Malthusian growth equation.

If b and l are piecewise continuous functions, then we can show that infinitely many complex solutions of (3) exist. If we denote them by $\{\varphi_n\}$, then the following facts hold.

(1) The φ_n occur in conjugate pairs, i.e., if φ_n satisfies (3) then so does $\bar{\varphi}_n$.
(2) $\operatorname{Re}\varphi_n < p^*$, for all n.
(3) $\operatorname{Re}\varphi_n \to -\infty$ as $n \to \infty$.

A formula can be derived for the constant B_∞. The details, which are somewhat involved, can be found in [1, p. 232 ff.]

$$B_\infty = \frac{\displaystyle\int_0^A h(t)e^{-p^*t}\,dt}{\displaystyle\int_0^A al(a)b(a)e^{-p^*a}\,da}. \tag{4}$$

Now we can show that the population approaches a *stable age distribution*. To this end, consider

$$\lim_{t\to\infty} e^{-p^*t}f(a, t).$$

From the formula for $f(a, t)$, we see that

$$\lim_{t\to\infty} e^{-p^*t}f(a, t) = B_\infty l(a)e^{-p^*a}$$

where B_∞ is the constant determined by (4). Therefore, for large times the population is approximately described by

$$e^{p^*t}B_\infty l(a)e^{-p^*a}. \tag{5}$$

If $p^* > 0$ the population increases with passing time, if $p^* < 0$ it declines and approaches zero. The expression (5) is known as the *stable age distribution* associated with the population. Notice that the time variation of the stable age distribution is determined by the real solution of the characteristic equation.

One of the consequences of the existence of a stable age distribution is that for large times, the proportion of the population in any age group remains constant. For example, the proportion of the population that is in the age bracket (a_1, a_2) is

$$\frac{\text{number with ages } a_1 < a < a_2}{\text{total population}} = \frac{\displaystyle\int_{a_1}^{a_2} f(a, t)\, da}{\displaystyle\int_0^\infty f(a, t)\, da}$$

which is approximately equal to

$$\frac{\displaystyle\int_{a_1}^{a_2} l(a) e^{-p^* a}\, da}{\displaystyle\int_0^\infty l(a) e^{-p^* a}\, da}$$

for large t.

The fact that the population approaches a stable age distribution is quite important, and many demographers' calculations are based on the stable age distribution.

Summary. The theoretical results that we have accumulated so far are easily summarized. Lotka's age dependent theory for the evolution of a female population is based on the renewal equation (1). This equation involves two functions that are determinable from data: $h(t)$, the contribution of the initial population to the births at time t, and $m(a) = b(a)l(a)$, the net maternity function that measures the viability and fertility of individuals.

If m is a piecewise continuous function that vanishes for large ages (say $m(a) = 0$ for $a \geq A$), then the population approaches a stable age distribution. In fact, in that case B can be written as

$$B(t) = B_\infty e^{p^* t} + R(t),$$

where p^* is determined from the characteristic equation (3) as the unique real solution of that equation for p. The remainder $R(t)$ is small when compared to $e^{p^* t}$ for large t, and the constant B_∞ is given by (4).

EXERCISES

1. The characteristic equation also arises in the formal solution of (1) using Laplace transforms. Derive this formal solution and show how the characteristic equation arises.

2. Since p^* is normally quite small, an approximate value for p^* can often be determined by replacing e^{-pa} in (3) by its Taylor expansion about $p = 0$ and then ignoring the terms of order p^3 and higher. Use this method to obtain a formula for an approximate value of p^*.

Project. In this project you are asked to use given fertility rates, life table, and initial

Table 2

Age Bracket	Number of Females ($\times 10^3$) in Initial Population	Number of Births per Female
[0, 5)	105	0
[5, 10)	100	0
[10, 15)	905	0.004
[15, 20)	805	0.298
[20, 25)	650	0.732
[25, 30)	560	0.512
[30, 35)	565	0.297
[35, 40)	620	0.157
[40, 45)	635	0.045
[45, 50)	580	0.002
[50, 55)	535	0
[55, 60)	465	0
[60, 65)	405	0
[65, 70)	300	0
[70, 75)	210	0
[75, 80)	135	0
[80, 85)	65	0
[85, 90)	15	0

age distribution to determine the intrinsic growth rate, stable age distribution, and projections of the population distribution at two specified times in the future. We will follow demographic custom and give data over five-year intervals. This suggests the approximation of taking the data to be constant over five-year intervals. For example, using the data in Table 1, we would define

$$
l(a) = \begin{cases}
0.76 & 0 \leq a < 5 \\
0.72 & 5 \leq a < 10 \\
0.69 & 10 \leq a < 15 \\
0.65 & 15 \leq a < 20. \\
\vdots
\end{cases}
$$

This approximation simplifies the integrals to finite sums.

Suppose that the initial age distribution is given by column 2 of Table 2 and the fertility rate is given by column 3.

(a) Determine the intrinsic growth rate. The formula derived in Exercise 2 may be used as a first approximation. (A good problem in numerical analysis is to use Newton's method to solve the characteristic equation for p. Newton's method and other methods are discussed in [4, ch. 3].)

(b) Evaluate the stable age distribution by using Eq. (4). (First $h(t)$ must be found for each t, and then the integrals in (4) must be evaluated. This is a lengthy but straightforward calculation).

(c) Determine $f(a, 5)$ and $f(a, 10)$.

4. Population Waves

Oscillations are common in natural phenomena. When given an impulse that forces it away from equilibrium, systems as diverse as an elastic spring, a bowl of jello, or water in a pan respond by oscillating for a period of time and eventually returning to an equilibrium condition. Under certain conditions, populations also exhibit oscillations. These oscillations are the topic of this section; a more detailed discussion, and applications to social and economic questions, may be found in [6].

4.1 Bernardelli Waves

In some populations, for example insect populations such as 13- and 17-year cicadas, the reproductive period is restricted to a very short time interval. Unfortunately, the analysis outlined above may not be valid in such cases because the maternity function can no longer be thought of as piecewise continuous. This situation will be illustrated by considering an example involving a maternity function of a more general type than that discussed previously.

Suppose that

$$m(a) = \sum_{j=1}^{k} m_j \delta(a - a_j),$$

where the m_j are positive constants and δ denotes the Dirac delta function. (The Dirac delta function is an example of a generalized function. It is interpreted through values of integrals in which it forms a part of the integrand; i.e., if g is a continuous function, then

$$\int_{-\infty}^{\infty} \delta(x - x_0)g(x)\,dx = g(x_0). \tag{6}$$

It is somewhat involved to describe generalized functions in a rigorous mathematical setting. Clearly, the delta function cannot be described by giving the value $\delta(x)$ for every real x. Indeed, we would have to write $\delta(x) = 0$ for $x \neq 0$ and $\delta(0) = \infty$. Still, the concept is quite simple: the delta function can be thought of as a device that "pops out" the value of an integrand at one point as in (6) and thereby states that the value of the integral depends only on the value of the integrand at one point, $x = x_0$.)

This maternity function indicates that individuals reproduce at ages a_j. For simplicity, suppose that $a_j = j\alpha$ where α is the length between breeding times. With this net maternity function the renewal equation becomes

$$B(t) = h(t) + \sum_{j=1}^{k} m_j B(t - j\alpha)H(t - j\alpha),$$

where H is the Heaviside function

$$H(x) = \begin{cases} 0, & x < 0, \\ 1, & x > 0. \end{cases}$$

Thus a collection of individuals born at time t will produce m_1 offspring at time $t + \alpha$, m_2 at time $t + 2\alpha$, etc. The characteristic equation corresponding to this choice of net maternity function is

$$1 = \sum_{j=1}^{k} m_j e^{-pj\alpha}. \tag{7}$$

Setting $v = e^{-p\alpha}$, we obtain

$$1 = \sum_{j=1}^{k} m_j v^j. \tag{8}$$

The right side of this equation is simply a polynomial in v with positive coefficients. Since we are concerned only with $v > 0$ (remember $v = e^{-p\alpha}$), since the polynomial is zero for $v = 0$ and since the first k derivatives of this polynomial are all positive for $v = 0$, we conclude that a unique solution v^* of (8) exists for $v > 0$. Therefore,

$$p^* = -(1/\alpha)\log v^*$$

satisfies (7). However, in contrast to the situation in Section 2, the numbers

$$p^* + (2\pi i n/\alpha), \qquad n = \pm 1, \pm 2, \cdots,$$

are also solutions of the characteristic equation (7) since $e^{2\pi i n} = 1$ for any integer n. Thus in this case the analog of the remainder R in (2) is not necessarily negligible in comparison with $e^{p^* t}$.

Consider, for example, the special case in which $k = 1$. Here, we have a population of individuals who can reproduce only once, when they reach age α. The renewal equation becomes

$$B(t) = \begin{cases} h(t), & 0 \leq t < \alpha, \\ m_1 B(t - \alpha), & \alpha \leq t. \end{cases} \tag{9}$$

This shows that for $0 \leq t < \alpha$

$$B(t + N\alpha) = m_1^N h(t).$$

If $m_1 = 1$, then each female will exactly reproduce herself when she reaches age α. Thus one expects the rate of additions to the population to merely repeat h in each time interval of length α. In fact,

$$b(t + N\alpha) = h(t), \qquad 0 \leq t < \alpha,$$

so that the rate of additions is a periodic function of t with period α. If $m_1 < 1 (> 1)$, then the rate of additions will oscillate with wave length α, but it will approach zero (∞) as $t \to \infty$.

If the rate of additions is periodic or nearly periodic, then the phenomenon is referred to as a *population wave*. Note that the wave length (period) of the oscillation in the rate of additions is the same as the age to reproduction. This feature will be observed in a more general setting later.

The example just studied is the analog for (1) of an observation made by Bernardelli in 1941 (see [8, p. 200]). He used a discrete (matrix) model. In particular, he showed that if the reproduction of the population is focused in one age bracket, then there is a population wave. Because of this, we refer to these phenomenal oscillations in the rate of additions caused by sharply restricted reproductive periods as Bernardelli Population Waves.

A maternity function like this one is rather extreme. While it may be relevant to some insect populations, it is not typical of most organisms. However, it does provide insight into population waves in more realistic models. We will pursue this point in the next section.

EXERCISES

3. Give a detailed proof that there is a unique solution $v^* > 0$ of Eq. (8).

4. Select several different functions h and graph the resulting function B of Eq. (9) for the three cases $m_1 > 1$, $m_1 = 1$, and $m_1 < 1$.

Project. Repeat Bernardelli's analysis by formulating a discrete model for the dynamics of the female population (see [8] and [5 chs. 2 and 3]). Hint: Let $(n_0, n_1, \cdots, n_N)$ denote the sizes of the populations in the age brackets,

$$[0, a_1), [a_1, a_2), \cdots, [a_N, a_{N+1}),$$

respectively, where the lengths of these intervals are equal to one reproduction interval, hereafter taken to be the unit of time. Let l_i be the proportion of individuals in $[a_i, a_{i+1})$ who survive one unit of time. Finally, let b_i denote the fertility of individuals in $[a_i, a_{i+1})$.

Then, if $(n'_0, n'_1, \cdots, n'_N)$ denotes the population sizes one unit of time later, we have

$$n'_0 = b_0 l_0 n_0 + b_1 l_1 n_1 + \cdots + b_N l_N n_N$$

$$n'_1 = l_0 n_0, n'_2 = l_1 n_1, \cdots, n'_N = l_{N-1} n_{N-1},$$

and we no longer account for those who were in $[a_N, a_{N+1})$.

These equations can be written more concisely by taking advantage of matrix notation:

$$\begin{bmatrix} n'_0 \\ n'_1 \\ n'_2 \\ \vdots \\ n'_N \end{bmatrix} = \begin{bmatrix} b_0 & b_1 & \cdots & b_{N-1} & b_N \\ l_0 & 0 & \cdots & 0 & 0 \\ 0 & l_1 & \cdots & 0 & 0 \\ \vdots & & & & \\ 0 & 0 & & l_{N-1} & 0 \end{bmatrix} \begin{bmatrix} n_0 \\ n_1 \\ n_2 \\ \vdots \\ n_N \end{bmatrix};$$

or, if we set

$$\vec{n} = \begin{bmatrix} n_0 \\ n_1 \\ \vdots \\ n_N \end{bmatrix}, \vec{n}\,' = \begin{bmatrix} n_0' \\ n_1' \\ \vdots \\ n_N' \end{bmatrix} \text{ and } \mathscr{L} = \begin{bmatrix} b_0 & \cdots & b_N \\ l_0 & & 0 \\ \vdots & & \vdots \\ 0 & \cdots & 0 \end{bmatrix}$$

then we can write the system as $\vec{n}\,' = \mathscr{L}\vec{n}$. After two units of time we have

$$\vec{n}\,'' = \mathscr{L}\vec{n}\,' = \mathscr{L}^2\vec{n},$$

etc. This discrete version of the Lotka theory is due to P. H. Leslie [8] who developed several properties of solutions by analyzing the coefficient matrix of this model.

The case which Bernardelli described is presented here by taking $b_0 = b_1 = \cdots = b_{N-1} = 0$ and $b_N > 0$. This requires no substantial analysis, and in fact

$$n_0' = b_N n_N, \qquad n_0'' = b_N n_N' = b_N l_{N-1} n_{N-1},$$

and so on, until after $N + 1$ units of time.

$$n_0^{(N+1)} = (b_N l_{N-1} \cdots l_0)n_0.$$

This equation is the discrete version of (9). If $b_N l_N \cdots l_0 = 1$, then each initial cohort exactly reproduces itself, and the rate of additions will be a periodic function.

4.2 Population Waves near Bernardelli Waves

Useful insight into population waves can be obtained by considering the Bernardelli waves as a limiting form. Specifically, let us consider a situation in which the net maternity is slightly "smeared out." For example, let

$$m_\Delta(a) = \begin{cases} m/\Delta, & \alpha - \Delta < a < \alpha, \\ 0, & \text{otherwise}, \end{cases}$$

where Δ is a small positive constant. It can be shown that as $\Delta \to 0$ this function behaves increasingly like the generalized function $m\delta(a - \alpha)$. In this case, reproduction takes place not only at age α, but in a short time interval preceding age α also. The solution in this case should approach a Bernardelli wave as $\Delta \to 0$.

Before proceeding with the analysis, think about what effect this "smearing out" of m should have on B. Should B still be periodic or nearly periodic? What should be the wavelength?

Proceeding, we find the characteristic equation in this case to be

$$1 = \frac{m}{\Delta} \int_{\alpha - \Delta}^{\alpha} e^{-pa}\,da = \frac{m}{p\Delta} e^{-p\alpha}[e^{p\Delta} - 1].$$

When $\Delta = 0$ the Bernardelli case results, and we have

$$1 = me^{-p_0\alpha},$$

from which we conclude that

$$p_{0,n} = (1/\alpha)\log m + (2\pi i n/\alpha), \qquad n = 0, \pm 1, \pm 2, \cdots.$$

We continue in the hope that the solutions of the characteristic equation for $\Delta > 0$ will be near these values in some sense. (This hope is justified by the implicit function theorem.)

Using these values as starting points, let us determine some of the characteristic roots of the full problem ($\Delta > 0$) by using Taylor's formula: Fix a value for n and look for a solution (characteristic root) of the form

$$p_n = p_{0,n} + \Delta p_{1,n} + (\Delta^2/2)p_{2,n} + \cdots.$$

Substituting this expression into the characteristic equation and equating like powers of Δ in the result, we obtain (after a mildly tedious calculation)

$$p_{1,n} = -(p_{0,n}/2\alpha), \qquad p_{2,n} = c + id,$$

where c and d are rather complicated expressions.

If $m = 1$ the calculations are easier. In this case,

$$p_{0,n} = 2\pi i n/\alpha, \qquad p_{1,n} = -2\pi i n/2\alpha^2,$$
$$2p_{2,n} = -(\pi^2 n^2/\alpha^5) + i(\pi n/\alpha^3).$$

Thus

$$p_n = (-\pi^2 n^2/2\alpha^5)\Delta^2 + 2\pi i n[(1/\alpha) - (1/2\alpha^2)\Delta + (1/4\alpha^3)\Delta^2] + E,$$

where the error term E includes all terms in the Taylor series which contain Δ^3 and higher powers of Δ. This expression contains a great deal of information. For the remaining argument we neglect the error term E. In fact, for small values of n the error term is proportional to Δ^3 while for large values of $\pm n$ the real part of p_n is large and negative and consequently plays a dominant role in the solution.

The solution of the renewal equation corresponding to the choice $b(a)l(a) = m_\Delta(a)$ has the form

$$B(t) = \sum_{n=-\infty}^{\infty} B_n \exp(p_n t), \qquad \bar{p}_n = p_{-n}.$$

Using Euler's formula $e^{a+ib} = e^a(\cos b + i\sin b)$ and the fact that B is real (i.e., $B_n = \bar{B}_{-n}$, the complex conjugate of B_{-n}), we see that B can be written as

$$B(t) = \sum_{n=0}^{\infty} B_n \exp(t \operatorname{Re} p_n)\cos(t \operatorname{Im} p_n),$$

where $B_0 = B_0$, $B_n = 2B_n$ for $n > 0$, $\operatorname{Re} p_n$ denotes the real part of p_n, and $\operatorname{Im} p_n$ denotes its imaginary part.

This calculation shows that the real part of p_n measures the growth or damping of the contribution of the nth term to $B(t)$ while the imaginary part measures the frequency of oscillations. As noted earlier, $\text{Re}\,p_n$ is large and negative for large values of n, and consequently $\exp(t\,\text{Re}\,p_n)$ is much less than one for such values of n and t not near zero.

Therefore, we may write

$$B(t) = B_0 \exp(t\,\text{Re}\,p_0)\cos(t\,\text{Im}\,p_0) + B_1 \exp(t\,\text{Re}\,p_1)\cos(t\,\text{Im}\,p_1) + \cdots.$$

Using the value of p_0 and the approximation developed above for p_1, we have

$$\text{Re}\,p_0 = 0, \qquad \text{Im}\,p_0 = 0, \qquad (\text{remember } m = 1)$$

$$\text{Re}\,p_1 = -\pi^2\Delta^2/2\alpha^5, \qquad \text{Im}\,p_1 = 2\pi[(1/\alpha) - (1/2\alpha^2)\Delta + (1/4\alpha^3)\Delta^2].$$

Therefore,

$$B(t) = B_0 + B_1 \exp\left[-\pi^2 t\Delta^2/2\alpha^5\right]$$
$$\cos\left[2\pi t((1/\alpha) - (\Delta/2\alpha^2) + (\Delta^2/4\alpha^3))\right] + \cdots, \tag{10}$$

which shows clearly that the solution will be very slowly damped (since for Δ near zero $\Delta^2 t$ changes very slowly) and it will have oscillations with frequencies $(1/\alpha) - (\Delta/2\alpha^2) + (\Delta^2/4\alpha^3)$. The coefficient B_1 is given by the formula

$$B_1 = \frac{\Delta \displaystyle\int_0^\infty h(t)e^{-p_1 t}\,dt}{m \displaystyle\int_{\alpha-\Delta}^\alpha ae^{-p_1 a}\,da}.$$

As a result, we see that the smearing out of the Bernardelli case leads to a slowly damped rate of additions that exhibits oscillations having wavelengths given approximately by

$$((1/\alpha) - (\Delta/2\alpha^2) + (\Delta^2/4\alpha^3))^{-1} \sim \alpha + \Delta/2 + \cdots. \tag{11}$$

In particular, for times when $\Delta^2 t$ is much smaller than one, the solution will appear to be periodic, while for large times the rate of additions will approach the constant B_0.

4.3 Summary and Conclusions

Lotka defined the *mean generation time* T of a population to be the value such that

$$e^{p^* T} = \int_0^\infty l(a)b(a)\,da.$$

The integral on the right-hand side of this expression is called the population's *net reproduction rate* (NRR) [7], and it gives the number of female progeny expected to be born to a female just born. In Section 4.1 we had

$$\text{NRR} = \int_0^\infty m(a)\,da = \sum_{j=1}^k m_j, \qquad p^* = -(1/\alpha)\log v^*,$$

where v^* was defined as the positive root of $\Sigma_{j=1}^k m_j v^j = 1$. Thus

$$T = \alpha \left(-\log \sum_{j=1}^k m_j\right)\Big/\log v^*$$

and we see that T is proportional to α. In fact, when $k = 1$, $T = \alpha$.

In Section 4.2 we had

$$\text{NRR} = \int_0^\infty m_\Delta(a)\,da = m, \qquad p^* = (1/\alpha)\log m.$$

Thus

$$T = \alpha.$$

On the other hand, the wavelength was calculated to be α in Section 4.1 and $\alpha + \left(\dfrac{\Delta}{2}\right) + \cdots$ in Section 4.2. This shows that the length of the population waves is closely related to the mean generation time in the examples that we have considered.

This observation carries over to more general net maternity functions. This is strikingly illustrated in the data presented by Keyfitz and Flieger where the generation time listed for most populations [7, ch. 7 table 7] is quite near the wavelength ($2\pi/y$ in their notation [7, ch. 16, end of table 8].

This is an entirely reasonable result: a drastic change in the birth rate should be repeated in successive generations, at multiples of one generation time in the future.

EXERCISES

5. Determine the terms c and d in the representation $p_{2,n} = c + id$.

6. Determine the coefficient of Δ^2 in the expansion (11).

7. Plot the function B given by (10) for $\alpha = 1$, $B_0 = 1$, $B_1 = 1$, $\Delta = 0.01$.

Project. As we have seen, oscillations in populations take place over time intervals that are proportional to the mean generation time. Therefore, to observe the oscillations in the population projections, several projections (typically 30 years in length for human populations) must be calculated. This is a major undertaking.

In order to illustrate this oscillatory phenomenon in populations while keeping the calculations at a reasonably simple level, let us consider an imaginary insect population. In particular, let us consider the (as yet undiscovered) five-cicadas. These live as adults for only four to six weeks, after remaining in a nonreproductive state for five years. Therefore, the analysis outlined in Section 4.2 is applicable, and we take $\alpha = 5$, $\Delta = 0.15$. Let the contribution to births by the initial population be described by

$$h(t) = \begin{cases} F/\Delta, & \text{for } 5 - \Delta \leq t \leq 5 \\ 0, & \text{otherwise.} \end{cases}$$

Finally, suppose that each initial cohort will exactly reproduce itself five years later, i.e., $m = 1$. It is estimated that the species has been in existence in its present form for 1500 generations.

The aim of this project is to describe the dynamics of the species over 1500 generations. This can be accomplished by evaluating the terms in the expression for B:

$$B(t) = B_0 + \sum_{n=1}^{\infty} B_n \exp(-\pi^2 n^2 \Delta^2 t/2\alpha^5) \cos\left(2\pi n t\left(\frac{1}{\alpha} - \Delta\varphi\right)\right),$$

where $\varphi = (1/2\alpha^2) - (\Delta/4\alpha^3)$. How many terms of the series should be retained? We could use the first two terms, but for $n = 2$ and $t = 5 \times 1500$ (years), we have the exponent approximately equal to -1.06, it follows that the second term contains a factor e^{-1}. We view this as negligible.

Note: If we were to consider an actual case, we could study the 17-year cicada for which $\alpha = 17$, $\Delta = 1/170$. In this case we would have to retain many terms in the series to achieve comparable accuracy.

Returning to the case of five-year cicadas, we will analyze the function

$$B(t) = B_0 + B_1 \exp(-\pi^2 \Delta^2 t/2\alpha^5) \cos\left[2\pi t\left(\frac{1}{\alpha} - \Delta\varphi\right)\right].$$

(a) Determine $\Delta\varphi$ and the coefficients B_0 and B_1.
(b) Study the emergence at times $t = 5N$ for $N = 1, \cdots, 1500$:

$$B(5N) = B_0 + B_1 \exp[-\pi^2 N(1.8 \times 10^{-5})] \cos[2\pi N(1 - 5\Delta\varphi)].$$

(c) Study the damping. Is it significant? What is the percentage of reduction after 1500 generations? How long will it take for the oscillations to die out? (Remember that we have ignored terms of order e^{-1} in the series expansion of B.)
(d) Study the periodicity of the solution. Is the solution nearly periodic during the first 1500 generations? The answer to this question is no. This model illustrates a "beat" phenomenon.
    To see this, observe that

$$\cos[2\pi N(1 - 5\Delta p)] = \cos 2\pi N \times \cos(10N\pi\Delta\varphi) = \cos(10N\pi\Delta\varphi),$$

and evaluate this function for $N = 1, 2, \cdots$. Note that it assumes many values between -1 and $+1$.

There are many other questions of interest. Mainly, features not accounted for in the model should be discussed, such as the following.

What effect does a variation in the environment have on the population?

How would predation on the population during the reproductive period affect the population's dynamics?

Certainly effects such as these are significant for the population. These are discussed in [3].

References

[1] R. Bellman and K. L. Cooke, *Differential-Difference Equations.* New York: Academic, 1963.

[2] F. Hoppensteadt, *Mathematical Theories of Populations: Demographics, Genetics and Epidemics.* CBMS vol. 20. Philadelphia, Society for Industrial and Applied Mathematics, 1975.

[3] F. Hoppensteadt and J. B. Keller, "Synchronization of periodical cicada emergences," *Science*, vol. 194, pp. 335–337, 1976.

[4] E. Isaacson and H. B. Keller, *Analysis of Numerical Methods.* New York: Wiley, 1966.

[5] N. Keyfitz, *Introduction to the Mathematics of Population.* Reading, Ma. Addison-Wesley, 1968.

[6] ——, "Population waves," in *Population Dynamics*, T.N.E. Greville, Ed. New York: Academic, 1972.

[7] N. Keyfitz and W. Flieger, *Population: Facts and Methods of Demography.* San Francisco, CA: W. H. Freeman, 1971.

[8] P. H. Leslie, "On the use of matrices in certain population mathematics," *Biometrika*, vol. 33, pp. 183–212, 1945.

[9] A. J. Lotka, "The stability of the normal age distribution," *Proc. Nat. Acad. Sci.*, vol. 8, pp. 339–345, 1922.

CHAPTER 2
Population Growth: An Age Structure Model

Robert E. Fennell*

1. Introduction

In this chapter we consider the problem of determining the future size and age distribution of a population. The methods presented are basic in the study of human population growth and are derived from the works of P. H. Leslie [5] and N. Keyfitz [3]. Many concepts studied in an undergraduate linear algebra course are applied and, in addition, special properties of matrices with nonnegative components are utilized. The assignments are essential for an understanding of the model and its predictions, some assignments require computer access and an elementary scientific programming ability.

   The first problem in a modeling project is the development of a reasonable concept of the system under consideration. Although populations may be viewed in many different ways, for purposes of this module a population is to be regarded as a collection of individuals subdivided into distinct age groups. We shall further restrict attention to the females in the population; incorporation of males into the model will require some modifications. The problem is to devise a model to describe the growth of the population. This description is to be based on the assumption of fixed fertility and mortality rates for each age group.

2. An Example

Consider an isolated population in which no migration occurs and suppose we are interested in the number of individuals at 15-year intervals in the age groups 0–15, 15–30, 30–45, 45–60, and 60–75. We will assume individuals

* Department of Mathematical Sciences, Clemson University, Clemson, SC 29631.

do not live past age 75 and the only reproductive age groups are the second and third. We wish to project future population sizes at 15-year intervals. This choice, which guarantees that individuals who survive progress to the next age group at the end of one period, greatly simplifies calculations.

Let $W_i(t)$ denote the number of individuals in the ith age group at time t, $W_i(0)$ denotes the initial population size and is assumed to be known. We desire a model to describe the behavior of the vector of population sizes

$$W(t) = \begin{pmatrix} W_1(t) \\ W_2(t) \\ W_3(t) \\ W_4(t) \\ W_5(t) \end{pmatrix}$$

for $t = 0, 15, 30, \cdots$.

The population of the first age group at time $t + 15$ is formed by births which occur during the interval between t and $t + 15$ and which survive to time $t + 15$. This number is given by

$$W_1(t + 15) = b_2 W_2(t) + b_3 W_3(t),$$

where b_2 and b_3 denote the number of births in a period, which survive to the end of that period, per individual.

For age groups two through five, we assume the size at time $t + 15$ is proportional to the size of the next preceeding age group at time. t. That is, for $i = 2, 3, 4$, and 5, we assume

$$W_i(t + 15) = s_{i-1} W_{i-1}(t),$$

where s_i denotes the proportion of individuals in the ith age group at time t who survive to the $(i + 1)$st age group at time $t + 15$. In order to project future population sizes the birth and survival rates b_2, b_3, and $s_i, i = 1, \cdots,$ 4 are assumed constant from period to period.

Using vector matrix notation, the growth model may be represented by

$$W(t + 15) = GW(t)$$

for $t = 0, 15, 30, \cdots$, where

$$G = \begin{pmatrix} 0 & b_2 & b_3 & 0 & 0 \\ s_1 & 0 & 0 & 0 & 0 \\ 0 & s_2 & 0 & 0 & 0 \\ 0 & 0 & s_3 & 0 & 0 \\ 0 & 0 & 0 & s_4 & 0 \end{pmatrix}.$$

This model allows one to project population growth in an iterative fashion. Since we may conclude inductively that the population growth is governed by the equation

$$W(15n) = G^n W(0)$$

for $n = 0, 1, 2, \cdots$, the matrix G is called a *growth matrix* or *projection matrix*.

EXERCISES

1. Discuss and criticize the assumptions leading to the model of this example. What factors influence fertility and mortality rates?

2. Consider a hypothetical population for which $b_2 = 1.5$, $b_3 = 1$, $s_1 = 0.98$, $s_2 = 0.96$, $s_3 = 0.93$ and $s_4 = 0.90$. Let $W_1(0) = 1000$, $W_2(0) = 900$, $W_3(0) = 800$, $W_4(0) = 700$, and $W_5(0) = 600$ and compute $W(15n)$ for $n = 1, \cdots, 20$. For each period and each age group, compute the growth rate $W_i(t + 15)/W_i(t)$. Also calculate the total population and the percentage of this total in each age group at the end of each period.

The Appendix contains a Fortran program for the calculations of Exercise 2. This exercise illustrates the property of the model that once an individual enters the population she progresses from age group to age group with given probabilities. Also the notion of an intrinsic rate of growth and of a stable age distribution are introduced. One should have observed that the rate of growth for each age group, $W_i(15(n + 1))/W_i(15n)$, approaches a constant as time increases and that the proportion of the total population in each age group also approaches a constant.

In order to explain these observations we partition the matrix G so that

$$G = \begin{pmatrix} A & \tilde{0} \\ B & C \end{pmatrix}$$

where

$$A = \begin{pmatrix} 0 & b_1 & b_2 \\ s_1 & 0 & 0 \\ 0 & s_2 & 0 \end{pmatrix}, \qquad \tilde{0} = \begin{pmatrix} 0 & 0 \\ 0 & 0 \end{pmatrix}$$

$$B = \begin{pmatrix} 0 & 0 & s_3 \\ 0 & 0 & 0 \end{pmatrix}, \qquad C = \begin{pmatrix} 0 & 0 \\ s_4 & 0 \end{pmatrix}.$$

EXERCISES

3. Show that

$$G^n = \begin{pmatrix} A^n & \tilde{0} \\ B_n & C^n \end{pmatrix}$$

where $B_n = \sum_{i=0}^{n-1} C^i B A^{n-1-i}$.

4. Show that the characteristic equation of A, $\det(a - \lambda I) = 0$, is given by $\lambda^3 - s_1 b_2 \lambda - s_1 s_2 b_3 = 0$.

5. Show that A^n has all components positive for some positive integer n. Letting

$$\tilde{W}(15n) = \begin{pmatrix} W_1(15n) \\ W_2(15n) \\ W_3(15n) \end{pmatrix}, \qquad W^*(15n) = \begin{pmatrix} W_4(15n) \\ W_5(15n) \end{pmatrix},$$

it follows that

$$\tilde{W}(15(n+1)) = A\tilde{W}(15n)$$

and

$$W^*(15(n+1)) = B\tilde{W}(15n) + CW^*(15n).$$

Thus the components of $\tilde{W}(15n)$ are independent of those of $W^*(15n)$. Since the fourth and fifth age groups are assumed to be nonreproductive, the observation that these age groups do not contributed to the future growth of the first three groups should be evident. Consequently, we will see that the growth behavior of the whole population may be explained in terms of the growth of the subpopulation consisting of the first three age groups.

3. Powers of a Nonnegative Matrix

For the population consisting of the first three age groups we have

$$\tilde{W}(15n) = A^n \tilde{W}(0),$$

and we see that an analysis of the behavior of $\tilde{W}(15n)$ depends on an understanding of the properties of A^n as n increases. The behavior of $\tilde{W}(15n)$ may be explained in terms of the following algebraic properties of A:

(1) A has a positive eigenvalue λ_1, which is a simple root of the characteristic equation of A;
(2) A has an eigenvector $x^{(1)}$ corresponding to λ_1, such that each component of $x^{(1)}$ is positive;
(3) for each nonzero vector x_0 with nonnegative components, a positive constant c depending on x_0 exists such that

$$\lim_{n \to \infty} A^n x_0 / \lambda_1^n = cx^{(1)}.$$

Convergence is to be interpreted as componentwise convergence.

These properties of the matrix A may be deduced from the general theory of nonnegative matrices. However, since the matrix A of the model is of a special form, the properties may be derived from elementary concepts.

Property 1 follows from the form of the characteristic equation of A, $f(\lambda) = 0$, (see Exercise 4). Since $f(0) = -s_1 s_2 b_3 < 0$ and $f(\lambda)$ approaches infinity as λ approaches infinity, at least one positive eigenvalue exists. That only one such root exists may be deduced by calculus methods or in more general problems by Descartes' Rule of Signs [2]. This rule states that the number of positive roots, counting multiplicities, of a real polynomial, arranged in descending powers of λ, is either equal to the number of variations of signs in the coefficients of $f(\lambda)$ or to that number less an even integer.

EXERCISE

6. Use calculus methods to verify that only one positive root exists for the characteristic equation of A. Verify Descartes' Rule of Signs (see the text by Dickson [2] for a proof).

An eigenvector $x^{(1)}$ corresponding to the eigenvalue λ_1 must satisfy the system of equations

$$Ax^{(1)} = \lambda_1 x^{(1)}.$$

Property (2) follows immediately upon solving this system of equations.

EXERCISE

7. If $x^{(1)}$ is a eigenvector vector corresponding to λ_1, show that $x_2 = (s_1/\lambda_1)x_1$ and $x_3 = (s_2 s_1/\lambda_1^2)x_1$ where the components of $x^{(1)}$ are x_1, x_2, and x_3.

Since one may choose the first component of $x^{(1)}$ arbitrarily, a characteristic vector corresponding to λ_1 is given by

$$x^{(1)} = \begin{pmatrix} 1 \\ s_1/\lambda_1 \\ s_1 s_2/\lambda_1^2 \end{pmatrix}.$$

Property (3) is more involved. We will deduce this property from a well-known result for stochastic matrices.

Theorem. *Let P be an $m \times m$ matrix with nonnegative components. Assume that each row sum of P is one and that P^n has all components positive for some positive integer n. Then a row vector z exists, all of whose components are positive, such that*

$$\lim_{n \to \infty} P^n = ez,$$

where e is the column vector with all components equal to one. Moreover, the sum of the components of z is one.

EXERCISE

8. Verify this theorem. The text by Roberts [7, p. 292] contains a proof.

Property (3) may be deduced from the following corollary.

Corollary. *Let A be an $m \times m$ matrix with non-negative components such that A^n has all components positive for some positive integer n. Assume that A has a positive eigenvalue λ_1 and a corresponding eigenvector $x^{(1)}$ with positive components. Then there is a row vector y with positive components such that*

$$\lim_{n \to \infty} A^n / \lambda_1^n = x^{(1)} y.$$

A proof of this corollary may be found in [1]; since this text may not be readily available, we include the details.

PROOF. Let D be the diagonal matrix with $d_{ii} = x_i^{(1)}$ and $d_{ij} = 0$ for $i \neq j$. Since $x^{(1)}$ has positive components, D^{-1} exists and is a diagonal matrix with diagonal components $1/x_i^{(1)}$. Also $De = x^{(1)}$ and hence

$$[D^{-1}(1/\lambda_1)AD]e = D^{-1}(1/\lambda_1)Ax^{(1)} = e.$$

Since $[D^{-1}(1/\lambda_1)AD]e$ is the vector each of whose components is the corresponding row sum of $D^{-1}(1/\lambda_1)AD$, we see that each row sum of $D^{-1}(1/\lambda_1)AD$ is one. Also $[D^{-1}(1/\lambda_1)AD]^n = D^{-1}(1/\lambda_1^n)A^nD$ and it follows that $[D^{-1}(1/\lambda_1)AD]^n$ has all components positive for n sufficiently large. By the theorem

$$\lim_{n \to \infty} D^{-1}(1/\lambda_1^n)A^nD = ez,$$

where z has positive components. Thus

$$\lim_{n \to \infty} (1/\lambda_1^n)A^n = DezD^{-1} = x^{(1)}y$$

and $y = zD^{-1}$ has positive components.   □

Property (3) may now be verified. By the Corollary one obtains for any vector x_0

$$\lim_{n \to \infty} A^n x_0 / \lambda_1^n = x^{(1)} y x_0,$$

where $c = yx_0$. Note that c is positive whenever x_0 is nonzero with nonnegative components. Thus

$$\lim_{n \to \infty} A^n x_0 / \lambda_1^n = cx^{(1)},$$

where $c = yx_0$. Note that c is positive whenever x_0 is nonzero with nonnegative components.

This completes the proof of properties (1), (2), and (3). It is interesting to note that λ_1 is the dominant eigenvalue of A, that is, if λ_i is an eigenvalue of A distinct from λ_1 then $|\lambda_i| < \lambda_1$. To verify this property, let z be an eigenvector corresponding to λ_i. Since $Az = \lambda_i z$ we conclude that $A^n z = \lambda_i^n z$ and $(1/\lambda_1^n)A^n z = (\lambda_i/\lambda_1)^n z$. By the Corollary

$$x^{(1)}yz = \lim_{n\to\infty} (\lambda_i/\lambda_1)^n z.$$

Since the limit exists and λ_1 is a simple root of the characteristic equation, we must have $|\lambda_i| < \lambda_1$.

The dominance of λ_1 aids in a more geometric understanding of Property (3) as the following exercise shows.

EXERCISE

9. Suppose A has distinct eigenvalues λ_1, λ_2, and λ_3 with $|\lambda_2| < \lambda_1$ and $|\lambda_3| < \lambda_1$. Let $x^{(1)}$, $x^{(2)}$, and $x^{(3)}$ be eigenvectors corresponding to λ_1, λ_2, and λ_3. Since any vector x_0 may be written as $x_0 = c_1 x^{(1)} + c_2 x^{(2)} + c_3 x^{(3)}$ for suitable scalars c_1, c_2, and c_3, show that

$$\lim_{n\to\infty} A^n x_0/\lambda_1^n = c_1 x^{(1)}.$$

Our explanation of the above properties of A follows the introduction given in [1]. For a more general survey of properties of nonnegative matrices the reader is referred to the text by Marcus and Minc [6].

4. Prediction and Implementation

An explanation of the growth patterns of the whole population in terms of the behavior of the first three age groups may now be given. We wish to explain the following basic properties of the growth model.

Property I. The population eventually grows at a constant rate.
Property II. The population age distribution approaches a constant distribution as time increases.

In Property I, we mean that for each age group the ratio $W_i(15(n + 1))/W_i(15n)$ approaches a constant as n increases. This relation for the population represented by the reduced model

$$\tilde{W}(15(n + 1)) = A\tilde{W}(15n)$$

follows from Property (3) of the preceding section. That is, for any nonzero initial population $W(0)$,

$$\lim_{n\to\infty} \tilde{W}(15n)/\lambda_1^n = \lim_{n\to\infty} A^n \tilde{W}(0)/\lambda_1^n = cx^{(1)}$$

where c depends on $\tilde{W}(0)$. Thus $W_i(15n)/\lambda_1^n$ converges to $cx_i^{(1)}$ and we see that $W_i(15(n + 1))/W_i(15n)$ converges to λ_1. Since the growth rate eventually approaches a constant, λ_1 is referred to as the *intrinsic growth rate*.

Property II refers to the fact that after a number of periods the proportion of the population in each age group becomes constant. To see that Property II holds for the reduced model, let

$$P(15n) = W_1(15n) + W_2(15n) + W_3(15n)$$

denote the total population size of the first three age groups at the end of the nth period. The proportion of the population in the ith age group is $\hat{W}_i(15n)/P(15n)$ for $i = 1, 2,$ and 3. Thus

$$\lim_{n \to \infty} W_i(15n)/P(15n) = \lim_{n \to \infty} \frac{W_i(15n)/\lambda_1^n}{P(15n)/\lambda_1^n}$$

$$= \frac{cx_i^{(1)}}{cx_1^{(1)} + cx_2^{(2)} + cx_3^{(1)}}$$

$$= \frac{x_i^1}{x_1^{(1)} + x_2^{(2)} + x_3^{(1)}}$$

where $x_1^{(1)}$, $x_2^{(1)}$, and $x_3^{(1)}$ denote the components of $x^{(1)}$. We see that the proportion of the population in the ith age group eventually depends solely on the eigenvector $x^{(1)}$. For this reason $x^{(1)}$ is referred to as the stable age distribution.

EXERCISE

10. Use the fact that Properties I and II hold for the reduced model to show that these properties hold for the original model

$$W(15(n + 1)) = GW(15n).$$

Notice that as a consequence of Property I, the size of each age group increases without bound if λ_1 is greater than one and approaches zero if λ_1 is less than one. Also notice that the limiting age distribution is independent of the initial population size.

We have shown that an analysis of the growth model for the whole population,

$$W(15(n + 1)) = GW(15n)$$

depends on the ability to calculate the dominant eigenvalue λ_1 and corresponding eigenvector $x^{(1)}$. The problem of finding λ_1 is that of finding a positive root of a polynomial equation, which we know beforehand has only one positive root. The Appendix contains a Fortran program for finding this root by Newton's Method. This method is an iterative procedure for approximating λ_1. Since the method requires an initial approximation to λ_1, the following result [2] is useful.

Let A be the matrix of the example and let m and M be the smallest and largest of the column sums of A. Then $m \le \lambda_1 \le M$.

To see that this result holds, let e^T denote the transpose of the column vector e with all components equal to one. Clearly, $e^T m \le e^T A \le e^T M$, where the inequality symbol indicates that the inequality holds between corresponding components of the vectors. Since $Ax^{(1)} = \lambda_1 x^{(1)}$, we have

$e^T A x^{(1)} = e^T \lambda_1 x^{(1)}$. Hence $m e^T x^{(1)} \leq \lambda_1 e^T x^{(1)} \leq M e^T x^{(1)}$ since all components of $x^{(1)}$ are positive. Since $e^T x^{(1)}$ is positive, we have $m \leq \lambda_1 \leq M$. A similar result holds for row sums.

We have previously shown that a stable age distribution is given by

$$x^{(1)} = \begin{pmatrix} 1 \\ s_1/\lambda_1 \\ s_1 s_2/\lambda_1^2 \end{pmatrix}.$$

EXERCISES

11. With G as in Exercise 2, compute the intrinsic growth rate λ_1 and the stable age distribution $x^{(1)}$. Use $x^{(1)}$ to approximate the eventual percentage of the total population in each age group (see Exercise 10). Compare the results of this exercise with the computations of Exercise 2.

12. What are the consequences of the intrinsic growth rate having the value one? What is the stable age distribution in this case? For the hypothetical population of Exercise 2, determine modifications of the birth rates b_2 and b_3 which lead to an intrinsic growth rate of $\lambda_1 = 1$.

5. Conclusion

Although the analysis in this chapter has been in terms of a particular example, the techniques apply to the conceptual model of a population given in the introduction. The population must be partitioned into age groups of equal length and predictions of future growth made at multiples

Age Group	Rate
5–10	0.00102
10–15	0.08515
15–20	0.30574
20–25	0.40002
25–30	0.28061
30–35	0.15260
35–40	0.06420
40–45	0.01483
45–50	0.00089

Table 1. United States Females Fertility Rates 1966 (Female Births/Individual/Period) [4]

Table 2. United States Females Survival
Rates 1966 [4]

Age Group	Rate	Age Group	Rate
0–5	0.99670	50–55	0.96258
5–10	0.99837	55–60	0.94562
10–15	0.99780	60–65	0.91522
15–20	0.99672	65–70	0.86806
20–25	0.99607	70–75	0.80021
25–30	0.99472	75–80	0.69239
30–35	0.99240	80–85	0.77312
35–40	0.98867		
40–45	0.98274		
45–50	0.97437		

Table 3. United States Females
Population 1966 (thousands) [4]

Age Group	Size	Age Group	Size
0–5	9,715	50–55	5,498
5–10	10,226	55–60	4,839
10–15	9,542	60–65	4,174
15–20	8,806	65–70	3,476
20–25	6,981	70–75	2,929
25–30	5,840	75–80	2,124
30–35	5,527	80–85	1,230
35–40	5,987	85+	694
40–45	6,371		
45–50	5,978		

Survival rates and population sizes for age
groups above 85 have been combined.

of this length. The assumption of fixed fertility and mortality rates provides a basis for the prediction of growth patterns. This assumption is questionable for human populations over a long period of time. We have assumed that fertility and mortality rates are given. For a discussion of the estimation of these parameters from census data one may consult the texts by Keyfitz [3] and Keyfitz and Flieger [4]. The latter reference contains demographic data for seventy countries including the data in Tables 1–3 for the United States. Also, these texts contain refinements and extensions of the model presented in this chapter.

EXERCISES

13. Perform Exercise 1 and 11 using the given data for United States females.

14. Derive an age structure model for United States males and females. One method
is to assume the female model holds, for each female birth there is also a male
birth, and survival rates for male groups are constant. How can one incorporate
migration into this model?

Appendix

A Fortran Program for Exercise 2

```
      C
      C THE ARRAY G IS INITALIZED WITH GIVEN RATE DATA
      C THE ARRAY WB IS INITIALIZED WITH INITIAL POP. DATA
      C THE ARRAYS W AND WC ARE WORKING ARRAYS
      C NL REPRESENTS THE NUMBER OF PERIODS CONSIDERED
      C
      C
1         DIMENSION G(5,5),W(5),WB(5),WC(5)
2         READ 1, NL
3       1 FORMAT (12)
4         READ 2,((G(I,J),J=1,5),I=1,5)
5       2 FORMAT (5F10.5)
6         READ 2,(WB(I),I=1,5)
7         PRINT 10
8      10 FORMAT ('1',' INITIAL GROWTH MATRIX')
9         DO 3 I=1,5
10      3 PRINT 11,(G(I,J),J=1,5)
11     11 FORMAT (' ',5F10.2)
12        PRINT 12
13     12 FORMAT (' ',' INITIAL POPULATION OF AGE GROUPS')
14        PRINT 13, (WB(I),I=1,5)
15     13 FORMAT (' ',5F10.2)
16        DO 6 N=1,NL
17        DO 5 I=1,5
18        W(I)=0.0
19        DO 4 J=1,5
20      4 W(I)=W(I)+G(I,J)•WB(J)
21      5 CONTINUE
22        P=0.0
23        DO 30 I=1,5
24     30 P=P+W(I)
25        DO 31 I=1,5
26        WC(I)=W(I)/P
27     31 WB(I)=W(I)/WB(I)
28        PRINT 14,N
29     14 FORMAT ('0',' PERIOD',13)
30        PRINT 19,P
31     19 FORMAT (' ',' TOTAL POPULATION',F25.2)
      C
      C W CONTAINS PROJECTED POPULATION FOR NEXT PERIOD
      C WC CONTAINS POPULATION DISTRIBUTION
```

```
      C WB CONTAINS GROWTH RATES FOR AGE GROUPS
      C
32       PRINT 16,(W(I),I=1,5)
33 16 FORMAT (' ',' POPULATION OF AGE GROUPS ',5F15.2)
34       PRINT 21,(WC(I),I=1,5)
35 21 FORMAT (' ',' POPULATION DISTRIBUTION ',5F15.5)
36       PRINT 23,(WB(I),I=1,5)
37 23 FORMAT (' ',' GROWTH RATE FOR AGE GROUPS',5F15.5)
38       DO 6 I=1,5
      C
      C WB IS INITIALIZED FOR NEXT PERIOD
      C
39  6 WB(I)=W(I)
40       STOP
41       END
```

A Fortran Program for Newton's Method:
$$f(x) = a_3 x^3 + a_2 x^2 + a_1 x + a_0.$$

```
      C
      C A3 A2 A1 A0 REPRESENT GIVEN COEFFICIENTS
      C
1        READ 1,A3,A2,A1,A0
2      1 FORMAT (4F10.5)
3        PRINT 2,A3,A2,A1,A0
4      2 FORMAT (' ',' POLYNOMIAL COEFFICIENTS ',4F10.5)
5        X1=1.0
6     10 X=X1
7        F=A3*X**3+A2*X**2+A1*X+A0
8        DF=A3*3*X**2+A2*2*X+A1
9        X1=X-F/DF
10       PRINT 3,X1
11     3 FORMAT (' ',' APPROXIMATE ROOT ',F10.5)
12       IF(ABS (X-X1).GT..0001)GOTO10
13       IF(F.GT..0001)GOTO10
14       STOP
15       END
```

Solutions to the Exercises

1. Many unanswered questions remain. How does one estimate birth and death rates? How does one allow for migration? How does one incorporate dependence of birth and death rates on environmental, political, social, and economic factors into the model?

2. (This exercise is essential for an understanding of the growth patterns predicted by the model.) One may wish to choose different values for birth and death rates. Since the eventual growth rate and population distribution are independent of the initial population size, it is interesting to assign different initial populations for the

same growth matrix. The growth rate using the given data is $\lambda_1 = 1.455$ and the eventual distribution is given by $(0.388, 0.261, 0.172, 0.110, 0.068)$.

3. Induction.

4. Notice the symmetry. If the model contains a larger number of age groups this symmetry carries over.

5. Answer 5.

6. Any text on the theory of equations contains a proof of Descartes' Rule of Signs. The problem may be solved by analyzing the signs of the derivative of the characteristic polynomial.

7. The solution of the linear system of equations is straightforward. Notice the symmetry.

8. This is a standard result for stochastic matrices. The reference cited contains a proof. Most texts on stochastic processes also contain a proof.

9. The student must know that eigenvalues corresponding to distinct eigenvectors are independent.

10. This exercise is essential. One should use the results for the reduced model and the relations $W_i(t + 15) = s_{i-1} W_{i-1}(t)$ for the latter age groups.

11. A computer program in Fortran for finding λ_1 is provided in the Appendix. It is interesting to investigate the sensitivity of this root to variations in the birth and or death rates. Here, $\lambda_1 = 1.45487$.

12. Let $b_2 + x$ and $b_3 + y$ denote modified birth and death rates. Compute the new characteristic equation. Assuming $\lambda_1 = 1$ is a root, one obtains that the point (x, y) must lie on the line $0.98x + 0.9408y = -1.4108$. We must also have $b_2 + > 0$ and $b_3 + y > 0$. Thus there are many choices of x and y which lead to an intrinsic growth rate equal to one.

13. This exercise requires extension of the model to a population subdivided into 18 age groups, five years in length. All previous techniques for the five age group examples carry over. The programs in the Appendix must be modified slightly. One should notice the symmetry in the results of Exercises 4 and 7 in solving for that characteristic equation and the stable age distribution.

14. The male–female model should be straightforward using a 36×36 growth matrix. One method incorporating migration into the model is to assume that in any period the number of migrants into an age group is proportional to the number of individuals entering that age group from the original population.

References

[1] E. J. Cogan et al, "Mathematical models," Dartmouth College Writing Group, Committee on the Undergraduate Program, Mathematical Association of America, 1958.

[2] L. E. Dickson, *New First Course in the Theory of Equations*. New York: Wiley, 1939.

[3] N. Keyfitz *Introduction to the Mathematics of Population*. Reading, MA: Addison-Wesley, 1968.

[4] N. Keyfitz and W. Flieger, *Population Facts and Methods of Demography*. San Francisco, CA: W. H. Freeman, 1971.

[5] P. H. Leslie, "On the use of matrices in certain population mathematics," *Biometrika*, vol. 20, Part 3, pp. 183–212, 1945.

[6] M. Marcus and H. Minc, *A Surey of Matrix Theory and Matrix Inequalities*. Allyn and Bacon, 1964.

[7] F. S. Roberts, *Discrete Mathematical Models*. Englewood Cliffs, NJ: Prentice-Hall, 1976.

Notes for the Instructor

This chapter has been prepared with the belief that discovery leads to understanding. For this reason fullest appreciation will be achieved by completing the assignments. Assuming the prerequisite of an understanding of basic concepts of linear algebra, this chapter is self-contained except for some reference work in Exercises 6 and 8.

A simple application of the model is presented in Section 2. Exercise 2 of this section illustrates the growth patterns predicted by the model and is essential. Section 3 contains a discussion of properties of nonnegative matrices. We suggest that Properties (1), (2), and (3) of this section be accepted on first reading and that one pass on to Sections 4 and 5. In Section 4 the results of Section 3 are used to explain the observations of Exercise 2. Finally, in Section 5 the reader is asked to apply the model to the population consisting of United States females. The Appendix contains Fortran programs required in Exercises 2 and 11. These programs require slight modifications in order to perform Exercise 12.

Objectives. Linear algebra concepts are used to analyze a basic demographic model.

Prerequisites. Basic concepts of linear algebra: basis, eigenvalues, eigenvectors, characteristic equation. An elementary scientific programming ability.

Remark. This model and its predictions may be presented in one class period. A theoretical analysis of the model, illustrating many concepts studied in an undergraduate linear algebra course, is included but requires more time. Assignments are essential for an understanding of the material and involve matrix manipulations, use of the computer to solve polynomial equations and to perform matrix multiplications, theorem proving, and library reference work. A section including comments for the instructor is provided along with an Appendix containing Fortran programs.

CHAPTER 3

A Comparison of Some Deterministic and Stochastic Models of Population Growth

Helen Marcus–Roberts*

1. Introduction

A debate which has involved philosophers for many years is whether the world is basically deterministic or whether there are elements of chance in the unfolding of natural processes. Whether to look at the world as deterministic or stochastic is a fundamental decision which faces the mathematical modeler. He is not necessarily making a philosophical decision by making this choice. We may be able to understand a fundamentally stochastic world by looking at it deterministically, or a fundamentally deterministic world by looking at it stochastically. In this module, we shall compare and contrast the difficulties involved in and the information obtainable from deterministic and stochastic models of some phenomena. We shall study alternate models of population growth, of increasing complexity, giving at each stage a deterministic and a stochastic model. We shall in the process make points about the tools and techniques of modeling and about the mathematics of population growth, which should be of interest in and of themselves.

This module will be organized in the following way. Section 2 is a brief discussion of the philosophy of model building, Section 3 explores probability generating functions, Section 4 discusses the derivation of the general system of differential equations for the pure birth process, and Section 5 presents models of population growth.

* Department of Mathematics and Computer Science, Montclair State College, Upper Montclair, NJ 07043.

2. Basic Philosophy of Model Building

Mathematical modelers are confronted with various philosophical and/or practical decisions before starting to model real world phenomena. We will briefly discuss three of these choices. First, is the choice between models that are used for prediction purposes only and consider only gross aspects (e.g., for control purposes as in setting hunting regulations) versus models in which parameters of the model give some insight or deeper understanding of the actual phenomena being modeled. Second, as we have mentioned is the choice between deterministic and stochastic models. Third, a choice between reality and tractable or do-able mathematics. We discuss these three choices in some detail.

2.1 Gross Aspects (Prediction) versus Meaningful Parameters

Modelers can derive models that can be used to give general predictions in which parameters do not relate specifically to the phenomenon being studied, or they can derive models incorporating assumptions about the phenomenon. Clearly, the use to be made of the model will dictate which type is desirable. As an example we consider some models of the growth of the number of malaria parasites in a host. Malaria was once one of the most devastating diseases, capable of destroying whole cultures. Malaria still occurs today in Africa and the Far and Middle East. Briefly, malaria is caused by a parasite that is carried by mosquitos who have ingested blood from an infected person or animal. The parasites undergo sexual reproduction in the mosquito and on its next meal the mosquito exchanges infected blood (with parasites) for normal blood. The parasites in the blood of the human host attack the red blood cells (rbc's) and undergo asexual reproduction. A single parasite in a red blood cell reproduces and forms 12–40 new parasites (depending on the species). The red blood cell bursts and releases the new parasites so they can start the process over by infecting more red blood cells. The process of the cells bursting is amazingly regular. All infected red blood cells burst about every 48 or 72 hours depending on the species of parasites. The regularity is fairly well established because every 48 or 72 hours there is a characteristic behavior of chills and fever spikes (this is a form of protein shock when the rbc's burst). If blood samples are drawn periodically it is possible to show rises and declines in the number of parasites. A typical graph of the number of parasites counted is given in Figure 3.1. We note many peaks and troughs. One of the classical models to predict the number of parasites on a given day was a *gamma function*. The gamma function is given by $y = cx^a e^{-bx}$, where x is the day, y is the number of parasites, and a, b, c are estimated from data.[1] The gamma function is strictly unimodal and is

---

[1] a, b, c are obtained as moment estimates as follows: $c = \bar{x}$(mean), $b = s^2$(variance), and $a = \Sigma(x_i - \bar{x})^3/n$.

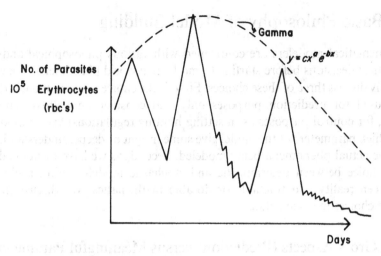

Figure 3.1. Typical Graph of Number of Malaria Parasites.

superimposed on Figure 3.1 by the dashed line. It is hard to believe that the gamma function can do more than lead to a very superficial prediction of the number of parasites. (Statistical χ^2—Goodness of Fit suggests that the gamma is not a good fit.)

Another approach to modeling the growth of malaria parasites would be to incorporate the cyclical nature of the process and thereby derive models in which the parameters are a significant part of the model. This can be done by using branching processes to model the growth of the parasites. See Marcus–Roberts and Roberts [7] for a first attempt to do this. In sum, the modeler must carefully consider the purposes and uses of his model and then choose between the two types. In this module we will consider models of population growth in which the parameters relate specifically to the phenomenon being modeled.

2.2 Deterministic versus Stochastic Models

Deterministic models of population growth are derived under the assumption that population growth is such that the future development of the population can be predicted *exactly* once its state at some initial time is specified. These models do not permit any random fluctuations; that is, a particular event such as a birth must occur with absolute certainty. In deterministic models, the population is assumed large enough and the factors determining individual birth and death rates are constant enough that the consequences of random fluctuations can be ignored. This would probably be true only for a very large population under highly idealized conditions, where we can ignore the noise or random aspects. For example, if we are dealing with millions of cells (red blood cells, or malaria parasites) in the human body, then being off by a few hundred cells is of little consequence.

Stochastic models of population growth are derived under the basic assumption that population growth is a random event; that is, an organism (cell or parasite) may reproduce during a given time period with a certain probability p, where $0 \leq p \leq 1$. No events occur with absolute certainty. We can build these ideas into the model by allowing chance or random fluctuations in the process. Some populations are small enough or variable enough that random fluctuations can be appreciable.

Schematically, we represent the difference between deterministic and stochastic models in Figure 3.2. Our figure illustrates an observation we shall make often in what follows, namely, that often the solution of a deterministic model turns out to equal the expected value of the stochastic analog. Thus the stochastic solution gives us, in a sense, more information than the deterministic solution (we shall discuss this further in Section 5); many modelers therefore consider it to be the better approach, regardless of one's philosophy of the world. Some people feel, on the other hand, that one goes to stochastic models only because one does not really understand the correct deterministic process! In Section 5, we will develop deterministic and stochastic models of simple growth in populations and compare the two.

2.3 Reality versus Tractable Mathematics

A lot of modeling of biological processes (and nonbiological phenomena) is a compromise between the biological phenomena and mathematics. If one wants the model to reflect the complexities of the process, one finds that the more closely the model is made to conform to nature, the more unmanageable it becomes from the mathematical point of view. (This drawback is somewhat tempered because of some of the sophisticated computers and computer techniques that now exist.) A compromise is often made between the extremes of a model that is so crude as to be unrealistic or misleading and a model that is too complex mathematically. We will try to demonstrate this point by introducing more and more realistic and complex biological assumptions into our model.

In Section 5, we will also present some alternate methods that can be used to answer the same mathematical questions arising from models of the types we are presenting. One of the methods of solution requires the knowledge of probability generating functions. Therefore, we will present a brief overview of probability generating functions and their uses in Section 3. We hope the reader who has never been exposed to this subject will find it interesting.

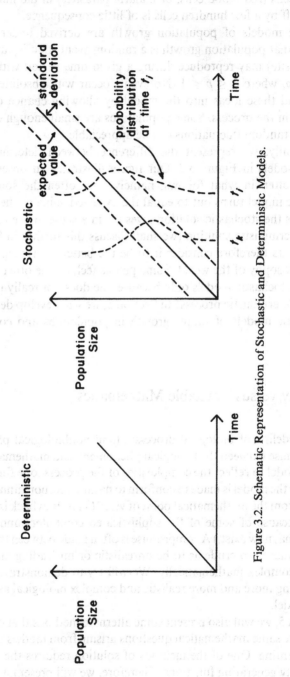

Figure 3.2. Schematic Representation of Stochastic and Deterministic Models.

3. Probability Generating Functions (pgf's)

3.1 Definition and Basic Facts

Definition. Let $a_0, a_1, a_2, \cdots$ be a sequence of real numbers. If

$$A(s) = a_0 + a_1 s + a_2 s^2 + a_3 s^3 + \cdots$$

converges in some interval $-s_0 < s < s_0$, then $A(s)$ is called the *generating function* of the sequence $\{a_j\}$.

Two points to note are (1) s is just a *dummy*, in effect a place holder (or indicator variable), and (2) if the sequence $\{a_j\}$ is bounded, then $A(s)$ will converge for at least $|s| < 1$. Consider the following examples.

(a) Let $\{a_j\}$ be 1, 1, 1, $\cdots$. Therefore,

$$A(s) = 1 + 1 \cdot s + 1 \cdot s^2 + 1 \cdot s^3 + \cdots$$

$$= 1 + s + s^2 + s^3 + \cdots$$

$$= \sum_{i=0}^{\infty} s^i$$

$$= \frac{1}{1 - s}, \qquad \text{if } |s| < 1.$$

The generating function for the sequence 1, 1, 1, $\cdots$ is $1/(1 - s)$.

(b) Let $a_0 = 1$, $a_1 = 1/1!$, $a_2 = 1/2!$, $a_3 = 1/3!$, $\cdots$, $a_k = 1/k!$, $\cdots$. Then

$$A(s) = 1 + \frac{1}{1!}s + \frac{1}{2!}s^2 + \frac{1}{3!}s^3 + \frac{1}{4!}s^4 + \cdots = e^s.$$

A very interesting special case occurs where the elements of the sequence $\{a_j\}$ are probabilities. All such sequences are bounded. Suppose X is a discrete random variable which takes on the values 0, 1, 2, $\cdots$, with certain probabilities $p_j = \Pr[X = j]$. Then the generating function

$$P(s) = \sum_{\text{all values}} p_j s^j$$

is called the probability generating function (pgf). Note that $P(s) = E[s^X]$. It turns out that $P(s)$ uniquely determines the probability density, i.e., knowing $P(s)$ defines the probabilities $\Pr[X = j]$.

We shall see in Section 4 that it is possible to start out with a set of assumptions and then find the probability generating function without knowing $\Pr[X = j]$. Probability generating functions, since they turn out to be unique, can then be used to determine the probability density, the mean and variance of the random variable, etc. In particular, given a pgf, the following information can be derived.

(a)
$$\frac{1}{j!}\frac{d^{j}P(s)}{ds^{j}}\bigg|_{s=0} = p_{j} = \Pr[X = j].$$

The reader should verify this fact. See Exercise 1 at the end of Section 3. The importance of this fact is that if we have the pgf for a discrete distribution, we know the distribution. No two distinct distributions can have the same pgf.

(b) To verify that we have an honest probability density (the sum of probabilities is 1), one shows that $P(1) = 1$, since

$$P(1) = \sum_{j=0}^{\infty} \Pr[X = j]s^{j}\big|_{s=1}$$

$$= \sum_{j=0}^{\infty} \Pr[X = j]$$

$$= 1.$$

(c) By taking appropriate derivatives of the pgf, it is quite easy to determine the mean μ and variance σ^{2}.

$$P'(1) = E[X] = \mu. \tag{1}$$

PROOF.

$$P'(s)\big|_{s=1} = \frac{dP(s)}{ds}\bigg|_{s=1} = \sum_{j=0}^{\infty} \Pr[X = j]s^{j-1}j\big|_{s=1}$$

$$= \sum_{j=0}^{\infty} \Pr[X = j]j$$

$$= E[X]$$

$$= \mu. \qquad\Box$$

$$P''(1) + P'(1) - (P'(1))^{2} = E[(X - \mu)^{2}]$$
$$= \sigma^{2}. \tag{2}$$

(The reader should verify (2). See Exercise 2, at the end of Section 3.)

3.2 The pgf's of Some Important Probability Distributions

We shall determine the pgf for various probability distributions which we shall encounter later, and also give examples of the uses of pgf's.

3.2.1. Binomial. The binomial distribution arises from the following:

(1) repeat an experiment n times under identical conditions (n identical trials);

(2) trials are independent;

(3) dichotomous outcomes (success $[S]$ or failure $[F]$);
(4) $\Pr[S] = p$ and is constant, and $\Pr[F] = 1 - p = q$.

We are interested in the probability of k successes in n trials, that is $\Pr[X = k]$. We have

$$\Pr[X = k] = \binom{n}{k}p^k q^{n-k}.$$

(Note that $\Sigma_{k=0}^n \binom{n}{k}p^k q^{n-k} = (p + q)^n = 1^n = 1$.) The pgf is given by

$$P(s) = \sum_{k=0}^n \binom{n}{k}p^k q^{n-k} s^k$$

$$= \sum_{k=0}^n \binom{n}{k}(ps)^k q^{n-k}$$

$$= (ps + q)^n.$$

Using the pgf, let us determine $\Pr[X = 2]$:

$$\frac{1}{2!}\frac{d^2 P(s)}{ds^2} = \frac{1}{2!}\frac{d^2}{ds^2}[(ps + q)^n]$$

$$= \frac{1}{2!}\frac{d}{ds}[n(ps + q)^{n-1}p]$$

$$= \frac{n(n - 1)}{2!}(ps + q)^{n-2}p^2.$$

Thus

$$\frac{1}{2!}\frac{d^2 P(s)}{ds^2}\bigg|_{s=0} = \frac{n(n - 1)}{2!}(p \cdot 0 + q)^{n-2}p^2$$

$$= \frac{n(n - 1)}{2!}q^{n-2}p^2$$

$$= \binom{n}{2}p^2 q^{n-2}.$$

Clearly, this method can be used to find the $\Pr[X = k]$ for $k = 0, 1, \cdots, n$. The mean of the binomial distribution, is gotten by first finding

$$P'(s) = \frac{d}{ds}(ps + q)^n$$

$$= n(ps + q)^{n-1}p$$

and evaluating $P'(s)$ when $s = 1$. That is,

$$\mu = P'(1) = n(p + q)^{n-1}p$$

$$= n(1)^{n-1}p$$

$$= np.$$

In fact, it is well-known that the mean number of successes in a binomial experiment is given by np.

To determine the variance of the binomial distribution we must determine $P''(1) + P'(1) - \{P'(1)\}^2$. First, we find $P''(1)$:

$$P''(1) = \frac{d^2}{ds^2}(P(s))\big|_{s=1} = \frac{d}{ds}(n(ps + q)^{n-1}p)\big|_{s=1}$$

$$= n(n - 1)(ps + q)^{n-2}p^2\big|_{s=1}$$

$$P''(1) = n(n - 1)(p + q)^{n-2}p^2$$

$$= n(n - 1)p^2.$$

Then the variance is given by

$$\sigma^2 = n(n - 1)p^2 + np - (np)^2$$

$$= n^2p^2 - np^2 + np - n^2p^2$$

$$= np - np^2$$

$$= np(1 - p) = npq.$$

Again it is well-known that the variance of a binomial distribution is given by npq.

3.2.2. Poisson. The Poisson probability distribution is a discrete distribution that counts the number of times an event occurs over time or in space. The number of times the event can occur is not bounded and hence $k = 0, 1, 2, \cdots$ (but observed values of k are usually small). The Poisson distribution is used as a model for random occurrences in space or time (for example, bombs over London, spatial distribution of plants in a field, and the distribution of accidents in a factory).

The Poisson distribution is given by

$$\Pr[X = k] = \frac{e^{-\lambda}\lambda^k}{k!}.$$

The Poisson distribution is sometimes referred to as the *binomial exponential limit*, since

$$\lim_{\substack{n \to \infty \\ p \to 0 \\ np \to \lambda}} \binom{n}{k}p^kq^{n-k} = \frac{e^{-\lambda}\lambda^k}{k!}.$$

The pgf for the Poisson is given by

$$P(s) = \sum_{k=0}^{\infty} \frac{e^{-\lambda}\lambda^k}{k!}s^k$$

$$= e^{-\lambda}\sum_{k=0}^{\infty} \frac{(\lambda s)^k}{k!}$$

$$= e^{-\lambda}e^{\lambda s}$$
$$= e^{\lambda(s-1)}.$$

Using the pgf of the Poisson, we can show that[2]

(i) $P(1) = e^{\lambda(1-1)} = e^0 = 1$ (as expected);

(ii) $P'(s) = \lambda e^{\lambda(s-1)}$ so that $P'(1) = \lambda = E[X] = \mu$;

(iii) $P''(s) = \lambda^2 e^{\lambda(s-1)}$ and $P''(1) = \lambda^2$, so that
$$\sigma^2 = P''(1) + P'(1) - (P'(1))^2$$
$$= \lambda^2 + \lambda - \lambda^2$$
$$= \lambda.$$

It is well-known that the mean and variance of the Poisson distribution are given by λ. Therefore, from the generating function of the Poisson, we see that the coefficient of $(s - 1)$ in the exponent is equal to the mean and variance. From the uniqueness of pgf's we know that if we derive pgf $e^{5(s-1)}$, we have a Poisson distribution with $\Pr[X = k] = e^{-5}5^k/k!$ and mean and variance $= 5$.

(iv) The reader should verify that

$$\frac{1}{k!} \cdot \frac{d^k P(s)}{ds^k}\bigg|_{s=0} = \frac{e^{-\lambda}\lambda^k}{k!}.$$

(See Exercise 4 at the end of Section 3.)

3.2.3. Geometric and Negative Binomial. The geometric and negative Binomial are often referred to as *waiting time distributions*. Let us consider an experiment where we have a fixed probability p of a success and $q = 1 - p$ is the probability of a failure, and the trials are independent. We perform the experiment and are interested in the probability that the first success occurs on the kth trial. Schematically,

Trial   1   2   3   4 $\cdots$ $k-1$ k

Outcome F F F F $\cdots$ F S.

$$\underbrace{\qquad\qquad\qquad\qquad\qquad}_{k-1} \qquad k = 1, 2, \cdots.$$

If we let random variable X denote the trial of the first success, then we are interested in

$$\Pr[X = k].$$

It follows that

$$\Pr[X = k] = q^{k-1}p, \qquad k = 1, 2, 3, \cdots,$$

and this is known as the geometric distribution. The pgf of the geometric distribution is given by

---

[2] The reader should try to compute mean and variance by the definition to appreciate how much easier the pgf approach is. (See Exercise 5 at the end of Section 3.)

$$P(s) = \sum_{k=1}^{\infty} q^{k-1}ps^k$$

$$= ps \sum_{k=1}^{\infty} q^{k-1}s^{k-1}$$

$$= ps \sum_{k=1}^{\infty} (qs)^{k-1}$$

$$= \frac{ps}{1-qs}.$$

(The reader should use the pgf to determine the mean μ, the variance σ^2, and $\Pr[X = k]$. See Exercise 6 at the end of Section 3.)

A logical extension of the geometric distribution is to wait for the mth success. Let us determine the probability that the mth success occurs on the $(k + m)$th trial. Schematically,

$$\begin{array}{cccccc}
\text{Trial} & 1 \ \ 2 \ \ 3 & \cdots & m + k - 1 & m + k \\
\text{Outcome} & & & & S.
\end{array}$$

$(m - 1)$ successes
and k failures

If we let the random variable X denote the trial of the mth success, we can determine the probability $\Pr[X = k + m]$ by noting that the number of successes in the first $m + k - 1$ trials follow a binomial distribution. Therefore, it follows that

$$\Pr[X = k + m] = \binom{k + m - 1}{m - 1} p^{m-1}q^kp$$

$$= \binom{k + m - 1}{k} p^{m-1}q^kp$$

$$= \binom{k + m - 1}{k} q^kp^m,$$

and

$$P(s) = \sum_{k=0}^{\infty} \binom{k + m - 1}{k} q^kp^ms^{k+m}$$

$$= \frac{(sp)^m}{(1 - qs)^m}$$

(by using the Maclaurin expansion). (The reader should use the pgf to determine μ, σ^2, and $\Pr[X = k + m]$. See Exercise 7.)

EXERCISES

1. Using the definition of a pgf,

$$P(s) = \sum_{j=0}^{\infty} \Pr[X = j]s^j,$$

verify that

$$\frac{1}{j!} \frac{d^j P(s)}{ds^j}\bigg|_{s=0} = \Pr[X = j].$$

2. Using the definition of a pgf and the fact that $E[X] = \mu$, verify that

$$E[(X - \mu)^2] = \frac{d^2 P(s)}{ds^2}\bigg|_{s=1} + \frac{dP(s)}{ds}\bigg|_{s=1} - \left(\frac{dP(s)}{ds}\bigg|_{s=1}\right)^2$$

$$= P''(1) + P'(1) - (P'(1))^2.$$

3. Using the definition $\mu = E[X] = \sum_{k=0}^{n} k \Pr[X = k]$, and

$$\text{Var}(X) = \sum_{k=0}^{n} (k - \mu)^2 \Pr[X = k] = \sum_{k=0}^{n} k^2 \Pr[X = k] - \mu^2,$$

derive the mean μ and variance σ^2 of the binomial. Compare these results to those determined by using pgf's.

4. Given the pgf $P(s) = e^{\lambda(s-1)}$ of a Poisson distribution, verify that

$$\Pr[X = k] = \frac{1}{k!} \frac{d^k P(s)}{ds^k}\bigg|_{s=0}.$$

5. Using the definition $\mu = E[X] = \sum_{k=0}^{\infty} k \Pr[X = k]$, and

$$\sigma^2 = \text{Var}(X) = \sum_{k=0}^{\infty} (k - \mu)^2 \Pr[X = k] = \sum_{k=0}^{\infty} k^2 \Pr[X = k] - \mu^2,$$

derive the mean μ, and variance σ^2, of the Poisson. Compare these results to those determined by using pgf's.

6. (a) Using the pgf $P(s) = sp/(1 - qs)$ of the geometric distribution,
      (1) determine $\Pr[X = k]$,
      (2) derive the mean μ,
      (3) derive the variance σ^2.
   (b) Using the definitions $\mu = E[X]$ and $\sigma^2 = E[(X - \mu)^2]$, derive μ and σ^2. Compare to the results obtained in (a).

7. Using the pgf $P(s) = (sp)^m/(1 - qs)^m$ of the negative binomial distribution, do Exercise 6.

4. Derivation of the General System of Differential Equations for the Pure Birth Process

In this section we develop the stochastic version of a general birth process. In Section 5 we will consider particular cases of the general birth process and compare and contrast them to deterministic analogs. We start by letting $X(t)$ be the size of the population at time t. The value of $X(t)$ will be governed by probabilistic laws. Technically, $X(t)$ is a random variable and $\{X(t); t \geq 0\}$ defines a stochastic process. The parameter t, which we interpret as time, is real and continuous, but the random variable $X(t)$ will have a discrete set of possible values, the nonnegative integers, corresponding to population sizes. Our main interest will be to determine the probability distribution

$$p_n(t) = \Pr[X(t) = n], \qquad n = 0, 1, 2, \cdots.$$

We will use the following notation in our development.

1. $o(h)$ is a quantity such that $\lim_{h \to 0} o(h)/h = 0$. That is, $o(h) \to 0$ more quickly than $h \to 0$.

2. E_n is the state of the system at some point in time t, where $t > 0$, if exactly n individuals are present at the end of the interval 0 to t. Therefore, we can say that $p_n(t)$ is the probability of being in state E_n at time t.

In deriving the basic system of differential equations for the pure birth process, we will be assuming that only births occur—no deaths. This is equivalent to saying that either an increase in the population occurs or nothing happens. Such assumptions are realistic, e.g., in the early stages of the development of a bacterial colony. Although the model does not have wide applicability, we want to use this simple case in order to make the comparisons between the stochastic and deterministic analogs. We will briefly discuss how to bring in death and other complications in Exercise 39 at the end of Section 5.4.

Our stochastic model will be derived by using the following postulates.

(1) Direct increases in the population from a state E_n are possible only to E_{n+1}. (An example of such a process is binary fission: $o{<}^0_0$.)
(2) If, at time t, the system is in state E_n, then the probability of an increase of one in the population in the ensuing short interval of time, t to $t + h$, is assumed to be $\lambda_n h + o(h)$. Here λ_n is the birth rate of the population when the system is in state E_n.
(3) If we assume that at time t, the system is in state E_n, then the probability of an increase greater than one organism in the ensuing short interval of time, t to $t + h$, is assumed negligible, i.e., $o(h)$.
(4) We assume that events in nonoverlapping time intervals are independent.

These four assumptions will be used to determine $p_n(t)$, the probability that at time t, the population size will be n, with $n > 0$. The whole process is easy to conceptualize by considering two adjacent (nonoverlapping) intervals of time $(0, t)$ and $(t, t + h)$. Schematically, we represent these two intervals by

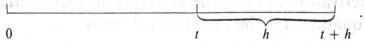

Specifically, we will start by considering the possible ways we can have a population of size n at time $t + h$, by considering what can happen in the intervals $(0, t)$ and $(t, t + h)$. Schematically, we find the following ways to attain a population of size n, where h is small.

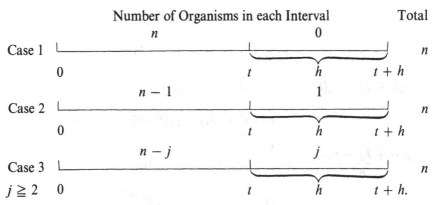

The following factors enable us to use this formulation.

(1) The events in the nonoverlapping time intervals are independent.
(2) The process has a lack of memory. That is, the only thing of interest in Case 1 is that at time t the population size is n, not what happened previously; in Case 2, the population size is $n - 1$ at time t, not what happened before time t, and similarly for Case 3.
(3) We have a time homogeneous process. That is the probability of a birth in a short interval of time depends only on the length of the interval and not on when it occurs. We are assuming that all forces governing the process remain constant so that the probability of an increment is the same for all short time intervals and is independent of the past development of the process.

For each of the three cases we can determine the probability that there will be n organisms at time $t + h$ by using our assumptions.

Case 1: Exactly n events occur in $(0, t)$ and none in $(t, t + h)$. This happens with probability

$$p_n(t)[1 - (\lambda_n h + o(h))].$$

Case 2: Exactly $n - 1$ events occur in $(0, t)$ and one in $(t, t + h)$. This happens with probability

$$p_{n-1}(t)[\lambda_{n-1} h + o(h)].$$

Case 3: Exactly $(n - j)$ events occur in $(0, t)$ and j in $(t, t + h)$, $j = 2, 3, \cdots, n$.

Since these events are mutually exclusive for each value of j, the probability that one of these events occurs is

$$\sum_{j=2}^{n} p_{n-j}(t)[o(h)].$$

Since all three cases are mutually exclusive, it follows that

$$p_n(t + h) = p_n(t)[1 - (\lambda_n h + o(h))] + p_{n-1}(t)[\lambda_{n-1} h + o(h)]$$

$$+ \sum_{j=2}^{n} p_{n-j}(t)o(h)$$

$$= p_n(t) - \lambda_n h p_n(t) + \lambda_{n-1} h p_{n-1}(t)$$

$$+ \sum_{j=1}^{n} p_{n-j}(t) o(h) - p_n(t) o(h)$$

$$p_n(t + h) - p_n(t) = -\lambda_n h p_n(t) + \lambda_{n-1} h p_{n-1}(t)$$

$$+ o(h) \sum_{j=1}^{n} p_{n-j}(t) - p_n(t) o(h)$$

$$\lim_{h \to 0} \frac{p_n(t + h) - p_n(t)}{h} = \lim_{h \to 0} \left[-\lambda_n p_n(t) + \lambda_{n-1} p_{n-1}(t) \right.$$

$$\left. + \frac{o(h)}{h} \sum_{j=1}^{n} p_{n-j}(t) - p_n(t) \frac{o(h)}{h} \right].$$

Using the definition of the derivative and taking limits we see that

$$p_n'(t) = -\lambda_n p_n(t) + \lambda_{n-1} p_{n-1}(t), \tag{3}$$

where $p_n'(t) = dp_n(t)/dt$. A similar analysis shows that

$$p_0'(t) = -\lambda_0 p_0(t). \tag{4}$$

Equations (3) and (4) are the basic system of differential equations for a pure birth process. Depending on the birth rate λ_n and initial conditions giving $p_n(0)$ for all λ_n, these equations may or may not be solvable. The λ_n correspond to different assumptions about the way the population size increases. Various techniques are available for solving Eqs. (3) and (4). We will discuss three methods:

(a) using the appropriate technique from the theory of differential equations and then solving by induction,
(b) using probability generating functions and partial differential equations,
(c) using Laplace transformations.

In Section 5, we will make various assumptions about the mode of population growth, and hence λ_n, and determine both the deterministic and stochastic solutions under the various assumptions. An assortment of techniques for solving the basic stochastic equations will be used.

5. Models of Population Growth

In this section we will present four different models for a pure birth process. Each model will have first a deterministic formulation and then a stochastic formulation, the latter based on the general birth process discussed in Section 4. We will not allow deaths. Each model will make a somewhat more complex assumption about the mechanism of growth than the previous model. It should become evident that as the assumptions get more complex so do the equations and, relatively speaking, so does the mathematics for solution. We will also show the different information we can obtain from the stochastic solution that we cannot obtain from the deterministic solution. We will not discuss the philosophical question about which is the correct mechanism.

5.1 Model I

5.1.1. Deterministic. Let us consider a population which only permits births (no deaths) and assume a constant birth rate λ per unit of time. We are saying that the population creates a new individual at the rate of λ per unit of time. A convenient example is the emissions of radioactive particles which occur periodically over time, but at a given rate. We introduce the following notation:

$$N_t \text{ is the population size at time } t$$

and

$$N_0 \text{ is the initial population size.}$$

N_t corresponds to our $X(t)$ of Section 4, but we use a different notation to emphasize the fact that N_t is not a random variable. In this case $N_0 = 0$. (Specifically, in the case of radioactive emissions, N_t would be the number of particles counted by a geiger counter in the interval $(0, t)$ or any interval of length t.) Based on our assumptions, we can conclude that if Δt is a short interval of time, then

$$N_{t+\Delta t} - N_t = \lambda \Delta t.$$

That is, the increase in the population size in a short interval of time Δt is just $\lambda \Delta t$, i.e., is proportional to the length of the interval. Applying the definition of the derivative, we see that since

$$\lim_{\Delta t \to 0} \frac{N_{t+\Delta t} - N_t}{\Delta t} = \lambda,$$

$$\frac{dN_t}{dt} = \lambda.$$

Hence using integration, we find

$$N_t = \lambda t + c.$$

Since $N_0 = 0$, it follows that

$$N_t = \lambda t.$$

We conclude that if the birth rate is λ per unit time, then at time t, the population size (or number of radioactive particles) will be exactly λt. Graphically, we have Figure 3.3.

If $\lambda = 3$ per minute, it follows that N_5 (where 5 means five minutes) is

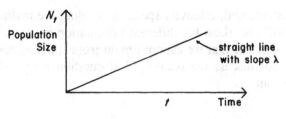

Figure 3.3

Table 1[†]

No. of Particles k	No. of Intervals with k Particles
0	57
1	203
2	383
3	525
4	532
5	408
6	273
7	139
8	45
9	27
$k \geq 10$	16
	2608.

† Source: Feller [4], original data
from Rutherford, Chadwick, and
Ellis, *Radiations from Radioactive
Substances*, Cambridge, 1920, p. 172.

3(5) or 15 particles, $N_{20} = 3(20)$ or 60 particles, and $N_{4.5} = 3(4.5)$ or 13.5 particles. Note that this method predicts noninteger numbers of particles. Basically, we predict the population size with a straight line through the origin with slope λ. The rate of change of population size is constant, but is larger or smaller depending on the value of λ.

If we consider the radioactive emissions example more carefully we might have a question. Is it reasonable to assume that exactly λ emissions will always exist per unit of time? If we had a geiger counter and counted the number of particles in several equal intervals, we would not have an equal number in each interval.

In a famous experiment, a radioactive substance was observed during 2608 time intervals of 7.5 seconds each and the number of particles reaching a counter was recorded for each period. The data are given in Table 1. We see that to assume that exactly λ particles will exist per unit of time seems very unreasonable. To assume an average number per unit of time and to assume that a certain number of particles will be emitted with a certain probability might be more reasonable. This would lead us to the stochastic analog.

5.1.2. Stochastic.

We have in Section 4 derived the general system of differential equations for a pure birth process, with a general birth rate λ_n. Modifying the assumptions of the model, and applying them to a pure birth process, we would set $\lambda_n = \lambda$, i.e., let the birth rate be constant and independent of time and the population size at time t. Then the probability that an event (a birth) occurs during a time interval $(t, t + h)$ is $\lambda h + o(h)$ for all n. Equations (3) and (4) of the basic system of differential equations become

$$p_n'(t) = -\lambda p_n(t) + \lambda p_{n-1}(t), \qquad n \geq 1 \tag{5}$$

$$p_0'(t) = -\lambda p_0(t). \tag{6}$$

5.1.2.1 Solution by Induction.

We will use two different methods to solve these differential equations. The first method is to solve (6), then (5) for $n = 1$ and then, by induction, solve it in general. Consistent with our assumptions about the process (spontaneous process, $N_0 = 0$ in the deterministic model), the initial conditions are

$$p_0(0) = 1, \qquad p_n(0) = 0, \qquad n \geq 1.$$

Let us rewrite (6) as

$$\frac{dp_0(t)}{dt} = -\lambda p_0(t).$$

This equation is of the form known as separable; therefore we can rewrite is as

$$\frac{dp_0(t)}{p_0(t)} = -\lambda \, dt.$$

Solving, we get

$$\ln p_0(t) = -\lambda t + c$$

and

$$p_0(t) = e^{-\lambda t} e^c.$$

However, when $t = 0$, $p_0(0) = 1$, and so

$$p_0(0) = e^{\lambda 0} e^c$$

$$1 = e^0 e^c$$

and

$$e^c = 1.$$

Therefore,

$$p_0(t) = e^{-\lambda t}.$$

We use this fact and substitute it into equation (5), getting

$$\frac{dp_1(t)}{dt} = -\lambda p_1(t) + \lambda e^{-\lambda t}.$$

If we rewrite this as

$$\frac{dp_1(t)}{dt} + \lambda p_1(t) = \lambda e^{-\lambda t}, \tag{7}$$

we find we have an ordinary first-order differential equation, that is, an equation of the form

$$\frac{dy(x)}{dx} + p(x)y(x) = q(x).$$

To solve such an equation, we have to determine the integrating factor $e^{P(x)}$ where $P(x) = \int_{x_0}^{x} p(s)\,ds$. Then the general solution is given by

$$y(x) = y(x_0)e^{-P(x)} + e^{-P(x)} \int_{x_0}^{x} q(m)e^{P(m)}\,dm.$$

Specifically for (7), using $x_0 = 0$ and $x = t$, we determine that

$$y(x) = p_1(t)$$
$$p(x) = \lambda$$
$$q(x) = \lambda e^{-\lambda t}.$$

Therefore, $P(t) = \int_0^t \lambda\,ds = \lambda t$. Thus

$$p_1(t) = p_1(0)e^{-\lambda t} + e^{-\lambda t} \int_0^t \lambda e^{-\lambda s}e^{\lambda s}\,ds$$

$$= p_1(0)e^{-\lambda t} + e^{-\lambda t} \int_0^t \lambda\,ds$$

$$= p_1(0)e^{-\lambda t} + e^{-\lambda t}\lambda t.$$

However, since $p_n(0) = 0$ for $n \geq 1$, $p_1(t) = \lambda t e^{-\lambda t}$.

We solve for $p_2(t)$ in the same way, that is, by substituting in Eq. (5) and solving. We get

$$\frac{dp_2(t)}{dt} + \lambda p_2(t) = \lambda^2 t e^{-\lambda t}.$$

We note that this is also an ordinary first-order differential equation. The integrating factor is again $e^{\lambda t}$, so we get that

$$p_2(t) = p_2(0)e^{-\lambda t} + e^{-\lambda t} \int_0^t \lambda^2 s e^{-\lambda s}e^{\lambda s}\,ds$$

$$= p_2(0)e^{-\lambda t} + e^{-\lambda t}\lambda^2 \int_0^t s\,ds$$

$$= p_2(0)e^{-\lambda t} + \frac{(\lambda t)^2}{2}e^{-\lambda t}.$$

Using the initial condition that $p_n(0) = 0$ for $n \geq 1$, we find that

$$p_2(t) = \frac{(\lambda t)^2}{2}e^{-\lambda t}.$$

If we solve for $n = 3$, we find that

$$p_3(t) = \frac{(\lambda t)^3}{3!}e^{-\lambda t}.$$

We shall now prove by induction that for all k,

$$p_k(t) = \frac{(\lambda t)^k}{k!}e^{-\lambda t}. \tag{8}$$

We know this is true for $k = 0$. Assuming this is true for $k = n$, let us show it is true for $k = n + 1$. We see that

$$\frac{dp_{n+1}(t)}{dt} + \lambda p_{n+1}(t) = \frac{\lambda^{n+1}t^n e^{-\lambda t}}{n!}.$$

This is also an ordinary first-order differential equation. The integrating factor is $e^{\lambda t}$, so we find that

$$p_{n+1}(t) = p_{n+1}(0)e^{-\lambda t} + e^{-\lambda t}\int_0^t \frac{\lambda^{n+1}s^n e^{-\lambda s}e^{\lambda s}}{n!}\,ds$$

$$= p_{n+1}(0)e^{-\lambda t} + e^{-\lambda t}\lambda^{n+1}\int_0^t \frac{s^n}{n!}\,ds$$

$$= p_{n+1}(0)e^{-\lambda t} + e^{-\lambda t}\frac{\lambda^{n+1}t^{n+1}}{(n+1)n!}$$

$$= \frac{(\lambda t)^{n+1}}{(n+1)!}e^{-\lambda t},$$

which proves (8).

If we refer to Section 3, we see that the probabilities given in (8) are similar to those given for the Poisson distribution. They are identical if we replace λt here by λ. Using (8) we can, for any birth rate λ, determine the probability of having a particular number of organisms (particles) at any point in time t. (See Table 2 and Figure 3.4.) Therefore, for any time t, it is possible to determine the likelihood of a particular number of organisms; we are no longer limited to saying exactly λ organisms will exist. We can also derive more information by knowing the probability distribution at any point in time. For any probability distribution it is possible to determine

Table 2. Value of $p_n(t)$ when $\lambda = 3$

$t = 1$	$t = 5$	
$p_0(1) = 0.04978$	$p_0(5) = 0.0000003$	$p_{21}(5) = 0.0298645$
$p_1(1) = 0.1493612$	$p_1(5) = 0.0000046$	$p_{22}(5) = 0.0203622$
$p_2(1) = 0.2240418$	$p_2(5) = 0.0000344$	$p_{23}(5) = 0.0132797$
$p_3(1) = 0.2240418$	$p_3(5) = 0.0001721$	$p_{24}(5) = 0.0082998$
$p_4(1) = 0.1680314$	$p_4(5) = 0.0006453$	$p_{25}(5) = 0.0049799$
$p_5(1) = 0.1008188$	$p_5(5) = 0.0019357$	$p_{26}(5) = 0.0028730$
$p_6(1) = 0.0504094$	$p_6(5) = 0.0048395$	$p_{27}(5) = 0.0015961$
$p_7(1) = 0.0216040$	$p_7(5) = 0.0103703$	$p_{28}(5) = 0.0008551$
$p_8(1) = 0.0081015$	$p_8(5) = 0.0194443$	$p_{29}(5) = 0.0004423$
$p_9(1) = 0.0027005$	$p_9(5) = 0.0324072$	$p_{30}(5) = 0.0002211$
$p_{10}(1) = 0.0008102$	$p_{10}(5) = 0.0486108$	$p_{31}(5) = 0.0001070$
$p_{11}(1) = 0.0002210$	$p_{11}(5) = 0.0662874$	$p_{32}(5) = 0.0000502$
$p_{12}(1) = 0.0000552$	$p_{12}(5) = 0.0828592$	$p_{33}(5) = 0.0000228$
$p_{13}(1) = 0.0000127$	$p_{13}(5) = 0.0956068$	$p_{34}(5) = 0.0000101$
$p_{14}(1) = 0.0000027$	$p_{14}(5) = 0.1024359$	$p_{35}(5) = 0.0000043$
$p_{15}(1) = 0.0000005$	$p_{15}(5) = 0.1024359$	$p_{36}(5) = 0.0000018$
$p_{16}(1) = 0.0000001$	$p_{16}(5) = 0.0960336$	$p_{37}(5) = 0.0000007$
$p_{17}(1) = 0.0000000$	$p_{17}(5) = 0.0847356$	$p_{38}(5) = 0.0000003$
	$p_{18}(5) = 0.0706130$	$p_{39}(5) = 0.0000001$
	$p_{19}(5) = 0.0557471$	$p_{40}(5) = 0.0000000$
	$p_{20}(5) = 0.0418103$	

the mean and variance. The mean of the Poisson distribution (8) was determined in Section 3 to be λt. The expected number of particles is thus λt. We recall that this is the prediction for the exact number of particles given in the deterministic analog. Often (but not always) the expected value of the stochastic analog is the same as the solution of the corresponding deterministic model. For the two cases given in Table 2, for $\lambda = 3$, at 1 minute the expected number of particles is 3, and when $t = 5$, the expected number of particles is 15. We also recall that for the Poisson, the variance is also λt. Thus the standard deviation (SD) is $\sqrt{\lambda t}$. This gives us more information than just knowing the mean.

In summary, for the stochastic version of the birth process with birth rate $\lambda_n = \lambda$, we have concluded that $p_n(t) = e^{-\lambda t}(\lambda t)^n/n!$, $E[X(t)] = \lambda t$; and SD$[X(t)] = \sqrt{\lambda t}$. Schematically, we get Figure 3.5. The stochastic solution therefore permits us to determine the expected number of particles as well as to get a feeling for the variability that would be expected in repeated realizations of the process. We see that as λ increases, the variability will also increase (as it will as t increases). That is, there will be greater deviation from the expected values. If we were to take the data in Table 1 and test the closeness of fit of the data to the prediction from the Poisson distribution, we would not have sufficient evidence to reject the Poisson as a reasonable model.

We saw that solving (5) can be somewhat tedious. In fact, if we extend

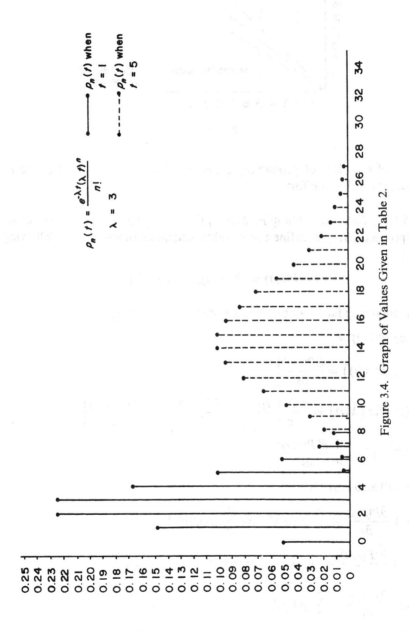

Figure 3.4. Graph of Values Given in Table 2.

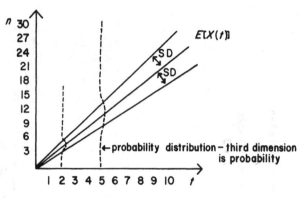

Figure 3.5

some of the ideas of probability generating functions, we will be able to solve, (5) with less effort.

5.1.2.2 *Solution by Use of Probability Generating Functions.* For a stochastic process $\{X(t)\}$ we define a probability generating function in the following way:

$$P(s, t) = \sum_{j=0}^{\infty} p_j(t)s^j = E[s^{X(t)}].$$

The following facts can be demonstrated. For all $t \geq 0$,

(a) $P(1, t) = 1$

(b) $E[X(t)] = \left.\dfrac{\partial P(s, t)}{\partial s}\right|_{s=1}$

(c) $\mathrm{Var}[X(t)] = \left.\dfrac{\partial^2 P(s, t)}{\partial s^2}\right|_{s=1} + \left.\dfrac{\partial P(s, t)}{\partial s}\right|_{s=1} - \left[\left.\dfrac{\partial P(s, t)}{\partial s}\right|_{s=1}\right]^2$

(d) $p_n(t) = \left.\dfrac{1}{n!}\dfrac{\partial^n P(s, t)}{\partial s^n}\right|_{s=0}.$

We will also make use of

(e) $\dfrac{\partial P(s, t)}{\partial s} = \sum_{j=1}^{\infty} jp_j(t)s^{j-1} = \sum_{j=0}^{\infty} jp_j(t)s^{j-1}$

(f) $\dfrac{\partial^2 P(s, t)}{\partial s^2} = \sum_{j=2}^{\infty} j(j-1)p_j(t)s^{j-2}$

(g) $\dfrac{\partial P(s, t)}{\partial t} = \sum_{j=0}^{\infty} p_j'(t)s^j.$

Utilizing these ideas, we will in some cases be able to solve equations (3) and (4) with much less effort. We will also be able to use the probability generating functions to derive the means and variances easily. Specifically, we reconsider (5) and (6):

$$p_n'(t) = -\lambda p_n(t) + \lambda p_{n-1}(t), \qquad n \geq 1 \tag{5}$$

$$p_0'(t) = -\lambda p_0(t). \tag{6}$$

How can we modify (5) so we can use probability generating functions? If we multiply (5) by s^n, we get

$$p_n'(t)s^n = -\lambda p_n(t)s^n + \lambda p_{n-1}(t)s^n.$$

If we next sum from $n = 1$ to ∞ and add (6), we get

$$\sum_{n=0}^{\infty} p_n'(t)s^n = -\lambda \sum_{n=0}^{\infty} p_n(t)s^n + \lambda \sum_{n=1}^{\infty} p_{n-1}(t)s^n. \tag{9}$$

We can rewrite the last term on the right as

$$\lambda s \sum_{n=1}^{\infty} p_{n-1}(t)s^{n-1} = \lambda s \sum_{m=0}^{\infty} p_m(t)s^m,$$

and therefore we can write (9) as

$$\frac{\partial P(s, t)}{\partial t} = -\lambda P(s, t) + \lambda s P(s, t),$$

or

$$\frac{\partial P(s, t)}{\partial t} = \lambda(s - 1)P(s, t). \tag{10}$$

This (partial differential) equation is of the form known as separable, so we can write (10) as

$$\frac{\partial P(s, t)}{P(s, t)} = \lambda(s - 1)\partial t$$

and we get

$$\ln P(s, t) = \lambda t(s - 1) + c$$
$$P(s, t) = e^{\lambda t(s-1)}e^c.$$

To determine the value of c, we have to determine the initial conditions for $P(s, t)$. We know that $p_0(0) = 1$ and $p_n(0) = 0$, and since

$$P(s, t) = \sum_{j=0}^{\infty} p_j(t)s^j$$

when $t = 0$, we get

$$P(s, 0) = p_0(0)s^0 + p_1(0)s^1 + p_2(0)s^2 + \cdots + p_k(0)s^k + \cdots$$
$$= p_0(0)s^0 + 0 \cdot s^1 + 0 \cdot s^2 + \cdots + 0 \cdot s^k + \cdots$$
$$= p_0(0)s^0$$
$$= 1 \cdot s^0$$
$$= 1.$$

Now

$$P(s, 0) = e^{\lambda(0)(s-1)}e^c$$

$$= e^0 e^c$$

$$= e^c.$$

Since $P(s, 0) = 1$, $e^c = 1$, and $c = 0$. Thus,

$$P(s, t) = e^{\lambda t(s-1)},$$

which is the pgf of a Poisson distribution with mean λt. We arrive at this conclusion in an easier way than by induction.

We will summarize this model (and all the others we present) in Section 5.5.

EXERCISES

8. For different values of λ, the birth rate, plot $N_t = \lambda t$. Discuss and interpret the differences in the various plots.

9. Discuss a process (or a few processes) for which $N_t = \lambda t$ might be a reasonable model.

10. If you are given data from a process which satisfies the conditions for the model $N_t = \lambda t$, discuss how you would determine the value of λ.

11. For the stochastic process, with $p_n(t) = e^{-\lambda t}(\lambda t)^n/n!$, determine the probabilities $p_n(t)$ for a range of values of t for a fixed value of λ. Plot the probabilities on a graph. Compare and interpret the differences.

12. For the stochastic process, with $p_n(t) = e^{-\lambda t}(\lambda t)^n/n!$, determine the probabilities $p_n(t)$ for a range of values of λ, for a fixed time t. Compare and interpret the differences.

13. Plot $E[X(t)]$ and SD $[X(t)] = \sqrt{\text{Var}[X(t)]}$ for different values of birth rate λ. Discuss the effect on $E[X(t)]$ and $\sqrt{\text{Var}[X(t)]}$ as λ gets larger.

14. Consider a process that might be modeled by the stochastic version of Model I and discuss.

5.2 Model II

A more realistic assumption about the way the population size increases is to assume that the birth rate is proportional to the population size. That is, each organism has a certain fixed probability of reproducing in the stochastic case, or each organism will produce a fixed number of organisms in the deterministic sense. This seems to be a more realistic assumption than the first model. However, this is still an extremely oversimplified model.

5.2.1. *Deterministic.* We will use the same notation as in Model I. Then our assumption about the birth rate λ per unit time being proportional to the population size can be expressed as

$$N_{t+\Delta t} - N_t = \lambda N_t \Delta t,$$

where Δt is a short interval of time. Since we are not permitting spontaneous generation, we must assume that $N_0 \neq 0$. For if $N_0 = 0$, then $N_{0+\Delta t} - N_0 = \lambda N_0 \Delta t$ would become $N_{0+\Delta t} - 0 = \lambda(0)\Delta t = 0$, or

$$N_{0+\Delta t} = 0,$$

and then $N_t = 0$, for all t. To determine N_t, we use the definition of the derivative, and find that

$$\lim_{\Delta t \to 0} \frac{N_{t+\Delta t} - N_t}{\Delta t} = \lambda N_t$$

$$\frac{dN_t}{dt} = \lambda N_t.$$

To solve, we write

$$\frac{dN_t}{N_t} = \lambda \, dt$$

$$\ln N_t = \lambda t + c$$

$$N_t = e^{\lambda t} e^c.$$

Using the initial condition, we have

$$N_0 = e^{\lambda \cdot 0} e^c$$

$$N_0 = e^c$$

$$N_t = N_0 e^{\lambda t},$$

and we see that in fact our assumptions lead to exponential growth. (We can modify this model in a very simple way to include deaths as well. If we assume the birth rate is a constant b and the death rate is a constant d, and define a net growth rate, $\lambda = b - d$, then we obtain the same formula for N_t.)

Let us assume that the population starts with 10^4 organisms, that is, $N_0 = 10^4$, and that the population doubles per unit time. Let us determine the birth rate λ, and then plot N_t. We are told that

$$N_0 = 10^4$$

and

$$N_1 = 2 \times 10^4,$$

giving $N_1 = 2N_0$. We have shown that

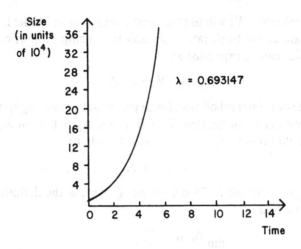

Figure 3.6

$$N_t = N_0 e^{\lambda t},$$

so that it follows that since $N_1 = 2N_0$

$$2N_0 = N_0 e^{\lambda 1}$$

$$2 = e^{\lambda}$$

$$\lambda = \ln 2$$

$$\lambda = 0.693147.$$

That is, organisms will reproduce at the rate of 0.693147 organisms per unit time. Therefore,

$$N_t = N_0 e^{0.693147 t}.$$

Plotting, we get Figure 3.6. If we were to plot this function on log paper, we would get a straight line.

Graphs like this are reasonable approximations for the growth of population of paramecia and amoeba over a short period of time if

(1) we are in a controlled environment with ideal conditions of temperature, unlimited food, etc.,
(2) we have neither predators nor death.

But its predictions are exact and allow no deviations.

As a second example, consider a population with $N_0 = 10^5$ that quadruples per unit time. Let us determine λ and plot N_t. We have

$$N_0 = 10^5,$$

$$N_1 = 4 \times 10^5,$$

$$N_1 = 4N_0,$$

$$N_1 = N_0 e^{\lambda(1)}$$
$$4N_0 = N_0 e^{\lambda}$$
$$4 = 1e^{\lambda}$$
$$\ln 4 = \lambda$$
$$\lambda = 1.38629,$$
$$N_t = N_0 e^{1.38629t}.$$

The graph for N_t is given in Figure 3.7.

In 1650, the world population was 0.5 billion (500,000,000) and it was growing at a rate of approximately 0.3% per year. If we assume that the growth rate ($\lambda = b - d$) remained constant, what was the doubling time? That is, how many years did it take for the population to reach 1 billion? This is equivalent to saying that

$$N_t = N_0 e^{0.003t},$$

where $N_t = 2N_0$. Therefore,

$$2N_0 = N_0 e^{0.003t}$$
$$2 = e^{0.003t}$$
$$\ln 2 = 0.003t$$
$$0.693 = 0.003t$$
$$t = 231.$$

That is, if the population grew at the rate of 0.3% per year, it would take 231 years for the population to double, or until the year $1650 + 231 = 1881$. In fact, it had doubled before 1850.

In 1970 the world population was 3.6 billion (3,600,000,000) and the rate of growth was 2.1% per year. If we could assume that the rate of growth

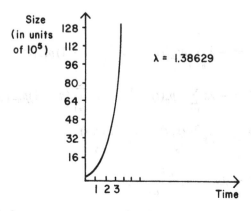

Figure 3.7

will remain constant, how many years would it take for the population to reach 7.2 billion? Using a similar analysis, we find that

$$N_t = N_0 e^{0.021t}$$

$$2N_0 = N_0 e^{0.021t}$$

$$2 = e^{0.021t}$$

$$\ln 2 = 0.021t$$

$$0.693 = 0.021t$$

$$t = 33 \text{ years.}$$

This is really frightening. From 1650 it took somewhat less than 200 years for the population to increase 0.5 billion, but from 1970 it might only take 33 years to increase 3.6 billion. The predictions depend on the assumption that the growth rate will be constant and exact every year, the major premise of the deterministic model.

5.2.2. Stochastic (Linear Birth Process). To find the stochastic analog of a birth process where the number of births is proportional to the population size, we will deal with equations (3) and (4), and we must determine the birth rate λ_n. For Model II, the appropriate birth rate λ_n can be expressed as λn, and we interpret λ as the rate at which a single organism will reproduce. We have $p_0(t) = 0$, for all t. Substituting in Eq. (3) we get

$$p'_n(t) = -\lambda n p_n(t) + \lambda(n - 1)p_{n-1}(t), \qquad n > 1. \tag{11}$$

In Model I we saw that solving equations such as (11) was easier using pgf's. To get these equations into the form required for pgf's, we proceed as in Section 5.1.2.2, and find

$$p'_n(t)s^n = -\lambda n p_n(t)s^n + \lambda(n - 1)p_{n-1}(t)s^n, \qquad n \geq 1,$$

$$p'_0(t)s^0 = -\lambda 0 p_0(t)s^0.$$

Hence

$$\sum_{n=0}^{\infty} p'_n(t)s^n = -\lambda \sum_{n=0}^{\infty} n p_n(t)s^n + \lambda \sum_{n=1}^{\infty} (n - 1)p_{n-1}(t)s^n$$

$$\frac{\partial P(s, t)}{\partial t} = -\lambda s \sum_{n=0}^{\infty} n p_n(t)s^{n-1} + \lambda s^2 \sum_{n=1}^{\infty} (n - 1)p_{n-1}(t)s^{n-2}$$

$$\frac{\partial P(s, t)}{\partial t} = -\lambda s \frac{\partial P(s, t)}{\partial s} + \lambda s^2 \frac{\partial P(s, t)}{\partial s}$$

$$\frac{\partial P(s, t)}{\partial t} = \lambda s(s - 1)\frac{\partial P(s, t)}{\partial s}. \tag{12}$$

Equation (12) is a linear partial differential equation of the first order and is solved by the Lagrange method. If we use the Lagrange method and assume that the initial population size is 1 and hence use the initial conditions

$$p_1(0) = 1, \qquad p_n(0) = 0, \qquad n > 1, \qquad p_0(t) = 0,$$

then we can show that

$$P(s, t) = \frac{se^{-\lambda t}}{1 - s(1 - e^{-\lambda t})}.$$

If we let $p(t) = e^{-\lambda t}$ and $q(t) = 1 - e^{-\lambda t}$, then we can write

$$P(s, t) = \frac{sp(t)}{1 - sq(t)}.$$

If we refer to Section 3, we note that for each t, this is the pgf of the geometric distribution with $p(t) = p$ and $q(t) = q$. Therefore, we find that $p_n(t)$ is the probability of having the first success on the nth trial if $p(t)$ is the probability of success and $q(t)$ is the probability of failure, and so

$$p_n(t) = e^{-\lambda t}(1 - e^{-\lambda t})^{n-1}.$$

Using the generating function we can find that $E[X(t)] = e^{\lambda t}$. (The reader is asked to verify this in Exercise 18 at the end of Section 5.2.) We note the expected value is equivalent to the deterministic solution when $N_0 = 1$. We can also show that $\mathrm{Var}[X(t)] = e^{\lambda t}(e^{\lambda t} - 1)$. (The reader is also asked to verify this in Exercise 18.)

For values comparable to the values of λ used in the deterministic analogues, we calculate $p_n(t)$, $E[X(t)]$, $\mathrm{Var}[X(t)]$ and $\mathrm{SD}[X(t)]$. (See Table 3 and Figure 3.8.) Note that as t increases, $\mathrm{SD}[X(t)] \sim E[X(t)]$. With $\lambda =$

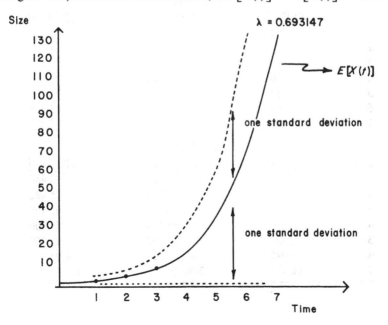

Figure 3.8. Mean and Standard Deviation in Model II.

Table 3. Value of $p_n(t)$ when $\lambda = 0.693147$

$t = 2$		$t = 5$	
$p_1(2) = 0.25$ $p_{13}(2) = 0.008$		$p_1(5) = 0.03125$ $p_{24}(5) = 0.01506$	
$p_2(2) = 0.188$ $p_{14}(2) = 0.006$		$p_2(5) = 0.03027$ $p_{25}(5) = 0.01459$	
$p_3(2) = 0.141$ $p_{15}(2) = 0.004$		$p_3(5) = 0.02933$ $p_{26}(5) = 0.01413$	
$p_4(2) = 0.105$ $p_{16}(2) = 0.003$		$p_4(5) = 0.02841$ $p_{27}(5) = 0.01369$	
$p_5(2) = 0.079$ $p_{17}(2) = 0.003$		$p_5(5) = 0.02752$ $p_{28}(5) = 0.01326$	
$p_6(2) = 0.059$ $p_{18}(2) = 0.002$		$p_6(5) = 0.02666$ $p_{29}(5) = 0.01285$	
$p_7(2) = 0.044$ $p_{19}(2) = 0.001$		$p_7(5) = 0.02583$ $p_{30}(5) = 0.01244$	
$p_8(2) = 0.033$ $p_{20}(2) = 0.001$		$p_8(5) = 0.02502$ $p_{31}(5) = 0.01206$	
$p_9(2) = 0.025$ $p_{21}(2) = 0.001$		$p_9(5) = 0.02424$ $p_{32}(5) = 0.01168$	
$p_{10}(2) = 0.019$ $p_{22}(2) = 0.001$		$p_{10}(5) = 0.02348$ $p_{33}(5) = 0.01131$	
$p_{11}(2) = 0.014$ $p_{23}(2) \sim 0$		$p_{11}(5) = 0.02275$ $p_{34}(5) = 0.01096$	
$p_{12}(2) = 0.011$		$p_{12}(5) = 0.02204$ $p_{35}(5) = 0.01062$	
		$p_{13}(5) = 0.02135$ $p_{36}(5) = 0.01029$	
		$p_{14}(5) = 0.02068$ $p_{37}(5) = 0.00996$	
		$p_{15}(5) = 0.02004$ $p_{38}(5) = 0.00965$	
		$p_{16}(5) = 0.01941$ $p_{39}(5) = 0.00935$	
		$p_{17}(5) = 0.01880$ $p_{40}(5) = 0.00906$	
		$p_{18}(5) = 0.01822$ $p_{41}(5) = 0.00878$	
		$p_{19}(5) = 0.01765$ $p_{42}(5) = 0.00850$	
		$p_{20}(5) = 0.01710$ $p_{43}(5) = 0.00824$	
		$p_{21}(5) = 0.01656$ $p_{44}(5) = 0.00798$	
		$p_{22}(5) = 0.01604$	
		$p_{23}(5) = 0.01554$	

Mean and Standard Deviation
$\lambda = 0.693147$

t	$E[X(t)]$	$\text{Var}[X(t)]$	$SD[X(t)]$
1	2	2	1.4142
2	4	12	3.464
3	8	56	7.483
4	16	240	15.492
5	32	992	31.496
6	64	4032	63.498
7	128	16,256	127.499

$\lambda = 1.38629$

t	$E[X(t)]$	$\text{Var}[X(t)]$	$SD[X(t)]$
1	4	12	3.464
2	16	240	15.492
3	64	4032	63.498
4	256	65,280	255.500
5	1024	1,047,552	1023.500
6	4096	16,773,120	4095.500
7	16,384	268,419,072	16,383.500

0.693147, there is a great deal of variation. With $\lambda = 1.38629$, the variation is really huge.

Returning to Eq. (12), if the initial population size is i ($i > 1$), then the initial conditions would be

$$p_i(0) = 1, \qquad p_j(0) = 0, \qquad j \neq i,$$

and the Lagrange method gives rise to the solution

$$P(s, t) = \left(\frac{s e^{-\lambda t}}{1 - s(1 - e^{-\lambda t})} \right)^i.$$

Once again, if we refer to Section 3, we find that this is the pgf of the negative binomial distribution. It follows that

$$p_n(t) = \binom{n-1}{n-i} (e^{-\lambda t})^i (1 - e^{-\lambda t})^{n-i},$$

$$E[X(t)] = i e^{\lambda t}$$

which is analogous to the deterministic solution $N_t = N_0 e^{\lambda t}$, and

$$\mathrm{Var}[X(t)] = i e^{\lambda t}(e^{\lambda t} - 1).$$

(The reader is asked to verify the formulas for $E[X(t)]$ and $\mathrm{Var}[X(t)]$ in Exercise 20 at the end of Section 5.2.)

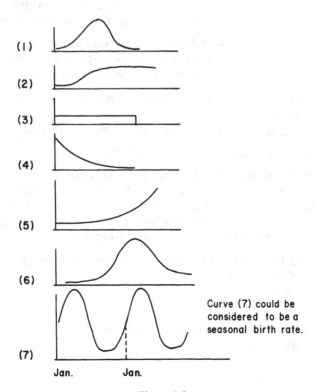

(1)

(2)

(3)

(4)

(5)

(6)

Curve (7) could be considered to be a seasonal birth rate.

(7)

Jan.   Jan.

Figure 3.9

Remark.[3] We can make this whole process more general by assuming that λ is actually a function of time $\lambda(\tau)$. It makes sense to assume that the birth rate will not be constant over time (that is, the birth rate λ is a function of time). It is possible to assume that $\lambda(\tau)$ can take on various functional forms as in Figure 3.9. In general, we can easily show that

$$P(s, t) = \frac{se^{-\int_0^t \lambda(\tau)\, d\tau}}{1 - s(1 - e^{-\int_0^t \lambda(\tau)\, d\tau})}$$

and therefore

$$p_n(t) = e^{-\int_0^t \lambda(\tau)\, d\tau}(1 - e^{-\int_0^t \lambda(\tau)\, d\tau})^{n-1}$$

$$E[X(t)] = e^{\int_0^t \lambda(\tau)\, d\tau}$$

and

$$\text{Var}[X(t)] = e^{\int_0^t \lambda(\tau)\, d\tau}(e^{\int_0^t \lambda(\tau)\, d\tau} - 1).$$

The treatment of the birth rate as a function of time really allows much more generality.

EXERCISES

15. Consider the model $N_t = N_0 e^{\lambda t}$. Suppose N_0 is not known exactly, but it is known that $10^2 \le N_0 \le 10^3$. Assume that $\lambda = 1$. Plot the graph of N_t for different values of N_0 (where $10^2 \le N_0 \le 10^3$), and consider the effect on the predictions of N_t.

16. Consider the model $N_t = N_0 e^{\lambda t}$. Suppose λ is not known exactly, but it is known that $0.5 \le \lambda \le 5$. Assume that $N_0 = 10$. Plot the graph of N_t for different values of λ (where $0.5 \le \lambda \le 5$) and consider the effects on the predictions of N_t.

17. The following table gives the population of the United States (exclusive of Alaska and Hawaii) in millions:

Year	1800	1820	1840	1860	1880	1900	1920	1940	1960
Population	5.3	9.6	17.1	31.4	50.2	76.0	105.7	131.7	178.5 .

(a) Assume the population of the United States was growing at a constant rate λ during 1800 to 1820. Use this value to predict the U.S. population in 1980.

(b) Predict the U.S. population in 1980 by finding estimates of λ for each consecutive 20-year period. Compare the predictions and explain any differences.

(c) Compare your predictions to the actual 1980 population.

18. Using the pgf $P(s, t) = se^{-\lambda t}/[1 - s(1 - e^{-\lambda t})]$, verify the following.
(a) $p_n(t) = e^{-\lambda t}(1 - e^{-\lambda t})^{n-1}$.
(b) $E[X(t)] = e^{\lambda t}$.
(c) $\text{Var}[X(t)] = e^{\lambda t}(e^{\lambda t} - 1)$.

19. Suppose we assume that $N_0 = 10^6$ and $N_1 = 0.5 \times 10^6$.
(a) Determine the value of λ.

---

[3] This remark may be omitted.

(b) Plot $N_t = N_0 e^{\lambda t}$.

(c) Determine $E[X(t)]$ and SD $[X(t)]$, in the stochastic analog.

20. Using the pgf $P(s, t) = \{se^{-\lambda t}/[1 - s(1 - e^{-\lambda t})]\}^i$, verify that

$$p_n(t) = \binom{n-1}{n-i}(e^{-\lambda t})^i (1 - e^{-\lambda t})^{n-i}$$

$$E[X(t)] = ie^{\lambda t}$$

$$\text{Var}[X(t)] = ie^{\lambda t}(e^{\lambda t} - 1).$$

21. Discuss a process that could be modeled by Model II.

22. Consider the stochastic version of Model II. Consider what happens to the predictions if i is not known exactly, but it is known that $10 \le i \le 10^2$. Assume $\lambda = 1$. Plot the graph of $E[X(t)]$, include SD $[X(t)]$ for different values of i, and consider the effect on the predictions for $E[X(t)]$ and SD $[X(t)]$.

23. Assume $i = 10$ and the parameter λ is unknown. If we can assume $0.5 \le \lambda \le 5$, plot the graph for $E[X(t)]$ and include SD $[X(t)]$ for different values of λ. Consider the effects on the predictions for $E[X(t)]$ and SD $[X(t)]$.

5.3 Model III

We now assume a process in which the birth rate decreases as the population size increases. We assume a maximum size k that the population can achieve. k is sometimes called the *carrying capacity* of the environment. Limitations of space or food restrict the size that the population can attain. This assumption may not be entirely realistic, but we will develop models for it to show how general the birth process is. The birth rate λ_n will be expressed as $\lambda_n = \lambda(k - n)$, i.e., it gets smaller as n approaches k. (For $n > k$, λ_n is defined to be 0.)

Thus

$$\lambda_0 = \lambda(k - 0)$$

$$\lambda_1 = \lambda(k - 1)$$

$$\lambda_2 = \lambda(k - 2)$$

$$\vdots$$

$$\lambda_{k-1} = \lambda(k - (k - 1)) = \lambda(1) = \lambda$$

$$\lambda_k = \lambda(k - k) = 0.$$

Then births can no longer occur. Schematically, we get Figure 3.10.

5.3.1. Deterministic. We express these assumptions as

$$N_{t+\Delta t} - N_t = \lambda(k - N_t)\Delta t,$$

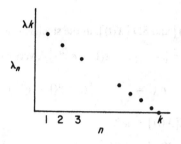

Figure 3.10

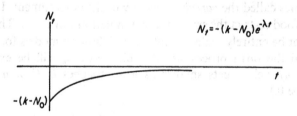

$$N_t = (k - N_0)e^{-\lambda t}$$

Figure 3.11

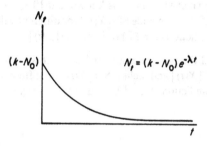

$$N_t = -(k - N_0)e^{-\lambda t}$$

Figure 3.12

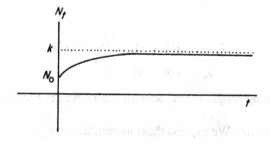

Figure 3.13

for Δt small and $N_t \le k$. Using the definition of the derivative, we get

$$\lim_{\Delta t \to 0} \frac{N_{t+\Delta t} - N_t}{\Delta t} = \lambda(k - N_t)$$

$$\frac{dN_t}{dt} = \lambda(k - N_t)$$

$$\frac{dN_t}{(k - N_t)} = \lambda\,dt$$

$$-\ln(k - N_t) = \lambda t + C$$

$$\ln(k - N_t) = -\lambda t + c$$

$$k - N_t = e^{-\lambda t}e^c$$

$$= c_1 e^{-\lambda t}$$

$$N_t = k - c_1 e^{-\lambda t}.$$

To determine the value of c_1 we note that

$$N_0 = k - c_1 e^{-\lambda(0)}$$

$$N_0 = k - c_1$$

$$c_1 = k - N_0, \qquad N_0 < k.$$

Thus

$$N_t = k - (k - N_0)e^{-\lambda t}.$$

We can sketch the curve defined by this equation in steps.

We first consider $N_t = (k - N_0)e^{-\lambda t}$, whose graph is shown in Figure 3.11. The curve for $N_t = -(k - N_0)e^{-\lambda t}$ is given in Figure 3.12. Finally, if we add k to get $N_t = k - (k - N_0)e^{-\lambda t}$, we are simply shifting the curve up, and we get Figure 3.13. As $t \to \infty$, the curve is asymptotic to $N_t = k$, which is the maximum population size.

We can rearrange $N_t = k - (k - N_0)e^{-\lambda t}$ into a more meaningful form. Multiplying out, we get

$$N_t = k - ke^{-\lambda t} + N_0 e^{-\lambda t}$$

$$= N_0 + k(1 - e^{-\lambda t}) + N_0 e^{-\lambda t} - N_0$$

$$= N_0 + k(1 - e^{-\lambda t}) - N_0(1 - e^{-\lambda t})$$

$$= N_0 + (k - N_0)(1 - e^{-\lambda t}).$$

Thus we can express the total population size N_t as the sum of the initial population size plus the number of new organisms.

As an example, consider $N_0 = 1$, $k = 30$, and $\lambda = 0.693147$. Then we show the predicted values of N_t in Table 4.

Table 4. $N_t = 1 + (30 - 1)(1 - e^{-0.693147t})$

Time (minutes)	N_t		
0.05	1 +	0.99	= 1.99
0.10	1 +	1.94	= 2.94
0.15	1 +	2.86	= 3.86
0.25	1 +	4.61	= 5.61
0.5	1 +	8.49	= 9.49
0.75	1 +	11.76	= 12.76
1	1 +	14.5	= 15.5
2	1 +	21.75	= 22.75
3	1 +	25.38	= 26.38
5	1 +	28.09	= 29.09
7	1 +	28.77	= 29.77
10	1 +	28.97	= 29.97
15	1 +	28.999	= 29.999
20	1 +	28.99999	= 29.99999
30	1 +	28.99999997	= 29.99999997

5.3.2. *Stochastic.* To find the stochastic analog of Model III, we simply let $\lambda_n = \lambda(k - n)$ and substitute it into Eqs. (3) and (4). We get from (3):

$$p_n'(t) = -\lambda(k - n)p_n(t) + \lambda(k - (n - 1))p_{n-1}(t),$$

and we can show from this that the pgf satisfies

$$\frac{\partial P(s, t)}{\partial t} = -\lambda k(1 - s)P(s, t) + \lambda s(1 - s)\frac{\partial P(s, t)}{\partial s}. \tag{13}$$

Equation (13) is a linear partial differential equation of the first order, which can be solved by the Lagrange method. We will present the solution by first assuming that the initial population size is 1, that is, $p_1(0) = 1$ and $p_n(0) = 0$, $n \neq 1$. Using the Lagrange method we find that

$$P(s, t) = s(e^{-\lambda t} + s(1 - e^{-\lambda t}))^{k-1}.$$

(If we write $p(t) = 1 - e^{-\lambda t}$ and $q(t) = e^{-\lambda t}$, then we see that the function $(q(t) + sp(t))^{k-1}$ is the pgf of a binomial distribution. The extra s in $P(s, t)$ is a factor that accounts for the initial population size.) We can determine the exact distribution by taking $(1/n!)\partial^n P(s, t)/\partial s^n|_{s=0}$, and we get

$$p_n(t) = \binom{k - 1}{n - 1}(1 - e^{-\lambda t})^{n-1}(e^{-\lambda t})^{k-n}.$$

(The reader should verify this fact. See Exercise 27 at the end of this Section.) Using the generating function, we discover that

$$E[X(t)] = 1 + (k - 1)(1 - e^{-\lambda t}),$$

which is equivalent to the deterministic solution, and

$$\text{Var}\,[X(t)] = (k - 1)(e^{-\lambda t})(1 - e^{-\lambda t}).$$

We can show that if the initial population size is i (in which case $p_i(0) = 1$ and $p_j(0) = 0$ when $j \neq i$), then

$$P(s, t) = s^i(e^{-\lambda t} + s(1 - e^{-\lambda t}))^{k-i}.$$

(We see that we again have a pgf for a binomial and s^i accounts for the initial population size.) The reader should determine $p_n(t)$ and $E[X(t)]$ and $\text{Var}\,[X(t)]$ from $P(s, t)$. See Exercise 28 at the end of this section.

EXERCISES

24. For the model $N_t = N_0 + (k - N_0)(1 - e^{-\lambda t})$, assume $N_0 = 1$, $k = 100$, and $\lambda = 0.693147$. Plot the graph of N_t.

25. Do Exercise 24, but assume $\lambda = 1.38629$. Compare and discuss the two plots of N_t.

26. Consider a range of values of λ, and for each, plot N_t (assume that $N_0 = 10$ and $k = 500$). Compare and discuss the plots of N_t.

27. Using the pgf $P(s, t) = s(e^{-\lambda t} + s(1 - e^{-\lambda t}))^{k-1}$, verify the following.
    (a) $p_n(t) = \binom{k - 1}{n - 1}(1 - e^{-\lambda t})^{n-1}(e^{-\lambda t})^{k-n}$.
    (b) $E[X(t)] = 1 + (k - 1)(1 - e^{-\lambda t})$.
    (c) $\text{Var}\,[X(t)] = (k - 1)e^{-\lambda t}(1 - e^{-\lambda t})$.

28. Using the pgf $P(s, t) = s^i(e^{-\lambda t} + s(1 - e^{-\lambda t}))^{k-i}$, do the following.
    (a) Determine $p_n(t)$.
    (b) Derive $E[X(t)]$.
    (c) Derive $\text{Var}\,[X(t)]$.

29. Consider a process that can be modeled by Model III, and discuss.

30. Consider the values of k and λ given in Exercise 24 and plot $E[X(t)]$ and $\text{SD}\,[X(t)]$. Assume $i = 1$.

31. Consider the values of k and λ, given in Exercise 25 and plot $E[X(t)]$ and $\text{SD}\,[X(t)]$. Assume $i = 1$. Compare the plots in Exercises 30 and 31.

32. Consider various values of λ, and for each, plot $E[X(t)]$ and $\text{SD}\,[X(t)]$, assuming $i = 10$ and $k = 500$. Compare and discuss the plots.

5.4 Model IV

This last model is developed to illustrate how some simple modifications in the process will lead to mathematical complexity. Interestingly, to develop realistic models of some phenomenon can be difficult because of the complexity of the mathematics. This is becoming less and less of a problem because of the sophistication and speed of electronic computers.

Model IV can be considered as a model for various processes, but we will only discuss two possibilities now.

(1) We will assume that each of the n organisms in the population would "normally" reproduce at the same rate λ but is subjected to the limitations of the carrying capacity of the system. Equivalently, as the population size increases the rate of growth per individual decreases. Symbolically, in the stochastic notation we can express this as a combination of our second and third models:

$$\lambda_n = \lambda n \left(\frac{k - n}{k} \right),$$

where k is the maximum population size. (We will use $(k - n)/k$ rather than $k - n$ because it makes obtaining solutions easier.) When n is small relative to k the birth rate λ_n is closer to λn. When n is large relative to k, the birth rate approaches 0. This birth rate can be generalized to

$$\lambda_n = \lambda n (Ak - Bn)/k.$$

(2) We can consider these assumptions as a simple model of an epidemic, where we assume the disease is contagious, and there are k people in all. Specifically, we will talk about $(k - n)/k$, the proportion of people who are susceptible. For the purposes of this model, we will also assume that once a person becomes infected they stay infected. So there are only two possible states, infective and susceptible, and a person can go from the susceptible state to the infective state, but not the other way. We are also assuming homogeneous mixing among infectives and susceptibles. Let k be the total population size, n the number of people who have the infection (number of infective). It follows that $k - n$ must be the number of susceptibles. Summarizing

λ_n	rate of infection given that n people are infected,
n	number of infectives,
k	total population,
$(k - n)/k$	proportion of susceptibles,
λ_n	$= \lambda n \left(\dfrac{k - n}{k} \right).$

If we look at λ_n, we find that we can interpret this to say when n is small, the rate of infection is high, since there are many susceptible contacts available to cause more infection. Since the number of infectives increases as the number of susceptibles decreases, the number of possible new cases decreases and so λ_n gets smaller.

Both processes are amenable to a deterministic and a stochastic solution.

5.4.1. Deterministic. The processes we have discussed can be expressed deterministically as

$$N_{t+\Delta t} - N_t = \lambda N_t \left(\frac{k - N_t}{k} \right) \Delta t$$

for small Δt. Using the definition of a derivative, we get

$$\frac{dN_t}{dt} = \lambda N_t \left(\frac{k - N_t}{k} \right).$$

Solving, we have

$$\frac{dN_t}{N_t(k - N_t)} = \frac{\lambda}{k} dt$$

$$\frac{dN_t}{kN_t} + \frac{dN_t}{k(k - N_t)} = \frac{\lambda}{k} dt$$

$$\frac{dN_t}{N_t} + \frac{dN_t}{k - N_t} = \lambda\, dt$$

$$\ln N_t - \ln (k - N_t) = \lambda t + c$$

$$\ln \frac{N_t}{k - N_t} = \lambda t + c$$

$$\frac{N_t}{k - N_t} = e^{\lambda t} e^c$$

$$\frac{N_t}{k - N_t} = c_1 e^{\lambda t},$$

letting $e^c = c_1$. We solve for N_t and get

$$N_t = \frac{k c_1 e^{\lambda t}}{1 + c_1 e^{\lambda t}}.$$

To evaluate c_1 we consider the initial conditions, and let $N_0 = i$. Then

$$N_0 = i = \frac{k c_1 e^{\lambda 0}}{1 + c_1 e^{\lambda 0}} = \frac{k c_1}{1 + c_1}$$

and

$$c_1 = \frac{N_0}{k - N_0}.$$

Substituting for c_1 in the equation for N_t, we get

$$N_t = \frac{k \left(\dfrac{N_0}{k - N_0} \right) e^{\lambda t}}{1 + \left(\dfrac{N_0}{k - N_0} \right) e^{\lambda t}}$$

$$= \frac{k N_0 e^{\lambda t}}{(k - N_0) + N_0 e^{\lambda t}}$$

$$= \frac{kN_0 e^{\lambda t}}{k + N_0(e^{\lambda t} - 1)},$$

which for convenience we rewrite as

$$N_t = \frac{kN_0}{ke^{-\lambda t} + N_0(1 - e^{-\lambda t})}$$

$$= \frac{N_0 k}{N_0 + (k - N_0)e^{-\lambda t}}.$$

This is the equation of the *logistic curve*, which is sometimes also known as the *sigmoid curve*. Let us sketch the curve.

(1) We recall that $N_0 = i$.
(2) As $t \to \infty$, the curve is asymptotic to

$$\lim_{t \to \infty} N_t = \lim_{t \to \infty} \frac{N_0 k}{N_0 + (k - N_0)e^{-\lambda t}} = k.$$

(3) (a) Where is the curve increasing or decreasing?
    (b) Is there a relative maximum or minimum?
    (c) Are there any inflection points?

To answer these questions, we could find the derivative by considering

$$\frac{dN_t}{dt} = \frac{d}{dt}\left(\frac{N_0 k}{N_0 + (k - N_0)e^{-\lambda t}}\right).$$

However, we already know that

$$\frac{dN_t}{dt} = \lambda N_t\left(\frac{k - N_t}{k}\right).$$

To determine where the curve is increasing or decreasing, we want to study if $dN_t/dt > 0$ or < 0. We can show quite easily that $dN_t/dt > 0$, if we can show that $N_t > 0$ and $N_t < k$, that is, $0 < N_t < k$. The equation

$$N_t = \frac{N_0 k}{N_0 + (k - N_0)e^{-\lambda t}}$$

can be rewritten as

$$N_t = \frac{k}{1 + \left(\dfrac{k - N_0}{N_0}\right)e^{-\lambda t}}. \tag{14}$$

If $k > N_0$, i.e., if we start out at a population below the carrying capacity k, then

$$\left(\frac{k - N_0}{N_0}\right)e^{-\lambda t} > 0$$

since $e^{-\lambda t} > 0$ and $(k - N_0)/N_0 > 0$. It follows from (14) that

$$1 + \left(\frac{k - N_0}{N_0}\right)e^{-\lambda t} > 1$$

and so $N_t < k$. Moreover, it is now easy to see from (14) that $N_t > 0$ since $k > 0$ and the denominator of (14) is greater than 1.

It follows that if $N_0 < k$, then

$$\frac{dN_t}{dt} = \lambda N_t \left(\frac{k - N_t}{k}\right) > 0,$$

since $0 < N_t < k$. Hence the curve is always increasing. Since $dN_t/dt > 0$, it follows that there can be no relative maximum or minimum.

Next, we must determine if there is an inflection point. The second derivative

$$\frac{d^2 N_t}{dt^2} = \lambda \left(\frac{k - N_t}{k}\right)\frac{dN_t}{dt} + \frac{\lambda N_t}{k}\left(-\frac{dN_t}{dt}\right)$$

$$= \frac{dN_t}{dt}\left(\lambda - \frac{\lambda N_t}{k} - \frac{\lambda N_t}{k}\right)$$

$$= \frac{dN_t}{dt}\left(\lambda - \frac{2\lambda N_t}{k}\right).$$

Therefore, $d^2 N_t/dt^2$ is equal to zero if either dN_t/dt or $\lambda - (2\lambda N_t/k)$ or both are equal to zero. We know that $dN_t/dt \neq 0$, and therefore we want to determine if a value of N_t exists for which $\lambda - (2\lambda N_t/k) = 0$.

$$\lambda - \frac{2\lambda N_t}{k} = 0$$

implies

$$\lambda = \frac{2\lambda N_t}{k}$$

$$N_t = \frac{k}{2}.$$

The last thing to do is determine the time when $N_t = k/2$. We find that

$$N_t = \frac{k}{2} = \frac{N_0 k}{N_0 + (k - N_0)e^{-\lambda t}}$$

$$1 = \frac{2N_0}{N_0 + (k - N_0)e^{-\lambda t}}$$

$$N_0 + (k - N_0)e^{-\lambda t} = 2N_0$$

$$(k - N_0)e^{-\lambda t} = N_0$$

$$e^{-\lambda t} = \frac{N_0}{k - N_0}$$

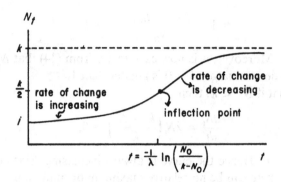

Figure 3.14

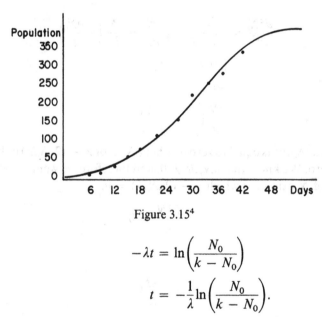

Figure 3.15[4]

$$-\lambda t = \ln\left(\frac{N_0}{k - N_0}\right)$$

$$t = -\frac{1}{\lambda}\ln\left(\frac{N_0}{k - N_0}\right).$$

The inflection point occurs when $t = (-1/\lambda)\ln(N_0/(k - N_0))$.

If we put all this information together, we get the curve for N_t given in Figure 3.14. In terms of the epidemic, we see that the number of new cases increases at a faster rate when $N_t < k/2$ (number of infectives is less than 1/2 the population) and then at a slower rate when $N_t > k/2$.

Figure 3.15 is a graph of the growth of a population of Drosophila under controlled experimental conditions. The data are fit very well by a logistic equation.

5.4.2. Stochastic. The stochastic analog of this process requires the use of $\lambda_n = \lambda n((k - n)/k)$. Substituting this birth rate into (3), we get

---

[4] Source: Batschelet [2]. The figure is reproduced from Lotka [6, p. 69] with the permission of Dover Publications. Data are attributed to R. Pearl and S. L. Parker.

$$p_n'(t) = -\lambda n\left(\frac{k-n}{k}\right)p_n(t) + \lambda(n-1)\left(\frac{k-(n-1)}{k}\right)p_{n-1}(t). \quad (15)$$

In terms of pgf's we get

$$\frac{\partial P(s,\,t)}{\partial t} = \lambda\left(\frac{k-1}{k}\right)s(s-1)\frac{\partial P(s,\,t)}{\partial s} + \frac{\lambda s^2(1-s)}{k}\frac{\partial^2 P(s,\,t)}{\partial s^2},$$

which is a linear partial differential equation of the second order. This is not readily amenable to a solution. We see how quickly the problem of analyzing a mathematical model has become mathematically complex. Instead of solving for $P(s,\,t)$, we can use Laplace transforms to solve (15) for $p_n(t)$. Because for some value of n, $k-n=0$, pertubation methods must be applied. We substitute $k_1 = k + \varepsilon$, for ε small, into (15) in place of k. Then $p_n^\varepsilon(t)$ is the corresponding probability. We can show that

$$p_n^\varepsilon(t) = \sum_{j=1}^{n}(-1)^{j+1}\binom{n-1}{j-1}\left(\frac{k_1-2j}{k_1-n}\right)\prod_{i=1}^{n}\frac{(k_1-i)}{(k_1-(i+j))}e^{-\lambda j[(k_1-j)/k_1]t},$$

$$n = 1, 2, \cdots, k.$$

In this form, it is not clear how to find a reasonable closed form for $E[X(t)]$ and $\mathrm{Var}[X(t)]$. It appears that even though for many models the $E[X(t)]$ of the stochastic model is equivalent to the deterministic solution, this is not always the case. It should be clear, however, that for given value of λ, and with the help of a computer, evaluating $p_n^\varepsilon(t)$, $E[X(t)]$, and $\mathrm{Var}[X(t)]$ would be easy. Thus the stochastic model can be worked out and predictions made.

One of the reasons we presented this model is to show how complex a model can become mathematically, when some relatively realistic assumptions are introduced.

EXERCISES

33. For the model

$$N_t = \frac{k}{1 + \left(\dfrac{k - N_0}{N_0}\right)e^{-\lambda t}},$$

assume $N_0 = 1$, $k = 100$, and $\lambda = 0.693147$, plot the graph of N_t. Determine the time when $N_t = k/2$.

34. Do Exercise 33, but assume $\lambda = 1.38629$. Compare and discuss the two plots of N_t.

35. Consider a range of values for λ, and for each plot N_t (assume that $N_0 = 10$ and $k = 500$). Compare and discuss the plot of N_t.

36. Discuss a process that might be modeled by the logistic curve.

37. Model IV can be used to model the number of people who will buy a new product (Polaroid camera, new model car). Discuss how to use Model IV. Interpret to what k, λ, and N_0 would correspond.

38. What modifications should be made in the formulation of the epidemic model to make it more realistic?

39. Consider how you would modify the general system of differential equations to account for deaths only or birth and death.

5.5 Summary

In this section we briefly summarize the four models we have discussed.

Model I:
(1) *Deterministic:* If $N_{t+\Delta t} - N_t = \lambda \Delta t$, then $N_t = \lambda t$.
(2) *Stochastic:* In a pure birth process with $\lambda_n = \lambda$,
 (a) $p_n(t) = e^{-\lambda t}(\lambda t)^n/n!$;
 (b) $E[X(t)] = \lambda t$;
 (c) $\mathrm{Var}\,[X(t)] = \lambda t$.

Model II:
(1) *Deterministic:* If $N_{t+\Delta t} - N_t = \lambda N_t \Delta t$, then $N_t = N_0 e^{\lambda t}$.
(2) *Stochastic:* In a pure birth process with $\lambda_n = \lambda n$,
 (a) if the initial population size i is 1, then
 (i) $p_n(t) = e^{-\lambda t}(1 - e^{-\lambda t})^{n-1}$,
 (ii) $E[X(t)] = e^{\lambda t}$,
 (iii) $\mathrm{Var}[X(t)] = e^{\lambda t}(e^{\lambda t} - 1)$;
 (b) If the initial population size is i, then
 (i) $p_n(t) = \binom{n-1}{n-i}(e^{-\lambda t})^i(1 - e^{-\lambda t})^{n-i}$,
 (ii) $E[X(t)] = ie^{\lambda t}$,
 (iii) $\mathrm{Var}\,[X(t)] = ie^{\lambda t}(e^{\lambda t} - 1)$.

Model III:
(1) *Deterministic:* If $N_{t+\Delta t} - N_t = \lambda(k - N_t)\Delta t$, then
 $N_t = N_0 + (k - N_0)(1 - e^{-\lambda t})$.
(2) *Stochastic:* In a pure birth process with $\lambda_n = \lambda(k - n)$ where the initial population size is i,
 (a) $p_n(t) = \binom{k-i}{n-i}(1 - e^{-\lambda t})^{n-i}(e^{-\lambda t})^{k-n}$;
 (b) $E[X(t)] = i + (k - i)(1 - e^{-\lambda t})$;
 (c) $\mathrm{Var}\,[X(t)] = (k - i)(e^{-\lambda t})(1 - e^{-\lambda t})$.

Model IV:
(1) *Deterministic:* If $N_{t+\Delta t} - N_t = \lambda N_t((k - N_t)/k)\Delta t$, then

$$N_t = \frac{k}{1 + \left(\dfrac{k - N_0}{N_0}\right)e^{-\lambda t}}.$$

(2) *Stochastic:* In a pure birth process with $\lambda_n = \lambda_n((k - n)/k)$,

$$p_n^{\varepsilon}(t) = \sum_{j=1}^{n} (-1)^{j+1}\binom{n-1}{j-1}\left(\frac{k_1 - 2j}{k_1 - n}\right)\prod_{i=1}^{n}\frac{(k_1 - i)}{(k_1 - (i + j))}e^{-\lambda j[(k_1 - j)/k_1]t},$$

$$n = 1, 2, \cdots, k.$$

References

[1] N. T. J. Bailey, *The Elements of Stochastic Processes.* New York: Wiley, 1964.
[2] E. Batschelet, *Introduction to Mathematics for Life Scientists.* New York: Springer-Verlag, 1971.
[3] D. R. Cox and H. D. Miller, *The Theory of Stochastic Processes.* New York: Wiley, 1965.
[4] W. Feller, *An Introduction to Probability Theory and its Applications,* Vol. I, 3rd ed. New York: Wiley, 1968.
[5] S. Karlin, *First Course in Stochastic Processes.* New York and London: Academic, 1966.
[6] A. J. Lotka, *Elements of Mathematical Biology.* New York: Dover, 1956.
[7] H. Marcus–Roberts and F. S. Roberts, "Malaria (models of the population dynamics of the malaria parasite)," this volume, chapter 5.

Notes for the Instructor

Prerequisites. Prerequisites for this chapter will depend on the use to which the chapter is put. The reader who just wants to get the overview without taking time to go through the mathematical details can get a lot out of this chapter with just a background in calculus (two semesters) and probability. Some of the details require more knowledge of differential equations and partial differential equations.

Remarks. This chapter is appropriate for probability, differential equations, and a modeling course. The deterministic models can be used in a calculus course.

Time. A quick overview can be accomplished in two hours, though this is not recommended. A detailed treatment could take several weeks.

CHAPTER 4

Some Examples of Mathematical Models for the Dynamics of Several-Species Ecosystems

H. R. van der Vaart*

Preface

The mathematics that is applied in this module spans several levels. First, calculus is called for throughout, especially the ability to find primitive functions. Second, extensive use is made of the isocline-and-arrow method; the background for this method is given in Appendix A, Sections A.1 and A.2. Third, for the study of differential equations in the neighborhood of singular points, the linearization method is used; this method is presented at length in Appendix A, Sections A.3 and A.4. Finally, Section 1.6 investigates certain aspects of difference equations. Most of the needed mathematics is developed in that section (see the cited literature for more information).

One can skip certain sections with relative ease, e.g., Section 1.6 or Section 2.3, but the instructor will be able to spot other possibilities as the work progresses. One can also skip some of the exercises that require more intricate mathematical work. One can choose between going over Sections A.3 and A.4 in detail, or just picking out the results. Finally, it should be said that our presentation proceeds in an analytic and geometric framework, but that the experience of past users indicates that supplementing this approach by work on analog or digital computers is quite effective, provided adequate guidance is available.

Depending on which of the above choices one makes, one may spend anywhere between four and ten weeks on this chapter. Besides Appendix A on certain mathematical tools, please note Appendix B (the bibliography) and Appendix C (the hints for solutions).

* Department of Statistics, North Carolina State University, Raleigh, NC 27650.

1. Introduction

1.1 Background

The term "ecosystem" was introduced by Tansley [63]. An ecosystem consists of a number of organisms (which may very well belong to many different species) and their environment, together with the interactions between the organisms *inter se* and between the organisms and their environment, all of which is contained in an often loosely defined and seldom isolated part of space. "Biogeocoenosis," a term coined by Sukachev, is perhaps more suggestive; it connotes a more or less complex interaction between biological community (biocoenosis) and habitat (biotope, expressed by the syllables "geo").

> "The individual ecosystems vary greatly in size and structure. The entire globe is an ecosystem, the only one which is not influenced by other ecosystems. An island, a forest, a pasture, a decaying tree stump with its moss and fungi, even a puddle on the path which is only temporarily inhabited, all such natural phenomena deserve to be called ecosystems. Thus, great variations exist not only in magnitude, duration and production, but also in the degree of dependence on other ecosystems." H. Ellenberg [12, p. 2].

Let us emphasize (cf. J. Balogh [6, p. 26]) that neither biocoenoses nor biotopes exist on their own in nature and that they are separated in our thinking only.

A long-standing effort in mathematical modeling of ecological problems concerns the variations in numbers of individuals belonging to the various species living together in an ecosystem or biogeocoenosis. The book by U. d'Ancona [3] provides a good entry to the older literature in this field. We will discuss some examples of such mathematical models, assuming that *no migration* takes place into or out of the ecosystem (that is, the theory is restricted to the case of no migration). We will also assume that the ecosystem has fixed spatial boundaries (as more or less suggested by Ellenberg's examples), so that we may equivalently describe events in terms of total numbers of individuals in the system or in terms of density (number of individuals per area or volume, as the case may be). There is obvious practical interest in the numerical aspects of population dynamics; think of insect pests, fishery research, population explosion, for example.

Between any two species in an ecosystem, any one of several relations may exist, such as:

(a) prey–predator (first species is eaten by second species) and host–parasite ("a small organism lives in or with and at the expense of a larger animal or plant," cf. W. C. Allee *et al.* [2, p. 253];

(b) cooperation ("helpful interactions between organisms," W. C. Allee *et al.*, [2, p.395]; or "mutually beneficial relationships between species," [2, p. 710], called mutualism by some authors, symbiosis by others;

(c) disoperation (harmful interactions between the organisms of the same or different species, cf. W. C. Allee *et al.*, [2, p. 395], e.g., most cases of competition where both want the same things from their surroundings.

1.2 Historical Beginnings of Mathematical Models in Ecosystem Dynamics

If one should be asked to provide the name of *one* scientist most intimately connected with the origin and development of the mathematical models to be discussed, one probably ought to mention Vito *Volterra*. According to the very informative biography of V. Volterra,[1] Volterra was interested in biological (and social) applications of mathematics as early as 1901. His active role in research in this area does not seem to have gotten underway before 1925, though, and was prompted by conversations with U. d'Ancona (also see d'Ancona [3, p. 52]) on the fluctuations of fish caught in the Adriatic Sea. In d'Ancona's words, however, "from the beginning Volterra attacked the problem in its general aspect." Indeed, the only trace of this motivation for Volterra's work seems to be the fact that one of this earliest papers on the subject, viz. a memoir (Variazioni e fluttuazioni in specie animali conviventi) of 142 papges, was published by the R. Comitato Talassografico Italiano (Memoria *131*, Venezia, 1972) which, according to its name, was concerned with matters of the sea. It would be interesting to compare the results of Volterra's (or indeed, anybody's) theory with the data that prompted its development. In the bibliography of d'Ancona [3], some publications by d'Ancona, all in Italian, are listed that probably provide such information (see also Županović, 1953, quoted on p. 259 of d'Ancona, loc. cit.).

Two other authors should be mentioned here for their substantial contributions to the early development of this field: Alfred J. Lotka and G. F. Gause (not to be confused with the mathematician C. F. Gauss). Some of *Lotka's* work actually preceded Volterra's; see Lotka [45, pp. 88–99, ch. 8] where some of his earlier work is also quoted. As for his motivation, it seems to have been more the desire for a general understanding of the "laws governing the distribution of matter among complexes of any specified kind" [44, p. 216] than such practical matters as were brought before Volterra by d'Ancona. Chemical systems were very much on Lotka's mind: see "monomolecular reactions" [44, p. 204] and "We have recognized the problem of chemical dynamics as a special case of a wider problem" [44, p. 216], from a paper whose first half discusses the relations between birth and death rates, age distributions, and life tables, problems of long-standing interest with students of human populations (demographers). *Gause* was a popula-

---

[1] Sir Edmund Whittaker, "Obituary Notices of Fellows of the Royal Society," 1941, reprinted in [68, pp. 5–39].

tion ecologist who conducted quite a few laboratory experiments. From the titles of some of his papers of 1934 and 1935 listed in Gause [17, bibliography] as well as from the overall thrust of the same book, it becomes apparent that he was quite interested in experimentally exploring Volterra's theory (also see Gause [18]). Among other things, he contributed greatly to the establishment of the idea that whenever two species compete against each other, one species often gains the upper hand completely (cf. Section 3.3 of this module).

1.3 A Partial List of More Recent Literature on the Subject

From the work begun by Lotka and Volterra until the present time, hundreds of papers have been published, either to further develop the mathematical theory, or to expound experimental work elicited by some phase of the mathematical theory (such as Gause's abovementioned work), or to set forth nonmathematized theoretical reflections on matters arising in this area.

If anybody wants to approach this vast body of literature, (s)he can rely on several books and surveys. Besides the books by Gause and d'Ancona already mentioned (both available in paperback), several other possibilities are suggested.[2]

J. Maynard Smith's *Mathematical Ideas in Biology* [52] cites only a few references, but Chapters 2 and 3 give an exposition that might help some students. *Models in Ecology* [53] by the same author emphasizes analysis of theoretical models; 87 references are given, some of which are concerned with observations.

M. Williamson [71] deals more with genetical aspects and has less on mathematical treatment than does Smith. A list of 286 references is provided.

D. B. Mertz [54] presents mainly nondeterministic observations and models of the flour beetle, with 102 references.

R. H. MacArthur's *Geographical Ecology; patterns in the Distribution of Species* [47, ch. 2] treats competition and predation.

The Dynamics of Arthropod Predator–Prey Systems [26] by M. P. Hassell contains a list of about 280 references, a majority of which represents observational work with a strong minority on theory; many models in the book are time-discrete.

R. M. May's 230 references [50] are mainly theoretical, with a strong minority on observational work.

The volume *Ecological Stability*, edited by M. B. Usher and M. H. Williamson [65] is a collection of 12 papers on various related subjects,

---

[2] The first five titles on this list should not give too many mathematical difficulties to undergraduate math majors; the next three are more advanced; the last title is definitely at the graduate level. The fourth and the eighth titles are biologically more demanding than the others.

theoretical and practical; each paper carrying its own list of references (between one and two pages long).

N. S. Goel et al. [21], a reprint of *Reviews of Modern Physics*, vol. 43, pp. 231–276, April 1971 is an attempt by a group of physicists to build a superstructure on the Volterra models.

A high density of relevant papers can be found in some issues of such journals as *The American Naturalist, Theoretical Population Biology, Acta Biotheoretica, Bulletin of Mathematical Biology* (formerly *Bulletin of Mathematical Biophysics*), *Journal of Theoretical Biology, Mathematical Biosciences, and Ecology.*

1.4 General Remarks about the Degree of Realism and the Mathematical Level of the Models To Be Discussed

In view of the overwhelming volume of literature in our subject area and the fact that the readers of this module are undergraduate students in mathematics, we obviously cannot hope to do much more than outline the early stages of this developing field. To acquaint the reader with the full spectrum of present-day research in these few pages is impossible. Some of the newer developments use mathematical tools that are fairly close to the ones we will use, but most of these developments, having gone in the direction of greater realism, require either more sophisticated mathematics or long computer programs (hence some knowledge of more sophisticated numerical methods). Thus we will have to do without the satisfaction of modeling the world, or a forest, or the tundra, or even that "simple" puddle in your backyard.

However, nothing shameful is to be found in retracing some of the steps that research mathematicians and biologists have taken during the last few decades. Many undergraduate physics courses do not even accomplish that sort of thing in physics, and ecosystems are rather complicated objects of research. The reader will reach a level at which he can recognize the concerns of many papers, e.g., in the *American Naturalist*, even if he will not (yet) be able to write those papers himself. The reader will also learn a few mathematical techniques that are very helpful in studying the behavior of solutions of (especially two-dimensional) systems of nonlinear ordinary differential equations of order one, which occur in several areas of applied mathematics.

An aspect of mathematical model building of which the reader should be advised, an aspect that is particularly obvious with such complex subjects as ecosystems, is the following. The very first model that Volterra put up (for a predator–prey system), while yielding some interesting results, was biologically trivial. The models that came after it cannot usually be solved analytically; they must be studied by qualitative methods or numerically, by means of a computer. Some people get discouraged when they realize that, in spite of all the work, such models are still elementary, biologically speaking. There is, of course, no reason for such discouragement. Research ecologists have worked with these models; the models have elicited a great deal of experimental work, intended either to refute or to expand them. This is the hallmark of the development of science: a continuing dialogue between experiments or observations on the one hand and theoretical considerations on the other, with the final "truth" being perhaps forever elusive. Many mathematicians find this situation distasteful, but whoever aspires to being a mathematician with applied interests in the life or social sciences had better adjust to the idea that any model he may propose of a real life situation may be criticized or rejected by a colleague, not because anything is wrong with his mathematics, but because his model does not satisfy that colleague on biological (or sociological) grounds.

In order that the reader may grow accustomed to the continual "threat" of criticism on the quality of whatever model he might be working with, we have scattered *discussion questions* throughout the module. In these the reader is invited to explore the weak points of the model discussed in the main text, to explain why (s)he thinks certain aspects are weak, and to set forth ways in which to improve the model, thus generating alternative models. If adequate computer facilities are available, groups of students could explore some of these "improvements" numerically. They might discover that the solutions to the improved systems show more realistic features, or that they look worse than the original systems. These discussion questions are, in a way, open-ended: they have no unique, correct answer but should serve to sharpen the reader's critical sense.

In the face of the critical attitude that this module seeks to develop in the reader, it is important not to lose sight of the fact that all major models discussed herein have actually been published in the research literature: none of them has been contrived for the special purpose of this project.

A final remark concerns the adduction of records of experiments or observations so that the reader may have numbers available against which to test this or that model. Unfortunately, graphs do seem to be preferred over tables by biology publishers. At this writing, the author still had not located one publication in which actual numbers were given: the tables given by Leigh [38, pp. 58–60] were read from certain graphs (as stated on pp. 53 and 56 of that article). The reader should glean his own numbers from these (or other) graphs. As for the problem of fitting any of the models under discussion to such data, the best the reader can do is eyeball them; optimal statistical methods for this purpose are the subject of active research, but a rough estimate can be obtained from looking at phase plane plots of the data.

1.5 Specific Remarks about the Mathematical Nature of the Models To Be Discussed

Our discussion will start with examples of mathematical models for systems consisting of only *two species* (to be expanded in some of the later sections). Such systems are rare in nature, but have been studied in the laboratory (e.g.,Gause [17] and Huffaker [30]). They have the pedagogical advantage that at least some of their mathematical properties can be handled by elementary means, because a two-dimensional space can be depicted easily on a piece of paper or on a blackboard. Thus they are accessible even to persons with a modest mathematical background. At the same time, in most real world situations, one must look at more than two species (e.g., see the discussion around equation (25) in Section 4. Some of the mathematical tools needed for the study of these larger, more general systems can be introduced during the discussion of the two-species models, others cannot. In any case, ecosystems of more than two species are not merely the frosting on the cake; in most real ecosystems they are very much the cake itself. The introductory nature of this module prompts the relative emphasis on two-species systems.

Another feature of our models which may be said to lack realism is that they are *deterministic*. They do not account for the many hard-to-control influences that characterize most biological experimentation and whose effects are clear from, among other things, the graphs in [17, figs. 24 and 25, pp. 106–107]. We have several reasons for restricting our discussion to deterministic models. *First*, the originators of the theory did it, probably on the example of the physical sciences, and countless papers have been, and still are, published in this vein. As was said before, this is an appropriate defense for an introductory discussion. *Second*, most of the stochastic models (note that the standard method coping mathematically with observations that are not "on the curve" is to incorporate probabilistic features) are mathematically intractable. Most of the work done on them has consisted of computer simulation (Monte Carlo) studies (e.g., Bartlett [7], Leslie and Gower [42], Leslie [41]) which took off from discrete models (see Discussion Question 1 in Section 1.6). Although this entire module does offer many opportunities for computer-oriented projects, we did not want to slant the main exposition in that direction. The literature (e.g., Reuter [59], Iglehart [32], Tsokos and Hinkley [64]) on mathematical and analytical work done on stochastic models amply demonstrates that this work is too advanced for our purposes. *Third*, the deterministic models often suggest problems to be studied by stochastic methods (cf. Feller [14], Neyman *et al.* [55], Mertz [54]). All in all, the deterministic model is a good port of entry but one must disembark if one is to see the land.

Finally, the great majority of the following models have the form of *differential equations*. This point has three main implications: (α) the models predict the immediate future on the basis of the *present*, not on the basis of any part of the past, (β) the *increment* of any of the state variables over a short time interval of length h is assumed to be a rather *special* type of *function* of h, and (γ) the models are basically *continuous*, rather than discrete. Let us discuss these points one at a time.

(α) The models may be regarded as a limiting case of a subset of the following category of models. If $x(t)$ represents the number of individuals of species 1 at time t and $y(t)$ represents the number of individuals of species 2 at time t, then the increase of both during the time elapsing between t and $t + h$ is assumed to depend on h, on $x(t)$, and on $y(t)$:

$$\begin{cases} x(t + h) - x(t) = F(h, x(t), y(t)) \\ y(t + h) - y(t) = G(h, x(t), y(t)) \end{cases}. \tag{1}$$

DISCUSSION QUESTION

1. Can you think of any reason(s) why, or of any example(s) in which, it might *not* be a good idea to express these changes (viz., $x(t + h) - x(t)$, and $y(t + h) - y(t)$) during the time interval from t to $t + h$ solely in terms of $x(t)$ and $y(t)$? In discussing this question, possibly for a one-species population such as the human population, try to think of relations between increments like $x(t + h) - x(t)$ and present as well as past population sizes. Any example where the link to the past seems quantitatively important would be a situation where the type of model in equation (1) should be viewed with suspicion and replaced by a model in which $F(\;)$ and $G(\;)$ depend also on values of $x(\;)$ and $y(\;)$ at times $<t$.

Remark 1. Models which do incorporate the past, such as

$$\begin{cases} x(t + h) - x(t) = F(h, x(t), y(t), x(t - \tau), y(t - \tau)) \\ y(t + h) - y(t) = G(h, x(t), y(t), x(t - \tau), y(t - \tau)) \end{cases},$$

are mathematically much more difficult than (1) (cf. Discussion Question 5 in Section 1.5). Even in the case of human populations, where omission of the past is quite suspicious, certain models of the form of (1) have satisfied demographers such as Pearl and Reed for a long time. So, with the same philosophy as expressed before, most of the discussions will refer to models of the form of (1).

(β) We will then assume that the functions $F(h, x, y)$ and $G(h, x, y)$ of (1) are of the form $h \cdot \varphi(x, y)$ and $h \cdot \psi(x, y)$, so (1) can be written in the form

$$\begin{cases} \dfrac{x(t + h) - x(t)}{h} = \varphi(x(t), y(t)) \\ \dfrac{y(t + h) - y(t)}{h} = \psi(x(t), y(t)) \end{cases}. \tag{2}$$

Remark 2. This assumption is similar to one made in all classical models of physics and chemistry. Yet, although it is natural to assume that $|x(t + h) - x(t)|$ is an increasing function of h, it is not clear why $|x(t + h) - x(t)|$ could not be proportional to $h^{1-\varepsilon}$ or to $h^{1+\varepsilon}$ ($\varepsilon > 0$), to name just two examples. In other words, although physics and chemistry have conditioned us to think, talk, and act in terms of *rates of change per time unit* (in fact, in terms of quantities such as $[x(t + h) - x(t)]/h$), this type of quantity does not necessarily provide the right kind of framework for ecological theory.

DISCUSSION QUESTION

2. Show that the next step in the modeling process (see (γ)) would result in the same equation (3) if we made the following weaker assumption about $F(h, x, y)$ and $G(h, x, y)$: $F(h, x, y) = h \cdot \varphi^*(h, x, y)$ and $G(h, x, y) = h \cdot \psi^*(h, x, y)$, provided $\lim_{h \to 0} \varphi^*(h, x, y) = ?$ and $\lim_{h \to 0} \psi^*(h, x, y) = ?$

(γ) Finally, again in analogy to physical and chemical models (a fine specimen of this kind of argument can be found in [15, vol. 1, sections 8–2, 8–3, and 9–5], where the traditional definition of speed is defended) it is argued that (1) should hold for any h, small or not-so-small, so that we may as well let $h \to 0$ and cast our model in the form of differential equations,

$$\left\{ \begin{array}{l} \dot{x}(t) = \varphi(x(t), y(t)) \\ \dot{y}(t) = \psi(x(t), y(t)) \end{array} \right\}. \tag{3}$$

Remark 3. This step is odious to many a biologist because his observations on populations are never made in a time continuum, but at separate moments of time, and because the number of individuals (represented by $x(t)$ and $y(t)$) is discrete and integer-valued. Mathematically speaking, the juxtaposition of discrete- and continuous-time models is not as harmless as one might think (see Section 1.6). Biologically speaking, one could argue that x and y represent the biomass[3] of these species, a continuous quantity (although observation consists of counting or estimating the number of individuals), or that they represent the average value (again, a continuous quantity) of discrete variables subject to relatively small random fluctuations superimposed on the broader sweep described by (3). In Section 1.6 we will give a few examples of the problems in comparing discrete and continuous-time models.

Once we accept the idea of differential equations as a category of models for ecosystems, the main question left with respect to model building is how to specify the functions $\varphi(\ )$ and $\psi(\ )$ in (3). We will begin with the observation that if species 1 were extinct at some moment in time, then $\dot{x}(t)$ must be zero from that moment on (no immigration!). The same is true for $\dot{y}(t)$. So

$$\left\{ \begin{array}{l} \varphi(0, y) = 0 \\ \psi(x, 0) = 0 \end{array} \right\}. \tag{4}$$

Although this can be achieved in various ways, one traditionally satisfies (4) by putting $\varphi(x, y) = x \cdot f(x, y)$ and $\psi(x, y) = y \cdot g(x, y)$, with $f(\ )$ and $g(\ )$ bounded. Thus (3) reduces to

---

[3] Although students of population dynamics readily propose the concept of biomass as a way out of the dilemma between discrete reality and continuous model, I do not know of an actual implementation of this concept. One could, for instance, use live weight, or dry weight, as measures of biomass.

$$\begin{cases} \dot{x}(t) = x(t) \cdot f(x(t), y(t)) \\ \dot{y}(t) = y(t) \cdot g(x(t), y(t)) \end{cases} \tag{5}$$

or, in abbreviated notation (remember that x and y *are* functions of t),

$$\begin{cases} \dot{x} = x \cdot f(x, y) \\ \dot{y} = y \cdot g(x, y) \end{cases}. \tag{5a}$$

In the following sections several choices of $f(\ ,\ )$ and $g(\ ,\ )$ will be discussed, according to the type of relations (prey–predator, cooperation, disoperation) between species 1 and 2.

Remark 4. Equation (4) is commonly, but not universally, adopted. Some publications discuss alternatives. In what follows, discussion questions and/ or remarks will draw attention to these exceptions.

As a first and very simple example of the principle expressed by (5) and also as preparation for further developments, let us take a very brief look at a model (in the spirit of (5)) for the growth of a population consisting of *one* species only (e.g., human populations), namely

$$\dot{x}(t) = x(t) \cdot f(x(t)), \quad \text{or} \quad \dot{x} = x \cdot f(x), \tag{5b}$$

where $f(x) = \dot{x}/x$ is the relative growth rate of the population. At an early date (in fact, after Malthus), demographers concluded that no (human) population was going to grow forever at a constant relative rate. They argued that some maximum population size K should exist that "the environment could carry" ($K = $ "carrying capacity" of the environment) and that the closer the population size would come to K, the smaller $\dot{x}/x$ should be. So $f(x)$ in (5b) should be equal to 0 if $x = K$ and equal to a decreasing function of x for $0 < x < K$. One of the simplest such functions is $f(x) = r(1 - x/K)$, which reduces (5b) to

$$\dot{x}(t) = rx(t)\left(1 - \frac{x(t)}{K}\right) \quad \text{or} \quad \dot{x} = rx\left(1 - \frac{x}{K}\right), \tag{5c}$$

the so-called *logistic* equation (e.g., see Gause [17, pp. 32–44]).

EXERCISES

1. Find $x(t)$ if $\dot{x}(t) = r \cdot x(t)$ for $t \geq t_0$, $x(t_0) = x_0$, and r is a constant (exponential or logarithmic growth).

2. Show that the function

$$x(t) = \frac{K}{1 + \dfrac{K - x_0}{x_0} e^{-r(t - t_0)}} \tag{5d}$$

is a solution of (5c) and takes the value x_0 at $t = t_0$ (hence is *the* solution of the

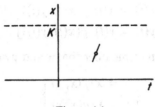

Figure 4.1

logistic equation that satisfies the initial condition $x(t_0) = x_0$. This solution is also defined for $t < t_0$.

3. For $r = 0.01$, $K = 800$, draw a graph of the function of t defined by (5d) for $t > t_0$ and $t < t_0$. Note that, within the context of our biological problem, $0 < x_0 < K$, but that the solution function (5d) is also defined for $x_0 > K$ and for $x_0 < 0$. Draw a graph of our function for these values of x_0 as well as for $x_0 \in]0, K[$.

4. One way of looking at a differential equation like (5c) is the following. Take any point in the $(t - x)$ plane; Equation (5c) allows you to calculate the slope $\dot{x}(t)$ of the solution curve which is supposed to pass through that point (Fig. 4.1). Suppose this is done (do it!) at a great number of points in the $(t - x)$ plane, and suppose a short line segment is drawn through each point in order to represent the corresponding slope at that point. In this way one obtains a picture strongly reminiscent of the old iron filings experiments in magnetism. Execute all this and compare the results with the graphs obtained in Exercise 3.

5. Compare two solution curves with the same r, K, and x_0, but different t_0 values. How do the two curves differ?

DISCUSSION QUESTIONS

3. From the form of (5d), the function of t seems to depend on four parameters, r, K, t_0, and x_0. Show that, in reality, only three parameters exist.

4. The specific choice, $r(1 - (x/K))$, for the function $f(x)$ of (5b) was made above for the somewhat flimsy reason that it is simple. Several rationalizations have been proposed in the past, none of them very convincing besides a reasonably good fit to data (e.g., see Pearl and Reed [56], quoted in [17]). An old (around 1839) argument by Verhulst postulated that in an agricultural society the relative rate of increase would be uninhibited until new farmland for farmers' sons would cease to be available, which would happen at a critical population size, say b. From that moment on, the relative rate of increase would diminish by an amount directly proportional to the excess of actual over critical population size. Show that this postulate leads to an expression for $f(x)$ of the above form—or does it?

5. Whatever processes cause a population's increase to slow down, it seems safe to assume that their effect is not instantaneous. Accordingly, replacing the logistic equation by

$$\dot{x}(t) = (r/K)x(t)(K - x(t - \tau)), \quad \text{for some } \tau > 0$$

has been proposed. This would express, albeit in a starkly simplified way, that the decrease of the relative rate of increase is governed by the population size in the past. Discuss how the presence of the term $x(t - \tau)$ compels you to modify the mathematical approach of Exercise 4. You should find that now you cannot draw a direction field as in Exercise 4 but have to construct every individual solution step by step, using its values at t and at $t - \tau$. How about the initial conditions? How would the solutions of the logistic equation compare with the solutions of the modified form for identical values of r and K? For some mathematical information, see Kakutani and Markus [34].

1.6 Discrete-Time versus Continuous-Time Models

In Remark 3 of Section 1.5 we alluded to problems with the comparison of discrete- and continuous-time models. These problems arise at two different levels, computing and model building. Mathematically speaking, the two are related, though not identical. An important difference between the two is the role of the step length. Discretization for *computational* purposes is caused by the fact that digital computers cannot represent continuous variables. No conceptual lower bound exists for the step length (although there is a *practical* lower bound), and so in many cases problems arising from discretization can be conquered satisfactorily by making the step length sufficiently small (so that the resulting approximation is "good enough").

Discretization for *modeling* purposes, as indicated in Remark 3 of Section 1.5, stems from the feeling that a model should exhibit the same discreteness as the object of study. Thus the step length is determined by the length of the period between observations, by the generation length, or by similar nonnegotiable quantities. Thus biologists will object to a smaller (or larger) step length than is natural in the context of their work. Therefore, problems arising from this kind of discretization cannot in general be attacked through diminishing the step length. We will list a few questions to enable the reader to discuss some aspects of these difficulties; for more information see H. R. van der Vaart [66]. A student project could easily grow from this topic. Some related questions are discussed in May [51]. More specialized aspects are studied in later work, such as Li and Yorke [43].

EXERCISES

1. The differential equation

$$\dot{x}(t) = \lambda x(t), \qquad x(0) = \xi,$$

has the solution

$$x(t) = e^{\lambda t} \cdot \xi.$$

The difference equation

$$x(t + h) - x(t) = h\lambda x(t), \qquad x(0) = \xi,$$

from which the differential equation arises as $h \downarrow 0$, has the solution

$$x(nh) = (1 + h\lambda)^n \cdot \xi,$$

which for $\lambda > 0$, $h > 0$ behaves as $e^{\lambda t} \cdot \xi$, but for $\lambda < 0$, $h > 0$ behaves very badly as soon as $|\lambda h| > 1$, and even worse as $|\lambda h| > 2$. Corroborate these statements.

2. The difference equation

$$x(t + h) - x(t) = (e^{\lambda h} - 1) \cdot x(t), \qquad x(0) = \xi,$$

as $h \downarrow 0$, yields the same differential equation as in Exercise 1. Show that the solution of this difference equation attains exactly the same numerical values at the appropriate times as the solution of $\dot{x} = \lambda x$, no matter what values λ and h have.

Remark 1. The preceding two exercises illustrate the general principle that more than one (in fact, many) difference equations exist, all of which will yield the same differential equation as $h \downarrow 0$, but whose solutions may behave quite differently from those of that differential equation, when the step length h is finite. The problem for the discrete-model builder is how to select the right difference equation; e.g., see Greenspan [24].

EXERCISE

3. Lest the reader think that decreasing the step length will always improve the degree to which the solutions of a difference equation approximate the solutions of the corresponding differential equation, a study should be made of the following difference equation:

$$x(t + 2h) - 4x(t + h) + (3 - 2\alpha h)x(t) = 0$$

or, equivalently,

$$\frac{1}{2h}[x(t + 2h) - 4x(t + h) + 3x(t)] = \alpha x(t).$$

(a) Show that if $x(\ )$ is differentiable, then the first member has the limit $-\dot{x}(t)$ as h tends to zero. (Hint: Use truncated Taylor series with remainder term $o(h)$). Thus this difference equation seems to be a candidate for generating approximate solutions for the differential equation $\dot{x}(t) + \alpha x(t) = 0$.

(b) Show that the condition $x(0) = \xi$ is not sufficient as initial condition, but the value of $x(\ )$ is needed at one more value of its argument, e.g., $x(h) = \eta$. (Now your calculator can find $x(2h)$, then $x(3h)$, etc.) Of course, if we want the solution to our difference equation to approximate the solution to $\dot{x}(t) + \alpha x(t) = 0$, $x(0) = \xi$, then we had better be careful in choosing the value η for $x(h)$. One might suggest $x(h) = \xi e^h$.

(c) Show that every solution to our difference equation is of the form,

$$c_1 \langle 2 - \sqrt{1 + 2\alpha h} \rangle^{t/h} + c_2 \langle 2 + \sqrt{1 + 2\alpha h} \rangle^{t/h}$$

for $t = 0, h, 2h, 3h, \cdots$; using our difference equation as a recurrence relation, we will find the values of $x(\ )$ at only these values of t.

(d) As $h \downarrow 0$, t fixed, the power in the first term has a limit, viz., $e^{-\alpha t}$ (prove!), which is encouraging (why?). However, the power in the second term does not have a limit for fixed t: it behaves asymptotically (for fixed t; $h \downarrow 0$) as

$$3^{t/h}e^{\alpha t/3}.$$

The quotient $\langle 2 + \sqrt{1 + \alpha h} \rangle^{t/h}/3^{t/h}$ has the limit $e^{\alpha t/3}$ as $h \downarrow 0$ for fixed t (prove!). This is the point made at the beginning of this exercise. Indeed, as $h \downarrow 0$ for fixed t, $3^{t/h}$ explodes; so things get *worse* in this case as the *step length h decreases*.

(e) The only way to avoid this disaster is to keep $c_2 = 0$, but in the practice of numerical analysis, this is impossible. Replacing a differential equation by a difference equation is done because digital computers can handle recurrence relations very well. In other words, in numerical work the solutions $c_1(\ldots)^{t/h} + c_2(\ldots)^{t/h}$ will not be used, but the computer will be given the values $x(0) = \xi$, $x(h) = \eta$, and then churn away. Now comes the clinch: even if η were "equal" to $\xi(2 - \sqrt{1 + 2\alpha h})$, still the computer, working with a finite word length (resulting in rounding-off error), will after some steps obtain values that do slightly differ from the ideal value $\xi \langle 2 - \sqrt{1 + 2\alpha h} \rangle^{t/h}$. Then this difference, however small, will *explode* according to the factor $3^{t/h}$, *faster* as h is *smaller*.

(f) The problem sketched in this exercise is part of the topic, "numerical stability of linear multistep methods"; e.g., see Lapidus and Seinfeld [37, section 3.2].

(g) Let us reiterate that the role of this discussion in the present context is to show that even when we can manipulate the step length in a difference equation that is supposed to approximate a certain differential equation, the approximation does not necessarily become better; in fact, it may get worse.

Now we will return to our original point: a difference equation which yields a certain differential equation when, after the fashion of all physical science models, its step length h goes to zero, may have solutions that for finite h have a wildly different behavior from the solutions of the ('limiting') differential equation.

EXERCISES

4. The differential equation

$$\dot{x}(t) = -[x(t)]^2, \qquad x(t_0) = \xi,$$

has the solution

$$x(t) = \frac{1}{\dfrac{1}{\xi} + t - t_0}.$$

Explore its behavior for $t > t_0$ as $\xi = 200$, $\xi > 0$, $\xi = 0$, and $\xi < 0$.
   The difference equation

$$x(t + h) - x(t) = -h[x(t)]^2, \qquad x(t_0) = 200, \qquad h = 0.01$$

can be written as

$$x(t + h) = x(t)[\quad ? \quad].$$

Compute $x(t_0 + 0.01)$, $x(t_0 + 0.02)$, $x(t_0 + 0.03)$, and $x(t_0 + 0.04)$, and compare your results with the solutions of the differential equation. Do the same with the difference equation,

$$\frac{1}{x(t + h)} - \frac{1}{x(t)} = h, \qquad x(t_0) = 200, \qquad h = 0.01.$$

Also show that both of these difference equations yield the differential equation $\dot{x} = -x^2$ when $h \downarrow 0$.

5. Show that the solution (see Exercise 2, Section 1.5) of the logistic equation

$$\dot{x}(t) = \rho x(t) \left\langle 1 - \frac{x(t)}{\alpha} \right\rangle, \qquad x(0) = \xi \in \,]0, \alpha[,$$

coincides at the points $t = 0, h, 2h, 3h$, etc., with the solution of

$$\frac{\alpha}{x(t + h)} - 1 = \left\langle \frac{\alpha}{x(t)} - 1 \right\rangle e^{-\rho h}, \qquad x(0) = \xi \in \,]0, \alpha[.$$

Also show that the latter equation can be written as

$$x(t + h) = \frac{\lambda x(t)}{1 + \beta x(t)},$$

with $\lambda = e^{\rho h}$, $\beta = \,?$

DISCUSSION QUESTION

1. The last equation of Exercise 5 has been used by Leslie [40] as the point of departure for a stochastized version of the discrete logistic model. Given $x(\ \ )$ at time t, he determined $x(t + h)$ as a value of a normal random variable with mean $\lambda x(t) \cdot [1 + \beta x(t)]^{-1}$ and variously chosen variances, all of which he took to be proportional to the mean of $x(t + h)$. With a table of random numbers and a calculator, experiment with different variances and compare the result with the corresponding deterministic logistic.

2. Predator–Prey

2.1 Lotka–Volterra Model

Consider an ecosystem consisting of two species of animals, one of which (the prey) is eaten by the other (the predator). Let x represent the number of prey and y the number of predators. Suppose for a moment that there are no predators in the system, just individuals of the *prey* species, with plenty of food and space. Then one could imagine that the prey population would increase according to the Malthusian (geometric-logarithmic-exponential) pattern:

$$\dot{x}(t) = x(t) \cdot \gamma_1 \tag{6a}$$

where γ_1 would be a positive constant, the relative rate of increase. Now allow some predators into the system. Encounters will occur between individuals of the prey species and individuals of the predator species. A certain fraction of these encounters will have fatal results for the prey. So $\dot{x}(t)$, the rate of increase of the prey population, must be less than $x(t) \cdot \gamma_1$, and the difference should be proportional to the number of encounters per time unit. Now it stands to reason that the number of such encounters during a short time interval starting at time t is a monotone increasing function of $x(t)$ itself (the number of prey individuals at time t), as well as of $y(t)$ (the number of predator individuals at time t). The only unresolved problem is the choice of a function of x and y, monotone in x and monotone in y, to represent the number of encounters per time unit. In analogy to chemical kinetics (e.g., see Boudart [8, pp. 42, 51]), Lotka [45, p. 88] assumed this function to be $x \cdot y$. Thus (6a) has to be amended and replaced by

$$\dot{x}(t) = x(t) \cdot [+\gamma_1 - py(t)]. \tag{6b}$$

So much for the prey. Now suppose for a moment that there are no prey animals in our system, just *predators*. These predator individuals, being without food, would starve. So their population would decline. Let us assume, somewhat rashly, that their decline would obey this description:

$$\dot{y}(t) = y(t) \cdot (-\gamma_2), \tag{6c}$$

where γ_2 is a positive constant. Now suppose there are also some prey individuals in the system. Then the predators would be doing better. In fact, they would be doing better in proportion to the number of encounters with prey animals. So the value of $\dot{y}(t)$ should be increased by an amount proportional to the number of encounters between predator and prey. According to Lotka's assumption this means that (6c) should be amended and replaced by

$$\dot{y}(t) = y(t) \cdot [-\gamma_2 + qx(t)] \tag{6d}$$

Remark 1. Volterra [67, p. 38] does not adduce chemical kinetics in defense of the terms $+qxy$ or $-pxy$. He does remark that the relative rate of increase should be less than $+\gamma_1$ for the prey (because of the predators) and greater than $-\gamma_2$ for the predator (because of the prey). Then he goes on to say that the simplest (albeit rather crude) way to achieve this is by subtracting a term proportional to $y(t)$ and adding a term proportional to $x(t)$, respectively.

Remark 2. One could also, and perhaps more impressively, argue that a population of $y(t)$ predator individuals needs a total feeding rate of $y(t) \cdot \gamma_2$, just to maintain itself at that level. Therefore, only the excess over that amount contributes to the growth of the predator population:

$$\dot{y}(t) = qx(t)y(t) - \gamma_2 y(t),$$

the same equation as (6d).

Remark 3. Equation (6a), representing the growth of the prey population in the absence of predators, lacks realism in that no prey population would keep growing exponentially. So we really need an expression that will not exhibit unlimited growth in the absence of a predator (or even in the presence of a predator). The traditional tool to represent a limited growth is the logistic. For a prey population without predators,

$$\dot{x}(t) = x(t) \cdot [+\gamma_1 - \delta x(t)]. \tag{6e}$$

The argument that led from (6a) to (6b) will now lead to

$$\dot{x}(t) = x(t) \cdot [+\gamma_1 - \delta x(t) - py(t)],$$

or, in abbreviated notation,

$$\dot{x} = x \cdot (+\gamma_1 - \delta x - py). \tag{6f}$$

A similar argument might suggest that (6d) be replaced by

$$\dot{y} = y \cdot (-\gamma_2 + qx - \zeta y) \tag{6g}$$

EXERCISES

1. The Volterra prey–predator equations are (6b) and (6d) together,

$$\begin{cases} \dot{x} = x \cdot (+\gamma_1 \quad\quad - py) \\ \dot{y} = y \cdot (-\gamma_2 + qx \quad\quad) \end{cases}, \tag{7}$$

with $\gamma_1 > 0$, $\gamma_2 > 0$, $p > 0$, and $q > 0$. We want to study some of the properties of the solutions of this system. In the first place show that a *scale change* of x and y ($x = \beta_1 x_1$, $y = \beta_2 x_2$) makes it possible to write (7) in the form

$$\begin{cases} \dot{x}_1 = x_1 \cdot (+\gamma_1 \quad\quad + \alpha_{12} x_2) \\ \dot{x}_2 = x_2 \cdot (-\gamma_2 + \alpha_{21} x_1 \quad\quad) \end{cases} \tag{8}$$

with γ_1 and γ_2 the same as before, and $\alpha_{21} = \alpha > 0$, $\alpha_{12} = -\alpha_{21} = -\alpha$. The same kind of transformation will play a role later in models for n species systems.

2. Apply the phase plane-isocline-arrow method (see Appendix) to (7), and see how it leads you to expect a more or less cyclic behavior. (See Figure 4.2.)

3. Equations (7) can be treated analytically, not to express x and y as functions of t, but to find a relation between x and y, which in turn determines a family of closed curves in the $(x - y)$ plane. In fact, show that (7) for all real values, $\square$, of t entails

$$\frac{\dot{x}(\square)[-\gamma_2 + qx(\square)]}{x(\square)} = \frac{\dot{y}(\square)[+\gamma_1 - py(\square)]}{y(\square)}.$$

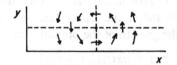

Figure 4.2

Show that integration of this equality from t_0 to t yields

$$\left(\frac{x(t)}{x_0}\right)^{-\gamma_2} \cdot \frac{e^{qx(t)}}{e^{qx_0}} = \left(\frac{y(t)}{y_0}\right)^{+\gamma_1} \cdot \frac{e^{-py(t)}}{e^{-py_0}} \tag{9}$$

Show for given (x_0, y_0) that this equation determines a closed curve.[4] Also make clear that with varying (x_0, y_0) this equation generates a family of cycles (closed curves), filling up the entire first quadrant. Thus the analytical work (which in this case was possible) confirms the quick-and-dirty graphical analysis mentioned in Exercise 2 in this section, as of course it should.

Remark 4. The reader has just become acquainted with a basic fact of life in mathematics as applied to the life sciences: most of the differential equations that one encounters there *cannot be solved* explicitly; most not even implicitly. This is frustrating to some people, but anybody going into applied mathematics must come to terms with it. After all, that is why *computers* were invented and built! Though one might think that mathematics as applied to physics has not had this problem, such is not the case. In the classical period of mathematical physics, each new differential equation was greeted by the creation, or rather canonization, of a new function (e.g., the functions of Mathieu, Lamé, Bessel, etc.). If you give a name (and a symbol) to a typical solution of the canonic form of a (linear) differential equation that you could not solve explicitly before that name and that symbol were given, then you can solve it "explicitly" afterward. So even the physicists in their classical period knew this problem. After the nonlinear equations came up (which happened very early in the development of mathematical biology, whereas it took a long time in mathematical physics), even the physicists stopped their name game; some of their research is now in the same situation as we are.

Remark 5. After the mathematical community realized that the list of special functions of mathematical physics would never end, more emphasis was put on determining certain properties of the collection of all solutions of a given (set of) differential equation(s) without first determining any kind of analytical expression for the solutions; viz., such properties as asymptotic behavior as time goes to infinity, the number and nature of singular points, the existence of periodic solutions, boundaries of regions of attraction of stable singular points, etc., variously called geometric or qualitative properties. Since the collection of all trajectories in the phase space (i.e., (x, y)-space in the above example) is called the *phase portrait* of the differential system, we may summarize the situation by saying that as the importance of nonlinear systems grew, the study of topological aspects of their phase portraits grew also. This is not to say that numerical solutions obtained by digital or analog computer are not useful or that analytical methods no longer play a role, but that nobody should feel frustrated if mathematical

---

[4] The proof is fairly long, although elementary. It is found in [3, p. 84]. This book was listed as essential, so there is little point in our reproducing the proof here.

models in ecology, biology, or any other field, are not solvable in closed form; the mathematical community has shed that frustration some time ago. Numerous textbooks exist which deal with such questions at various levels, e.g., Brauer and Nohel [9] (undergraduate level); Hurewicz [31] (slightly more advanced); Aggarwal [1] (seniors); Andronov *et al.* [4] (advanced, but excellent).

EXERCISES

4. The amended Volterra prey–predator equations (including logistic terms) are (6f) and (6g) together,

$$\begin{cases} \dot{x} = x \cdot (+\gamma_1 - \delta x - py) \\ \dot{y} = y \cdot (-\gamma_2 + qx - \zeta y) \end{cases},$$

(10)

where $\gamma_1, \gamma_2, \delta, \zeta, p, q$ represent positive numbers. In Exercise 1 you showed that a scale change in x and y could transform the matrix of coefficients of x (or x_1) and y (or x_2) of (7) into a skew-symmetric matrix,

$$\begin{pmatrix} 0 & \alpha_{12} \\ \alpha_{21} & 0 \end{pmatrix}$$

with $\alpha_{12} = -\alpha_{21}$. This is entirely impossible for (10). Why?

5. Apply the phase plane-isocline-arrow method (see Appendix) to (10), distinguishing two main cases,

$$\frac{\gamma_2}{q} < \frac{\gamma_1}{\delta}, \qquad \frac{\gamma_2}{q} > \frac{\gamma_1}{\delta},$$

and the limiting case in between: $\gamma_2/q = \gamma_1/\delta$.

6. Follow the work you did in Exercises 2 and 5 by the study of the matrix of the linear systems that approximate the given nonlinear systems in the neighborhood of each of their singular points (see Sections A.3 and A.4 of Appendix A). Do you find any contradictions?

7. A different way of finding a result equivalent to the one found in Exercise 3 takes off from the transformed equations (8) in Exercise 1. First determine (ξ_1, ξ_2) as the solution of

$$\begin{cases} +\gamma_1 \qquad\qquad + \alpha_{12} x_2 = 0 \\ -\gamma_2 + \alpha_{21} x_1 \qquad\qquad = 0 \end{cases}.$$

Since (see Exercise 1) $\gamma_1 > 0$, $\gamma_2 > 0$, $\alpha_{21} > 0$, and $\alpha_{12} < 0$, it follows that both ξ_1 and ξ_2 are positive. Show that (8) can be rewritten in the form

$$\begin{cases} \dot{x}_1/x_1 = \alpha_{12}(x_2 - \xi_2) \\ \dot{x}_2/x_2 = \alpha_{21}(x_1 - \xi_1) \end{cases}.$$

(11)

Multiply the first equation (11) by $(x_1 - \xi_1)$ and the second equation (11) by $(x_2 - \xi_2)$, and add the resulting equalities, using the fact that $\alpha_{12} + \alpha_{21} = 0$:

$$\frac{\dot{x}_1}{x_1}(x_1 - \xi_1) + \frac{\dot{x}_2}{x_2}(x_2 - \xi_2) = 0.$$

(11a)

Upon integration find

$$x_1(t) - \xi_1 \log x_1(t) + x_2(t) - \xi_2 \log x_2(t) = \text{constant} \qquad (11b)$$

or, equivalently,

$$[e^{v_1(t)} - v_1(t)]\xi_1 + [e^{v_2(t)} - v_2(t)]\xi_2 = \text{constant}, \qquad (11c)$$

where $x_i = \xi_i e^{v_i}$ $(i = 1, 2)$.

Remark 6. The first member of (11b) is a constant of motion or a first integal. This result is essentially equivalent to (9) (see Exercise 3), although the present method is easier to generalize to systems of more species. This result also shows (as did (9)) that the systems defined by (7), and (8) are conservative. This has excited some people with a physics background (Kerner [35], Goel *et al.* [21]), because they saw an opportunity to apply methods of classical and statistical mechanics to these ecosystem models. Unfortunately, models that are even slightly more realistic (such as (10)—see Exercise 4 and Remark 3) are no longer conservative, so that at present the usefulness of these efforts is doubtful. Equally unfortunate is that nobody has managed to find any biological meaning whatever for the constant of motion of (11b): Kerner himself conceded this during a conference on theoretical biology (cf. Jacobs [33, p. 155]).

Discussion Questions

1. The reader should explore why the integration method(s) discussed in Exercises 3 and 7 do not help in the case of equation (10). This does not, of course, mean that no solution curves $\langle x(t), y(t) \rangle$ exist, but that they (or rather, their projections onto the (x, y)-plane) cannot be represented by simple analytical expressions.

2. In Exercise 5 you found that the two main cases exhibit a major difference in phase portrait, a major difference also in biological outcome. If you told a biologist about this result, he would ask: What do these inequalities (viz. $\delta/\gamma_1 \gtrless q/\gamma_2$) mean biologically? What would your answer be?

3. In Hirsch and Smale [27], an excellent text on differential equations, Figure 4.3 is given as the phase portrait of (7). Any comments?

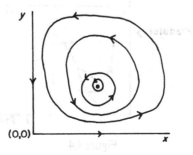

Figure 4.3

2.2 Critique of the Lotka–Volterra Model and Proposed Improvements

Experiments performed (a.o., by Gause [17]) to check the theoretical prediction of oscillations, have shown that in the case of homogeneous environments (such as occur easily in laboratory experiments) the predator species will often succeed in finishing off the prey species, contrary to the theory. However, if an environment is made sufficiently complex (or inhomogeneous), so that the prey species has a safe refuge, at least temporarily, then oscillations do occur (for instance, see Huffaker [30], or Flanders and Badgley [16]). This caused MacArthur and Connell [46] to come up with isoclines of the type discussed in the following Exercises 1 and 2.

EXERCISES

1. Show that the portion of the vertical isocline pointed out by the broken arrow in Figure 4.4 does make it impossible for the predator to run the prey into the ground.

2. According to further specification, the vertical isocline would, moreover, bend its rightmost end downwards (see Figure 4.4). What biological realism, if any, would be added by this bend?

Kolmogorov [36] did not so much criticize the Lotka–Volterra model as propose a generalization of it, in a direction somewhat different from (10). Again with x for the number of prey and y for the number of predators, he proposes

$$\left\{ \begin{array}{l} \dot{x} = K_1(x) \cdot x - L(x) \cdot y \\ \dot{y} = \qquad\qquad K_2(x) \cdot y \end{array} \right\}. \tag{12}$$

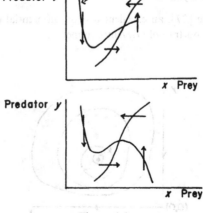

Figure 4.4

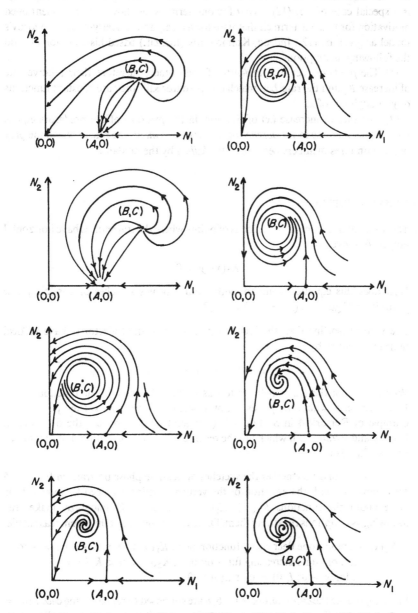

Figure 4.5. From Kolmogorov [36, p. 105]. Note: His N_1 Is Our x; His N_2 Is Our y.

Exercise

3. Show that the Lotka–Volterra model (8) is indeed a special case of (12). Also show that the amended model which included logistic crowding terms (see Eq. (10)) is a special case of Eq. (12) *except* for one term. Show how the abovementioned motivation for this one term clashes with the assumptions underlying Kolmogorov's model as given by (12). Indeed, Kolmogorov (loc. cit.) based his equation (12) on the following assumptions:

(1) The *predators* act *independently* of each other; therefore their relative rate of increase K_2 and the rate L at which one predator kills prey are constant functions of y, though not of x.

(2) The rate of increase $(\dot{x})$ of the prey in the *presence* of the predators equals their rate of increase in the *absence* of the predators *minus* the rate at which the prey population loses members because of the *killing* by the predators.

Discussion Questions

1. The horizontal isocline (i.e., the locus of points where the trajectories have horizontal tangents) is given by

$$K_2(x) \cdot y = 0.$$

How does this equation compare with Kolmogorov's sketches of possible phase portraits in Figure 4.5 ($N_1 = x; N_2 = y$)?

2. The vertical isocline (i.e., the locus of points where the trajectories have vertical tangents) is given by

$$K_1(x) \cdot x - L(x) \cdot y = 0.$$

Whether or not the y axis belongs to this isocline depends on the function $L(\ )$. How? The case where the y axis is not a part of the vertical isocline provides an example of Remark 4 in Section 1.5. (For another example see the diagrams in Holling and Ewing [29], which are the result of machine simulation, not of a model such as Eq. (3).)

3. Before we can discuss whether the sketches of possible phase portraits in Figure 4.5 are compatible with the equation of the vertical isocline, we need to know a little more about the functions $K_2(\ )$, $K_1(\ )$, and $L(\ )$. Kolmogorov makes the following assumptions regarding them. Discuss whether or not they seem reasonable.

$K_1(x)$ is a monotone decreasing function of x; $K_1(0) > 0 > K_1(+\infty) > -\infty$.
$K_2(x)$ is a monotone increasing function of x; $K_2(0) < 0 < K_2(+\infty)$.
$L(x) > 0$ for $x > 0$; $L(0) = 0$ or $L(0) > 0$.

In the Figure 4.5 the cases numbered 2, 6, 8 are supposed to represent the case $L(0) = 0$; the others, $L(0) > 0$. Check if the sketches do well by the vertical isocline. Also check the location of the singular points, as well as their nature (by the linearization method). For the saddle points among them, find the two asymptotic directions of trajectories passing through them. Finally, in cases 1, 3, 4, 5, 7 check the angles under which the trajectories hit the y axis.

Re this last point, Kolmogorov notes that as the equations are written the trajectories would go on to negative x values, which is biologically impossible. Therefore, he writes, one should interpret the equations in this way: once the trajectory has hit the y axis, the first equation stops action and from there on only the second equation acts, for $x = $ constant $= 0$.

Leslie [40, p. 20] objects to equation (7) on grounds related to those named in Section 2.1, Remark 3: no allowance is made for intraspecific competition (which is easily remedied by inserting negative terms, $-x^2$ and $-y^2$) and, more seriously, there is "no upper limit to the relative rate of increase of the predator." (This objection still holds against the amended Lotka–Volterra equations (10), although for any given x there is such an upper limit; then again, x itself is variable.) So Leslie wants the relative rate of increase of the predator to equal a constant diminished by a certain term; this term, since the predator species fares worse as the ratio of predator individuals to prey individuals grows, Leslie proposes to choose proportional to y/x. Therefore, his equation is

$$\left\{ \begin{aligned} \dot{x} &= x \cdot (r_1 - a_1 x - b_1 y), & \text{for the prey} \\ \dot{y} &= y \cdot \left(r_2 - a_2 \frac{y}{x} \right), & \text{for the predator} \end{aligned} \right\}. \tag{13}$$

EXERCISE

4. Sketch the phase portrait of this equation. Is it biologically more acceptable than the phase portrait of Eq. (10)? What happens around the points of the y axis? What are the singular points? Execute the linearization analysis in their neighborhoods, where possible.

DISCUSSION QUESTIONS

4. If you find the phase portrait of Eq. (13) to be less acceptable than that of Equation (10), can you then pinpoint a flaw in Leslie's argument?

5. Leslie [40] also touches on the topic we mentioned in Section 1.5, Remark 3 and in Section 1.6: the preference that many biologists have for discrete over continuous models. An additional reason for Leslie's interest in discrete models is the fact that he wants to represent numerically random agents influencing the ecosystem along the lines indicated in Section 1.6, Discussion Question 1. So how does Leslie choose a discrete model for a prey–predator system? He does so in analogy to the discretization of the logistic introduced in Section 1.6, Exercise 5. Just as

$$\dot{x}(t) = \rho x(t) \left(1 - \frac{x(t)}{\alpha} \right)$$

was (rigorously) replaced by

$$x(t + h) = \frac{\lambda x(t)}{1 + \beta x(t)},$$

so the first of the equations in (13) is (approximately) replaced by

$$x(t + h) = \frac{\lambda_1 x(t)}{1 + \alpha_1 x(t) + \beta_1 y(t)} \tag{14a}$$

and the second of the two is replaced by

$$y(t + h) = \frac{\lambda_2 y(t)}{1 + \alpha_2 [y(t)/x(t)]}. \tag{14b}$$

The role of the isoclines is now played by the locus of points (ξ, η) in the phase plane such that $x(t) = \xi$ implies that $x(t + h) = \xi$ (vertical isocline), or that $y(t) = \eta$ implies that $y(t + h) = \eta$ (horizontal isocline). Compare the isoclines, thus defined, for (14a) and (14b) with the isoclines (in the usual sense) for (13).

Another obvious reason for criticizing any and all of the predator–prey models discussed so far is that the food of the prey is not represented. This may be all right if the food of the prey is plentiful, but casts doubt on the realism of these models, especially if the prey itself is a predator of some other species. Also, an oddity lies in Volterra's modeling of a food chain: it has strange difficulties if the chain consists of an odd number of species. These difficulties disappear for the most part if the food of the prey is also represented in the model, even if the food consists of plants. Poletaev [57] and Êman [13] are among the authors that have explicitly addressed these problems. Êman proposed several models that (at the same level of crudeness as the original Volterra models) took explicit account of the *environment* of the predator and prey species: e.g., plants and soil. For a discussion of one or two models of this type, see Section 4.

Looking back to the first few pages of Section 2.1, we see clearly that the arguments for the interaction terms being proportional to $x \cdot y$ were not strong: an analogy to chemical kinetics, a remark that this choice is simple (though crude). It is no wonder that Kolmogorov suggested the qualitative investigation of more general models. On the other hand, by changing these interaction terms, one may achieve the explicit solvability of the equations. For instance, Gomatam [22] published a paper on the model (cf. (7)):

$$\left\{ \begin{array}{l} \dot{x} = +\gamma_1 x - b_1 x \log y \\ \dot{y} = -\gamma_2 y + b_2 y \log x \end{array} \right\}, \tag{15}$$

and on the model (cf. (10)):

$$\left\{ \begin{array}{l} \dot{x} = x(+\gamma_1 - b_{11} \log x - b_{12} \log y) \\ \dot{y} = y(-\gamma_2 + b_{21} \log x - b_{22} \log y) \end{array} \right\}. \tag{16}$$

EXERCISE

5. After substitutions $\log x = \xi$ and $\log y = \eta$, these equations reduce to linear equations and can be solved explicitly. Do so and discuss the properties of the corresponding solutions for $x(t)$ and $y(t)$ as compared to the results obtained on the original Lotka–Volterra models of (7) and (10).

None of these devices, however, are truly agreeable to a biologist for the simple reason that they do not reflect any biological knowledge or data concerning predator–prey interaction. Correspondingly, Holling, in a detailed paper which also discusses some older attempts in this area [28], conducted an experimental study of the interaction of one particular predator species and one particular prey species. As an example of the approach to modeling that biologists really like, this is a good paper to study.

A brief discussion of some points made by Watt [70] seems useful. (This paper is mainly on parasites rather than predators, but both parasites and predators have to find their victims before they can attack them, whether for the purpose of egg-depositing or eating, so his remarks are relevant for the discussion on interaction.) The Lotka–Volterra assumption that the number of prey attacked per time unit is proportional to $x \cdot y$, the product of the prey density and the predator density, Watt finds implausible for at least two reasons. *First*, it implies that for given predator density y, the number of prey attacked is directly proportional to the prey density x, no matter how many prey exist. This is unsatisfactory, if only because even the biggest glutton can eat only so much: any digestive system can process only a certain amount of food per time unit. Also, as hunger decreases a predator will search and attack less vigorously, etc. *Second*, the Lotka–Volterra assumption postulates that for given prey density x, the number of prey attacked is directly proportional to the predator density y, no matter how many predators are about. In other words, the prey-searching and attacking behavior of the predator individuals is not modified by increasing predator density: the predators are assumed to act independently of one another, no matter how many of them exist. Watt (loc. cit.) quotes many experimental studies showing that this assumption does not hold in the case of parasites, and the same is is bound to be true for predators. (Several alternatives have been discussed in the literature. Relatively accessible is May [50], available in paperback. Other references, which may or may not be accessible to the reader, are Holling [28], Watt [69], [70], Royama [61], *Problemy Kibernetiki*, especially vol. 25 [58].)

The *first* objection of the preceding paragraph may be answered by replacing the Lotka–Volterra cross-product $x \cdot y$ by $\mathscr{K} \cdot y \cdot (1 - e^{-\beta x})$ (used by Gause, Ivlev, and others; note that for small x this function $\sim x \cdot y$). This expression puts an upper bound on the number of encounters between any one predator and individuals of the prey species when the prey grows abundant. Of course, the replacement of $x \cdot y$ by $k \cdot x \cdot y/(b + x)$ would give similar service. The *second* objection may be answered similarly by replacing $x \cdot y$ by $c \cdot x \cdot (1 - e^{-dy})$ (used by Nicholson and Bailey, and others; what is the situation for small y values?).

DISCUSSION QUESTION

6. The reader should construct some alternative predator–prey models with the above building blocks and investigate their properties by the methods used before (isocline-arrow and linearization at singular points).

Another way to make our models more lifelike would be to account for inhomogeneities. The habitat of a real population is not homogeneous: for instance, the prey will often have hideaways, places where the predator has difficulty moving about. The populations are not homogeneous: age differences, differences in hunger condition, genetic differences, differences between the sexes. Each of these possibilities have been considered by one or more authors. One will find references in the journals cited in Section 1.3.

An obvious necessity is to discuss ecosystems consisting of more than two species: outside the laboratory, two-species ecosystems are virtually non-existent. We should also emphasize that species may enter into other relationships besides that of predator and prey. Section 3 will briefly discuss a few of those other relationships. Section 4 will mention some of the problems in the study of more than two species. The Section 2.3 will indicate a more qualitative approach to predator–prey theory than any other section.

2.3 General Remarks about the Predator–Prey Model

One is sometimes required to come up with a mathematical model for a situation the mechanism of which is relatively unknown. As an example of what one might be able to accomplish in such situations, let us try to draw *conclusions* regarding the functions $\varphi(x, y)$ and $\psi(x, y)$ (and/or their ratio) in the general equations (3):

$$\begin{cases} \dot{x} = \varphi(x, y) \\ \dot{y} = \psi(x, y) \end{cases} \tag{17}$$

merely *from* the very general observation that a small prey population cannot sustain as large a predator population as a large one, and that a large predator population eats more prey than a small one.

Thus, again with x the number of prey and y the number of predators, let us look at the rightmost vertical line in Figure 4.6. This line represents a number of different predator–prey systems, all with a sizable, though not excessive, number of prey, but with a varying number of predators, ranging from a very few (down) to many (up). A system at point a is a paradise for prey (very few predators), so the number of prey will increase somewhat; but it is maybe even more a paradise for the predator (abundant food supply), so the number of predators will increase as well. The system will move as indicated by the arrow at a. The reader can argue the other arrows, at points b through f: systems with more and more predators are less and less of a paradise for the prey. At c the prey can just hold their own against the predator; beyond c the prey population will decrease as kills exceed births. As we look at systems with still more predators, a point f will come where the predators do not find enough food to increase, and their population just holds the line. At point g the number of predators begins to decline, as starvation takes effect.

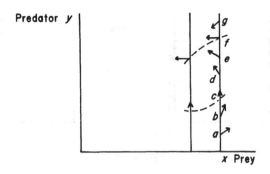

Figure 4.6

Now look at the line to the left of the one just discussed. There is less prey, so point c, as well as point f, will be reached earlier: fewer predators will now be able to prevent the prey population from increasing, and the predator population will fail to find enough food at a lower predator density.

EXERCISE

1. What is the value of $\varphi(x, y)$ at any of the points c (where $\dot{x} = 0$), and of $\psi(x, y)$ at any of the points f (where $\dot{y} = 0$)? What can you say about the values of $\psi(x, y)$ at c and of $\varphi(x, y)$ at f?

Evidently, points of type c make up the vertical isocline (where $\dot{x} = 0$) and those of type f make up the horizontal isocline (where $\dot{y} = 0$). The above argument suggests that in the right-hand part of the (x, y)-diagram the horizontal isocline should be above the vertical isocline and that both should tend to go to the left and down. This argument needs supplementation in two ways.

In the *first* place, the presentation was somewhat biased. On the one hand, in a collection of predator–prey systems, which all have a sizable, though not excessive, prey population but different sizes of predator populations, the systems with a large predator population clearly provide both species with a less attractive environment. The predators do not have enough to eat, and the prey have a good chance of being killed. So as we consider different ecosystems with the same prey density, but with more and more predators, the rate of increase of both predator and prey populations will decline until both species are actually decreasing (viz., if the system has a large prey population as well as a large predator population). A question remains, however, as to which of the two species will be the first to hit zero rate of increase. As is seen immediately, Figure 4.6 constitutes the second of these two possibilities (see the following remark).

Remark 1. The arrows in Figure 4.7 have the same role as in the Appendix on the phaseplane, isocline and arrow method: a horizontal arrow indicates

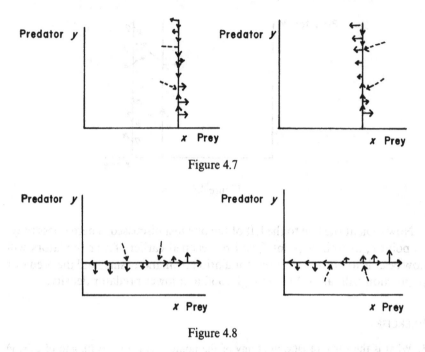

Figure 4.7

Figure 4.8

increase or decrease of the prey population (x = prey); a vertical arrow indicates increase or decrease of the predator population (y = predator); their lengths represent the relative size of $\dot{x}$ and $\dot{y}$, and the course of the system is determined by the resultant. Now compare Figure 4.6 and the second diagram in Figure 4.7.

In the *second* place, we need to supplement the argument around Figure 4.6 with a second collection of predator–prey systems. All systems in this collection will have a fairly small predator population, but their prey populations will have different sizes. A system with few predators but relatively many prey will see both predators and prey increasing. However, as we look at systems with fewer and fewer prey, both species will see their rate of increase go down, until both species are decreasing (viz., if the system has a small prey population as well as a small predator population). Again, two possibilities exist (Figure 4.8).

We should point out that, in both parts of the figure, to consider portions of the phase plane close to the coordinate axes (x = 0 and/or y = 0) is fairly unrealistic. With numbers close to zero, a better chance exists for "random influences" to step in, so the deterministic approach is not as valid here.

In conclusion, we find at least four possible cases of relative positions of the vertical and horizontal isoclines. These four possibilities are represented in the diagrams of Figure 4.9. The two lines that occurred in Figures 4.7 and 4.8 are repeated here, along with the crucial arrows located at the points indicated by the broken arrows in the two preceding figures. They indicate points of the horizontal and vertical isoclines.

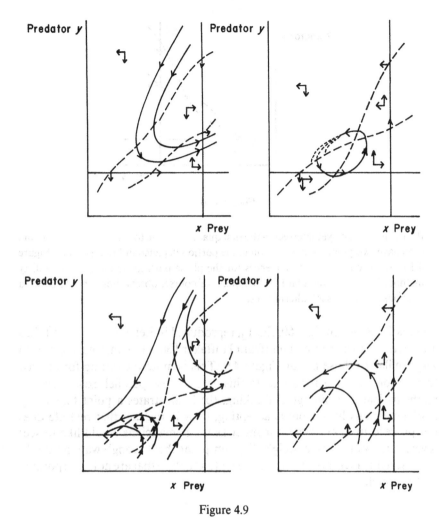

Figure 4.9

EXERCISE

2. Comment on the apparent nature of the singular points, if any, in Figure 4.9.

DISCUSSION QUESTIONS

1. The reader should explain those arrows that are not on the isoclines.

2. Two of the four possibilities depicted in Figure 4.9 are biologically unacceptable: which two? Why? The other two seem to suggest oscillations, damped or not, one (strong damping) or more. Show how the diagrams in Figure 4.9 lead to these statements.

3. The reader should ponder the following point: the unspecific, qualitative arguments presented so far have not given any unambiguous clue as to the location of certain parts of the isoclines in Figure 4.9. For instance, in the first and fourth diagrams

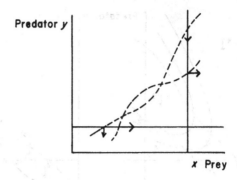

Figure 4.10

the isoclines might yet intersect in the first quadrant, close to the *x* axis, or they could even have two points of intersection in the portion depicted in Figure 4.9 (see Figure 4.10). Inquire into the consequences for the phase portrait by the quick-and-dirty method. For any given real life ecosystem, of course, observations should be used to choose between such alternatives.

Remark 2. Rosenzweig ([60, fig. 1], reproduced in Leigh [39, fig. 7–5]) has used actual experimental data (from Huffaker [30]) to construct a diagram very similar to those in our Figure 4.9. This is quite interesting for at least two reasons. (a) It shows that in this case a close parallel exists between mathematical and biological thinking. (b) It illustrates a point that many mathematicians have trouble accepting, namely the fact that real life does not proceed in as clear-cut a manner as mathematicians would like to see: several arrows in Rosenzweig's diagram point the "wrong" way, no doubt because many factors influence the real life situation that are not incorporated in the model.

3. Mutualism and Competition

3.1 Preliminary Remarks

Mutualism (Allee *et al.* [2, p. 245], May [50, pp. 25–26]), commensalism [2, p. 243], [50], and competition [50] may be explained as follows.

(a) Commensalism is a relation between two species in which one species profits and the other species neither profits nor suffers.
(b) Mutualism is a relation between two species in which both species profit.
(c) Competition is a relation between two species in which both species suffer.

Certainly this scheme is a simplification: it omits the infinite variations which live ecosystems abundantly provide. Competition especially is a subject on which much more can be said ([2, pp. 368, seqq.]; more literature is listed in Section 3.3 of this module). However the definitions given are sufficient for constructing the simple Volterra-type models.

3.2 Mathematical Models in the Volterra Tradition

The reader is invited to regard this section as one long discussion question and to analyze the following models by the methods discussed previously (i.e., phase plane-isocline-arrow analysis and linearization). As before, the parameters in these models are all understood to be positive, with one exception: the a_{ii} may be read as either equal to zero (no "crowding" between the individuals of species i), or positive ("crowding" exists). The reader should also explain these models in terms of the definitions given in Section 3.1:

commensalism
$$\left\{\begin{aligned} \dot{x} &= x(\varepsilon_1 - a_{11}x) \\ \dot{y} &= y(\varepsilon_2 + a_{21}x - a_{22}y) \end{aligned}\right\} \tag{18}$$

mutualism
$$\left\{\begin{aligned} \dot{x} &= x(\varepsilon_1 - a_{11}x + a_{12}y) \\ \dot{y} &= y(\varepsilon_2 + a_{21}x - a_{22}y) \end{aligned}\right\} \tag{19}$$

competition
$$\left\{\begin{aligned} \dot{x} &= x(\varepsilon_1 - a_{11}x - a_{12}y) \\ \dot{y} &= y(\varepsilon_2 - a_{21}x - a_{22}y) \end{aligned}\right\}. \tag{20}$$

The reader will find that with all $a_{ii} = 0$ the behavior of these models is rather unrealistic (populations explode). When analyzing these models with all $a_{ii} > 0$, the reader should find that the model for commensalism necessarily shows a point $S = (x, y)$ with $x > 0$, $y > 0$, such that all solution curves tend to S as time increases. The model for mutualism shows either the same situation or a population explosion of both species, depending on whether $(a_{11}/a_{12}) > (a_{21}/a_{22})$ or $(a_{11}/a_{12}) \leqq (a_{21}/a_{22})$. The model for competition shows four possibilities, depending on the disposition of the .two (horizontal and vertical) isoclines: all solutions tend (i) to a point in the interior of the first quadrant, (ii) to a point on the x axis, (iii) to a point on the y axis, or (iv) a combination of (ii) and (iii). The reader should find the inequalities that must be satisfied by the parameters to provide the conditions for each one of these four possibilities. The reader should also make a sustained effort to make some biological sense out of the dichotomizing inequalities that govern the mutualism and competition models. Generally speaking, they concern each species helping or hurting itself less or more than the other one. Further, the reader should investigate whether he would want to improve on these models in some way reminiscent of the discussions in Section 2.5 or in any other way.

Remark 1. Some people consider the results concerning competition unrealistic. There is no reason for this. In fact, ample experimental confirmation of these results is available. Ecosystems exist, both in the laboratory and outside, that have been observed to exhibit the behavior predicted for some parameter values, viz., one species of the two disappears and the other stays. The behavior predicted by possibility (iv) has been extensively investigated in the Tribolium experiments (e.g., see Mertz [54], or Neyman, *et al.* [55]): the observations show that the fate of the Tribolium system depends on the initial ratio of the densities of the two species. Roughly speaking, the species that is more numerous at the beginning stands a better chance of surviving. The model goes a long way in explaining this behavior: just stochastize it, in the spirit of Discussion Question 1 in Section 1.6.

EXERCISE

1. Investigate the behavior of the following alternative model for competition (from Gilpin and Ayala [19]):

$$\begin{cases} \dot{x} = r_1 x[1 - (x/K_1)^{\theta_1} - ay] \\ \dot{y} = r_2 y[1 - bx - (y/K_2)^{\theta_2}] \end{cases}, \tag{21}$$

where r_i, K_i, θ_i, a, b are all positive. Note the qualitative similarity between the phase portraits of Eqs. (20) and (21). The same four types of cases can be distinguished with respect to (21) as were distinguished with respect to (20), again on the basis of the relative disposition of the horizontal and vertical isoclines. However, an important difference exists between the two equations for case (i) (stable coexistence between the two species), and this difference is the reason why Gilpin and Ayala proposed the equation in the first place. For (21), case (i), the quadrangle formed by the four singular points need *not* be *convex*, whereas for (20), case (i), this quadrangle *is* necessarily *convex*. The point is that certain extensive experiments contradicted this convexity. The reader will explore conditions under which this convexity does not happen for (21), case (i). These facts played an important role in some recent discussions concerning the competitive exclusion principle (cf. Section 3.3 and Gilpin and Ayala [19]).

3.3 The Competitive Exclusion Principle

The four cases distinguishable in the competition model have given rise to a famous concept that has led to numerous experimental and some theoretical investigations and that still commands much attention in ecology. As the reader has noticed, three of the four possible cases of the Volterra model for competition between two species indicate the survival of one species and the extinction of the other. In one of these three cases it is not always the same species that survives: which one survives depends on which was the more numerous to begin with ("more numerous" in a technical sense: the question is on which side of a certain separatrix the initial point is located). Curiously enough, the first of the four cases was for a long time disregarded. Especially after the publication of Gause [17], who also added some experimental evidence, the so-called competitive exclusion principle (sometimes called Gause's principle) took a firm hold in the ecological literature. The scope of the present discussion does not allow us to pursue in detail the ups and downs of this principle ("two competing species cannot coexist," where one has to carefully define what is competing and what is coexisting). However, the history of this principle could easily serve as a paradigm of some of the ways in which a mathematical model, even a crude one, may be eminently useful, as well as some of the things that should not be expected of a mathematical model for biological problems, at least not yet.

If one looks over Gause [17], Hardin [25], Ayala [5], Gilpin and Justice [20], Stewart and Levin [62], Gomatam [23], and the literature cited by these authors, one realizes that an enormous amount of experimental work was elicited by this principle, which in turn was originated by (20). (Even though some utterances of the principle were made at an earlier date, the work really began after Gause [17], whose work was an explicit response to Volterra's publications.) In the earlier years most of this work tended to confirm the principle, but as ecologists probed deeper into the concept of competition, they started distinguishing situations in which the principle might not apply, either because of conceptual problems ("Can this situation be labeled competition?") or because of certain features of the ecosystem. Many questions came up; genetical differences, partitioning of the physical space into different habitats, larvae having needs different from adults, degree of competition (one resource shared, others not), etc. The eventual result seems to be that the original model (equation (20)) is seldom valid or applicable in a numerical sense (though valid in a broad, qualitative way), and that the concept of competition has expanded into a host of (sub)concepts. Still, to have elicited so much work is not a bad performance for one simple model.

Remark 1. One of the points that drew attention recently was illustrated in Exercise 1 of Section 3.2: observations have been made of coexisting competing species, conforming to the positions of singular points as described by Eq. (21), rather than by (20) (cf. Gilpin and Justice [20] and Gilpin and Ayala [19]).

4. Some Remarks on *N*-Species Systems

Models for *n*-species systems in the Volterra tradition have the following appearance:

$$\dot{x}_i = x_i\left(\varepsilon_i + \sum_{j=1}^{n} a_{ij}x_i\right), \qquad i = 1, 2, \cdots, n,$$

where the ε_i and a_{ij} may be positive or negative. Some special cases of this general setup have been studied more than others.

Let species 1 prey on species 2, which in turn preys on species 3, which in turn ..., all the way down to species n, which is prey to species $n - 1$, without itself preying on any other species. (Note that this last point is somewhat unrealistic; soon we will receive heavier punishment for it than you might expect.) In the tradition of (7), Volterra modeled such linear chains of predators by

$$
\left.
\begin{aligned}
\dot{x}_1 &= x_1(-\gamma_1 && + \alpha_{12}x_2) \\
\dot{x}_2 &= x_2(-\gamma_2 - \alpha_{21}x_1 && + \alpha_{23}x_3) \\
\dot{x}_3 &= x_3(-\gamma_3 && - \alpha_{32}x_2 && + \alpha_{34}x_4) \\
\dot{x}_4 &= x_4(-\gamma_4 && - \alpha_{43}x_3 && + \alpha_{45}x_5) \\
\dot{x}_5 &= x_5(+\gamma_5 && - \alpha_{54}x_4)
\end{aligned}
\right\} \quad (22)
$$

where, for convenience, we have taken $n = 5$ and where all γ_i and all displayed α_{ij} are positive (see d'Ancona [3]). By a change of scale one can always achieve that the matrix of the $\pm\alpha_{ij}$ is skew-symmetric; see Exercise 2 to follow. We shall assume that this is already the case. Then the following argument is well-represented in the literature. Let $(p_1, p_2, p_3, p_4, p_5)$ be the point in $(x_1, x_2, x_3, x_4, x_5)$-space at which the five right-hand members of (22) have the value zero with all $p_i > 0$. Let us write δ_i for γ_i $(i = 1, 2, 3, 4)$ and δ_5 for $-\gamma_5$. Let us write a_{ij} for α_{ij} $(i < j)$ and for $-\alpha_{ij}$ $(i > j)$. Let A be the matrix of the a_{ij}, A being skew-symmetric, as mentioned. Then the vector $\vec{p}$ satisfies the equation

$$
A\vec{p} = \vec{\delta}. \tag{23}
$$

Equations (22) can now be written

$$
\dot{x}_i/x_i = \sum_j a_{ij}(x_j - p_j),
$$

from which the reader may derive, by the same methods as indicated in Exercise 7, Section 2.1:

$$
\sum_{i=1}^{n} [x_i(t) - p_i \log x_i(t)] = \text{constant} \tag{24a}
$$

or, equivalently,

$$
\sum_{i=1}^{n} [e^{v_i(t)} - v_i(t)]p_i = \text{constant}, \tag{24b}
$$

where $x_i = p_i e^{v_i}$ $(i = 1, 2, \cdots, n)$. Thus we have found a function of x_i which remains constant through time, i.e., a "constant of motion" or "first integral." This result is an n-species analog of (11b) and (11c).

EXERCISE

1. A fatal flaw exists in the above derivation. This derivation depends on a vector $\vec{p}$ satisfying (23), where A is a skew-symmetric matrix. Show that an $n \times n$ skew-symmetric matrix is singular if n is odd. Also show directly that, for A as defined by (22), no vector $\vec{p}$ satisfies (23) (unless $\gamma_1, \gamma_3, \gamma_5, \alpha_{12}, \alpha_{32}, \alpha_{34}, \alpha_{54}$ satisfy a certain equality, which defines a thin set in parameter space). Thus the theory leading to (24) works only for ecosystems consisting of an *even* number of species interacting in a linear predator–prey chain! This is the heavy punishment, promised in the second paragraph of this section, for the lack of realism in model (22): it can *not* apply to *odd*-numbered systems.

The existence of the constant of motion (24) has had the same result as was discussed in Section 2.1, Remark 6. To the objections that were discussed there and in Section 2.2, add those brought up in the review of [21] in *Science* (June 2, 1972, p. 1007). We will raise a few critical points in the following exercises so that the reader may "discover" some of these objections.

EXERCISES

2. Show that in (22) one can find a unique set of proportions $\beta_1 : \beta_2 : \beta_3 : \beta_4 : \beta_5$ such that for $j = i + 1, i = 1, 2, 3, 4$,

$$\alpha_{ij}\beta_j = A_{ij} = \alpha_{ji}\beta_i.$$

If subsequently $x_i/\beta_i = X_i$, then the new equations in X_i have a skew-symmetric matrix as promised; show! It has been suggested that the X_i measure species i ($i = 1, 2, 3, \cdots$) in "comparable" units. Do you like this suggestion? What should be the physical or biological nature of these units?

3. Show that as soon as species 1 preys not only on species 2, but also on species 3, no set of proportions $\beta_1 : \beta_2 : \beta_3 : \beta_4 : \beta_5$ can be found that would give us a system of equations with a skew-symmetric matrix, *unless* the coefficients α_{ij} satisfy some very precise conditions (in the form of strict equalities). It seems highly unlikely that many ecosystems exist that would satisfy such equalities. This means that as soon as the predator–prey relations no longer form a linear chain ($1 \rightarrow 2 \rightarrow 3 \rightarrow 4 \rightarrow 5$) but have some extra link (e.g., $1 \rightarrow 2 \rightarrow 3 \rightarrow 4 \rightarrow 5$), then a *constant of motion would not exist*, generally speaking.

4. Show that as soon as two among our species compete against each other or are mutually advantageous to each other, we cannot possibly have a skew-symmetric matrix, not even if the chain of relations is linear (e.g., $1 \rightarrow 2 \rightarrow 3 \rightarrow 4$–5, with 4 and 5 related by competition or mutualism).

5. Show that as soon as logistic crowding terms are introduced in even one species, no amount of scale changing can achieve a skew-symmetric matrix. (Remember that a matrix A is skew-symmetric iff $A = -A^T$.)

6. So a linear chain of predator–prey relations is the only case for which it has been proven that a skew-symmetric matrix can always be achieved.

7. The biologically unacceptable fact that according to the model only even numbers of species could live in a steady state evaporates if one adds plants and soil. This was proposed by Poletaev [57] and Éman [13], whose work was quoted in Section 2.2 (in the paragraph following Discussion Question 5 in Section 2.2). A very simple example of a model of such a biogeocoenotic system is provided by the following equations:

$$
\begin{aligned}
\text{(predators)} \quad & \dot{x} = x(-\gamma_1 && + \alpha_{12}y) \\
\text{(prey)} \quad & \dot{y} = y(-\gamma_2 - \alpha_{21}x && + \alpha_{23}z) \\
\text{(plants)} \quad & \dot{z} = z(-\gamma_3 && - \alpha_{32}y && + \alpha_{34}u) \\
\text{(soil nutrients)} \quad & \dot{u} = \gamma_{41}x + \gamma_{42}y + \gamma_{43}z - \alpha_{43}uz.
\end{aligned}
\tag{25}
$$

Try and recover the thinking behind every term in (25). Investigate whether or not these equations admit an equilibrium point with x, y, z, and u all strictly positive. Do the same for a model with one more species in it. Would the parameters need to satisfy any special conditions in order that such an equilibrium point may exist? Equations (25) are crude, of course (no crowding terms for instance). Specifically, cross-products such as $\alpha_{12}xy$ can be given a semblance of credibility by a chemical kinetics type of argument: animals move around and collide (as in collision theory); but a cross-product such as $\alpha_{43}uz$ is even harder to defend: plants do not move around. However, the idea of drawing plants and soil into the model is basically sound, obviously, and it is interesting that this is enough to get rid of the odd–even paradox.

8. The reader can now construct a large number of Volterra (or even fancier) models, to represent one predator species living from two prey species (competing or mutualistic), or to represent two predator species competing for one prey, etc. Fishery models may be constructed with man as the predator, etc. The possibilities are endless, but it is rather difficult to do analytical mathematical work on these models. One will often have to take recourse in computers. One many gain some insight in the severity of the mathematical problems by looking at Coppel [11], who confesses that a satisfactory classification of systems of two differential equations with quadratic terms has not even been achieved yet. These are equations of the oversimplified type that present research is leaving behind! Therefore, further development of this field does depend on numerical methods, although room will always be found for clever qualitative analysis of these differential systems. To single out meaningful problems, mathematicians should consult extensively with interested ecologists. Added in proof: more on systems with quadratic terms in H. R. van der Vaart, "Conditions for periodic solutions of Volterra differential systems," Bull. Math. Biol. vol. 40, pp. 133–160, 1978.

Appendix A

A.1 Phase Plane, Isoclines, Arrows

Most mathematical models in this module are *autonomous* systems of ordinary differential equations:

are those of the particular authors, and do not necessarily reflect the views of NSF, MAA, the editors, or any others involved in these project activities.

There are many other individuals who contributed in some way to the realization of these four volumes, and it is impossible to acknowledge all of them here. However, there are two individuals in addition to the authors, editors and people named above who should receive substantial credit for the ultimate appearance of this publication. Katherine B. Magann, who had provided many years of dedicated service to CUPM prior to the closing of the CUPM office, accomplished the production of the report *Case Studies in Applied Mathematics.* Carolyn D. Lucas assisted in the running of the 1976 MAA Workshop, supervised the production of the resulting sixty modules, and served as managing editor for the publication of these four volumes. Without her efforts and perseverance the final product of this major project might not have been realized.

July 1982   W. F. Lucas

$x_i, y_i)$ is (x_i, y_i). The projection of the solution curve through the point (t_0, x_0, y_0) consists of all points (x_i, y_i) for which

$$x_i = x_0 + (t_i - t_0)a, \qquad y_i = y_0 + (t_i - t_0)b.$$

These points all belong to the line (in the (x, y) plane):

$$\frac{x - x_0}{a} = \frac{y - y_0}{b}, \qquad \text{or} \qquad (x - x_0)b = (y - y_0)a.$$

The slope of any such line at the point $(x, y) = (\xi, \eta)$ is obviously b/a, which ratio equals the value of $\dot{y}/\dot{x}$ as determined by equation I (at the point (ξ, η)). Finally, note that all solution curves in (t, x, y) space that pass through any of the points (t_0, x_0, y_0) with fixed (x_0, y_0) and variable t_0 (each value of t_0 giving rise to one solution curve!) are parallel and have one and the same projection onto the (x, y) plane. This final property is very much a consequence of system I being autonomous. It enables us to find out the states (x, y) through which the system is going to move or has moved (we call both together the "life history of the system"), simply by looking at the projection of the pertinent solution curve(s). If the point (x_0, y_0) belongs to the system's life history, then the pertinent solution curve(s) should contain some point (t, x_0, y_0), and the pertinent projection should contain the point (x_0, y_0). The cylinder erected on any such projection with generators parallel to the t axis is filled with congruent solution curves, which can be obtained from each other by suitable translations parallel to the t axis.

Remark 1. In the case of system I the two-vector valued *functions* determined by the equations

$$(I') \begin{cases} x = x_0 + (t - t_0)a \\ y = y_0 + (t - t_0)b \end{cases}$$

are called *solutions*, the *curves* in (t, x, y) space determined by the same equations are called *solution curves* (straight lines in this case), and the *projections* of these curves onto the (x, y) plane are called *orbits, trajectories,* or *paths*. In the case of system I the orbits are determined by

$$(x - x_0)b = (y - y_0)a,$$

which describes the life history of such systems. Note that this equation is obtained from (I') by the elimination of t. Further, the (x, y) plane itself is denoted as *phase plane*. Since the ratio $\dot{y}/\dot{x} = b/a$ has, for system I, the same value at every point of the phase plane, the concept of isocline (see Remark 2 to follow) degenerates here.

Solutions II'. Again choose numerical values for a, b, t_0, x_0, y_0, and plot the solution curves in (t, x, y) space. The result is somewhat harder to visualize than it was for I', but it is quite feasible. Again, if we compare all solution curves that pass through points (t_0, x_0, y_0) with fixed (x_0, y_0) and variable t_0 (each value of t_0 giving rise to one solution curve!), we see that these curves have parallel directions at points (t, x_0, y_0). In fact, these curves can be obtained from each other by suitable translations parallel to the t axis. Thus we can use their common projection (viz., the orbit through (x_0, y_0)) to find out the life history of each solution curve that passes through some point (t, x_0, y_0) (t arbitrary, (x_0, y_0) fixed). As before, we find the equation of this orbit by eliminating t from the equations II':

$$\left(\frac{x}{x_0}\right)^b = \left(\frac{y}{y_0}\right)^a.$$

The reader should explore the shape of this curve, for the time being only for $0 < a < b$ (other cases later). Simply solve for y and plot in the (x, y) plane. (Note that all points of the curve are in the same quadrant as the point (x_0, y_0): why? This also follows from the equations II'.) Also find the derivative of y as a function of x, at the point (ξ, η):

$$\frac{dy}{dx} = \frac{b}{a}\frac{\eta}{\xi}.$$

Remember, the point (ξ, η) is on the orbit defined by $(x/x_0)^b = (y/y_0)^a$! This equation for dy/dx can easily be obtained from the original system (II):

$$\frac{dy}{dx} = \frac{\dot{y}}{\dot{x}} = \frac{b}{a}\frac{\eta}{\xi}.$$

Remark 2. Without first finding explicit expressions for the solutions I' or II', one can still obtain a fairly good insight in the shape of the orbits by plotting the slopes of the (tangent lines to the) orbits at a sufficiently large number of points in the phase plane.[5] This process can be made a lot easier by making use of isoclines. An *isocline* is the locus of all those points (x, y) in the phase plane at which the slope of the orbit passing through (x, y) has a given value.

Exercise

2. Consider the system

$$\left\{\begin{matrix} \dot{x} = x \\ \dot{y} = 2y \end{matrix}\right\}.$$

The slope of the orbit through the point (ξ, η) has, at that same point, the value

$$\frac{dy}{dx} = \frac{\dot{y}}{\dot{x}} = \frac{2\eta}{\xi}.$$

The locus of all points where that slope is $+1$ is given by

[5] This is one of the alternative approaches mentioned in the beginning of Section A.1.

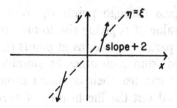

Figure 4.11

$$\frac{2\eta}{\xi} = 1.$$

The locus of all points where that slope is $+2$ is given by

$$\frac{2\eta}{\xi} = 2.$$

So $\eta = \frac{1}{2}\xi$ is the isocline corresponding to the slope $+1$, etc. Find the isoclines corresponding to the slopes $\frac{1}{4}, \frac{1}{2}, 3, -\frac{1}{4}, -\frac{1}{2}, -3$. Then draw these isoclines, and through some of their points draw (carefully!) short line segments to represent the tangent lines to the orbits at these points. (These drawings should be on a fairly large scale in order to achieve reasonable accuracy.) Now you can sketch a few orbits since you have now enough information on their directions at various and sundry points. Note that the abovementioned short line segments can be provided with *arrows* to indicate the direction in which time increases along the orbit. (E.g., if (ξ, η) is in the first quadrant, then $\dot{x} = \xi > 0$ and $\dot{y} = 2\eta > 0$, and so at (ξ, η) an orbit moves up and to the right as time progresses. If (ξ, η) is in the third quadrant, it is the other way around; see Figure 4.11.)

Also note that none of the above isoclines coincides with or is even tangent to an orbit!

Definitions. Before going on, we will write three definitions.

Solutions. Given a system of (ordinary) (autonomous) differential equations

$$\dot{\vec{x}} = \vec{f}(\vec{x}) \quad \text{or} \quad \begin{cases} \dot{x}_1 = f_1(x_1, x_2) \\ \dot{x}_2 = f_2(x_1, x_2) \end{cases},$$

where x_1 and x_2 represent two *unknown* functions of t, a *solution* is a fully specified two-vector valued function of t,

$$\vec{x} = \vec{\Phi}(t) \quad \text{or} \quad \begin{cases} x_1 = \Phi_1(t) \\ x_2 = \Phi_2(t) \end{cases},$$

such that substitution of $\vec{\Phi}(t)$ for $\vec{x}$ reduces the above differential equation to an identity in t. A curve in (t, x_1, x_2) space that is defined by a solution $\vec{x} = \vec{\Phi}(t)$ is called a *solution curve*.

EXERCISE

3. Check the claim that II′ is the solution of II against the definition of solution just given.

Remark 3. We have seen earlier that solutions depend on so-called initial conditions: if the value of the solution must be $\vec{x}_0$ at time t_0, then it is often useful to incorporate this condition into the notation:

$$\vec{x} = \vec{\Phi}(t; t_0, \vec{x}_0) \quad \text{or} \quad \begin{cases} x_1 = \Phi_1(t; t_0, x_{01}, x_{02}) \\ x_2 = \Phi_2(t; t_0, x_{01}, x_{02}) \end{cases}$$

where $\vec{\Phi}(t_0; t_0, \vec{x}_0) = \vec{x}_0$.

Orbits, Trajectories, or Paths. These are curves in the phase plane (here, the (x_1, x_2) plane), which geometrically are projections of solution curves and which analytically are determined by eliminating t from the two above equations $x_1 = \Phi_1(t; \cdots)$ and $x_2 = \Phi_2(t; \cdots)$, or, equivalently, by regarding these two equations as the parametrization of some curve (viz., the orbit) in the (x_1, x_2) plane.

Remark 4. If the solutions of a differential system are available in explicit form, there is no special problem in studying the orbits. If the solutions are not available, then it may happen that the equation of the orbits can be found (see Section 2.1, Exercise 3), although this is relatively rare. If this is not the case either, then we can choose between several alternative methods (and often use them all) for studying the orbits. The easiest of these is the quick-and-dirty *isocline and arrow method.* Its basis is the formula which we have already applied:

$$\frac{dx_2}{dx_1} = \frac{\dot{x}_2}{\dot{x}_1} = \frac{f_2(x_1, x_2)}{f_1(x_1, x_2)},$$

which gives the direction of the tangent line to any orbit at any point (except, of course, at singular points).

Isoclines. Given the differential system

$$\begin{cases} \dot{x}_1 = f_1(x_1, x_2) \\ \dot{x}_2 = f_2(x_1, x_2) \end{cases},$$

the curve which in (x_1, x_2) plane is defined by

$$(\cos \theta) \cdot f_2(\xi_1, \xi_2) = (\sin \theta) \cdot f_1(\xi_1, \xi_2),$$

is called the isocline corresponding to the slope $\tan \theta$; it is the locus of all points (ξ_1, ξ_2) such that the orbit through (ξ_1, ξ_2) has a tangent line at that point with slope $\tan \theta$.

Remark 5. In general an isocline is not an orbit; *in general* an orbit and an isocline have no common tangent lines at their points of intersection (though there are exceptions to this rule!). Among the continuum of isoclines two are of outstanding importance in most problems: the isocline corresponding to

$\theta = 0$ and the one corresponding to $\theta = \pi/2$; this is, the locus of points where the orbits have a horizontal direction (x_2 stationary; $\dot{x}_2 = 0$), and the locus of points where the orbits have a vertical direction (x_1 stationary; $\dot{x}_1 = 0$). For examples and applications see Section A.2 as well as many exercises in the main text of this chapter.

A.2 The Quick-and-Dirty Isocline-and-Arrow Method

At the beginning of this method stands the drawing of two isoclines, one corresponding to $\theta = 0$ and the other to $\theta = \pi/2$.

EXERCISE

1. For the following systems of differential equations find the equations for both the ($\theta = 0$) isocline and the ($\theta = \pi/2$) isocline, and sketch them.

$$\text{I} \quad \left\{ \begin{array}{l} \dot{x} = +px + \beta y \\ \dot{y} = -\beta x + py \end{array} \right\}, \quad p > 0, \beta > 0$$

$$\text{II} \quad \left\{ \begin{array}{l} \dot{x} = -px - \beta y \\ \dot{y} = +\beta x - py \end{array} \right\}, \quad p > 0, \beta > 0$$

$$\text{III} \quad \left\{ \begin{array}{l} \dot{x} = \quad\quad \beta y \\ \dot{y} = -\beta x \end{array} \right\}, \quad \beta > 0$$

$$\text{IV} \quad \left\{ \begin{array}{l} \dot{x} = \quad -\beta y \\ \dot{y} = +\beta x \end{array} \right\}, \quad \beta > 0$$

$$\text{V} \quad \left\{ \begin{array}{l} \dot{x} = -\lambda_1 x \quad\quad\quad + y^2 \\ \dot{y} = \quad\quad -\lambda_2 y + x^2 \end{array} \right\}, \quad \lambda_1 > 0, \lambda_2 > 0$$

$$\text{VI} \quad \left\{ \begin{array}{l} \dot{x} = x(+\gamma_1 - \delta x - py) \\ \dot{y} = y(-\gamma_2 + qx - \zeta y) \end{array} \right\} \left\{ \begin{array}{l} \gamma_1 > 0, \gamma_2 > 0, \delta > 0 \\ \zeta > 0, \ p > 0, q > 0 \end{array} \right\}.$$

In order to gain profitable information from these isoclines concerning the shape of the orbits we supplement our diagrams with a few easily derived items:

(α) For each of the six given differential equation systems, note that the value of $\dot{x}$ is negative on one side of the ($\theta = \pi/2$) isocline ($\theta = \pi/2$ iff $\dot{x} = 0$) and positive on the other side. Therefore, one can draw a horizontal arrow pointing left wherever $\dot{x} < 0$ and a horizontal arrow pointing right wherever $\dot{x} > 0$. In fact, one can organize this in a systematic fashion. First, note that in each of the six cases the two isoclines partition the phase plane into a number of subsets S: four in the first four cases, five in the fifth case and eleven in the sixth case. Second, there are always a few among those subsets S for which it is very easy to determine the sign of $\dot{x}$; e.g., for system I, $\dot{x} > 0$ at any point in the first quadrant. Third, as long as the functions $\varphi(\ \ )$ and $\psi(\ \ )$ in

$$\begin{cases} \dot{x} = \varphi(x, y) \\ \dot{y} = \psi(x, y) \end{cases}$$

are continuous (and they are in all cases discussed in this module), the sign of $\dot{x}$ must obviously be the same at all points inside any given subset S. Indeed, $\varphi(x, y)$, being continuous, cannot change sign without passing the value 0 and so the sign of $\dot{x}$ stays the same from one point to another point unless you have to cross the ($\dot{x} = 0$) isocline once (or thrice, etc.) in order to get from the first point to the second. Fourth, it is helpful to, whenever you cross the ($\dot{y} = 0$) isocline, put an arrow on that isocline, pointing left or right, as the case may be (note that the sign of $\dot{x}$ does not change when you cross the ($\dot{y} = 0$) isocline). Fifth, again because of the continuity of $\varphi(\ \ )$, it is clear that the value of $\dot{x} = \varphi(x, y)$ approaches 0 as the point (x, y) approaches an ($\dot{x} = 0$) isocline (one could express this by making the arrows shorter, but one may as well just keep it in mind for future reference).

EXERCISES

2. In each of the six diagrams that resulted from Exercise 1, draw all the horizontal arrows, $\rightarrow$ or $\leftarrow$, according to the specifications in (α).

3. In the following system $\dot{x}$ never changes sign, not even when crossing the ($\dot{x} = 0$) isocline:

$$\begin{cases} \dot{x} = (px + \beta y)^2 \\ \dot{y} = -\beta x + py \end{cases}.$$

Why not?

(β) Go over every sentence in the above paragraph marked (α) and see how it is changed when our concern is the sign of $\dot{y}$ instead of $\dot{x}$.

EXERCISE

4. In each of the six diagrams that you worked on in Exercise 2, draw all the vertical arrows, $\uparrow$ or $\downarrow$, according to the specifications listed under (β).

(γ) Finally, the arrows $\uparrow$ and $\rightarrow$ in a certain subset S mean that in that subset the orbits move up and to the right as time passes; similarly, for the

other three possibilities. Using this information, including the directions in which the isoclines must be crossed, one can start sketching the orbits: flattening them as you approach a ($\dot{y} = 0$) isocline, making them steeper as you approach an ($\dot{x} = 0$) isocline. (Why?).

EXERCISE

5. Do all the sketching of orbits you can in the six diagrams of Exercise 4. Note that certain conclusions suggest themselves strongly from these sketches, although one would try and find confirmation from some more precise argument. For example,

- for system I, the orbits seem to spiral outward from the origin;
- for system II, the orbits seem to spiral inward toward the origin;
- for systems III and IV, the orbits seem to go around in circles about the origin (draw some isoclines with different θ);
- for system V, the origin seems to be an attractor (no spirals!), and the point $((\lambda_1 \lambda_2^2)^{1/3}, (\lambda_1^2 \lambda_2)^{1/3})$ seems to be a saddlepoint;
- for system VI, two cases are to be distinguished: the slanted parts of the isoclines intersecting in the first, or in the fourth, quadrant. In the first case the origin and the point $(\gamma_1/\delta, 0)$ seem to be saddle-points, the point $(0, -\gamma_2/\zeta)$ a repulsor, and the point in the interior of the first quadrant an attractor (with or without spirals; that is not too clear).

A.3 Linear Systems

The quick-and-dirty isocline and arrow method is *global*. One can usually sketch orbits both far from and close to the origin or any singular point.

Remark 1. A *singular point* is any point in the phase plane that is an orbit in itself: if a system is at any singular point, it will stay there (mathematically speaking; however, if the singular point is unstable, then an analog computer would eventually get away from it, either because it would not ever get precisely there to begin with, or because electronic noise would throw it off). Singular points are found by requiring that both $\dot{x}$ and $\dot{y}$ equal zero, $\varphi(x, y) = 0 = \psi(x, y)$, cf. (A1).

The easiest way to confirm or refute the suggestions made by the quick-and-dirty method, and also to supplement those suggestions, is *linearization*. The basic idea of linearization is to study the *local* behavior of the orbits of a given system in the neighborhood of any of its singular points by studying the uniquely defined *linear system* which under certain conditions *approximates* the *given system*.

Remark 2. Linearization is not always meaningful, e.g., at the origin in the system

$$\begin{cases} \dot{x} = a_{11}x^2 + 2a_{12}xy + a_{22}y^2 \\ \dot{y} = b_{11}x^2 + 2b_{12}xy + b_{22}y^2 \end{cases}.$$

Linearization is not always decisive (see below), and it gives only local results. Thus limit cycles, for instance, need other methods to prove or disprove their existence, but such will be outside the scope of this chapter.

In order to understand this linearization method, we had better first take a look at *linear systems*. We will restrict ourselves to *two-dimensional*, autonomous systems:

$$\dot{\vec{x}} = A\vec{x} \tag{A2}$$

or

$$\begin{cases} \dot{x} = a_{11}x + a_{12}y \\ \dot{y} = a_{21}x + a_{22}y \end{cases}. \tag{A2a}$$

Obviously (why?), this system has only one singular point, the origin (that is, provided the matrix A is nonsingular). A linear system with singular point $\vec{p} = (p, q)$ is

$$\dot{\vec{x}} = A(\vec{x} - \vec{p})$$

or

$$\begin{cases} \dot{x} = a_{11}(x - p) + a_{12}(y - q) \\ \dot{y} = a_{21}(x - p) + a_{22}(y - q) \end{cases}. \tag{A2b}$$

The behavior of the second system follows directly from that of the first. So we will worry only about (A2). Note that we are restricting ourselves to autonomous systems, so A is a *constant matrix*. Also note that in general A is *not symmetric*.

The basic strategy for studying the solutions and orbits of (A2) consists of studying only a few special cases (i.e., a few special, canonical matrices A) and showing that the general case can be reduced to one of the canonical cases by means of a suitable linear transformation—much like the study of conics and quadrics in analytic geometry. The linear transformations work as follows. Let P be a constant nonsingular matrix. Define the unknown vector-valued function $\vec{z}(t)$ in terms of the unknown vector-valued function $\vec{x}(t)$ by

$$\vec{z}(t) = P\vec{x}(t) \Leftrightarrow \vec{x}(t) = P^{-1}\vec{z}(t) \Leftrightarrow \dot{\vec{z}}(t) = PAP^{-1}\vec{z}(t);$$

and all we need to do is to choose P so that PAP^{-1} is one of a few canonical matrices. The choice of the matrix P and the resulting type of special matrix PAP^{-1} depend on the eigenvalues of A.

Definition. *Eigenvalues* (or characteristic values, or latent roots) of any matrix A are defined as the roots of the polynomial equation

$$\det(A - \lambda I) = 0,$$

or, since A is a 2×2 matrix,

$$\begin{vmatrix} a_{11} - \lambda & a_{12} \\ a_{21} & a_{22} - \lambda \end{vmatrix} = 0, \text{ or } \lambda^2 - (a_{11} + a_{22})\lambda + a_{11}a_{22} - a_{12}a_{21} = 0.$$

In all applications in this module, the elements of the matrix A are real. Therefore, the eigenvalues are either real or conjugate complex. In fact, we will distinguish between the following cases:

(1) eigenvalues real and different
(2) eigenvalues real and equal
(3) eigenvalues pure imaginary and different
(4) eigenvalues complex and different
} both eigenvalues nonzero.

(5) one eigenvalue zero, one nonzero   } one eigenvalue zero.
(6) both eigenvalues zero   } both eigenvalues zero.

Canonical representatives of these six possibilities will now be discussed, roughly in order of complexity.

(6) Here we have to distinguish between two cases.

(a)
$$\begin{bmatrix} \dot{z}_1 \\ \dot{z}_2 \end{bmatrix} = \begin{bmatrix} 0 & 0 \\ 0 & 0 \end{bmatrix} \begin{bmatrix} z_1 \\ z_2 \end{bmatrix}.$$

Every point of the phase plane is a singular point!

(b)
$$\begin{bmatrix} \dot{z}_1 \\ \dot{z}_2 \end{bmatrix} = \begin{bmatrix} 0 & 1 \\ 0 & 0 \end{bmatrix} \begin{bmatrix} z_1 \\ z_2 \end{bmatrix}$$

This is a more interesting case. The reader will have no difficulty in showing that every point of the z_1 axis ($z_2 = 0$) is a singular point; that all orbits outside the z_1 axis are parallel to the z_1 axis, moving to the right (as $t \uparrow +\infty$) above the z_1 axis, and to the left below. The solution functions are obviously defined by

$$\vec{z}(t) = \begin{bmatrix} 1 & t \\ 0 & 1 \end{bmatrix} \vec{z}(0).$$

Prove!

(5)
$$\begin{bmatrix} \dot{z}_1 \\ \dot{z}_2 \end{bmatrix} = \begin{bmatrix} \lambda & 0 \\ 0 & 0 \end{bmatrix} \begin{bmatrix} z_1 \\ z_2 \end{bmatrix}$$

Every point of the z_2 axis in the phase plane is a singular point; the orbits are horizontal half-lines (do apply also the isocline and arrow method!).

(3)
$$\begin{bmatrix} \dot{z}_1 \\ \dot{z}_2 \end{bmatrix} = \begin{bmatrix} 0 & \beta \\ -\beta & 0 \end{bmatrix} \begin{bmatrix} z_1 \\ z_2 \end{bmatrix} \text{ or } \begin{Bmatrix} \dot{z}_1 = \beta z_2 \\ \dot{z}_2 = -\beta z_1 \end{Bmatrix}.$$

The orbits can be obtained very quickly by multiplying the first equation by z_1 and the second by z_2. Then add

$$z_1 \dot{z}_1 + z_2 \dot{z}_2 = 0.$$

So the orbits are circles around the origin:

$$z_1^2(t) + z_2^2(t) = z_1^2(t_0) + z_2^2(t_0).$$

Alternatively, we can study the value of $dz_2/dz_1 = -z_1/z_2$; so the slope of the orbit at the point (z_1, z_2) is orthogonal to the slope of the line through the origin and the point (z_1, z_2) (brush up that analytic geometry!).

Alternatively, we can combine the two equations into one:

$$\ddot{z}_1 = -\beta^2 z_1,$$

with the general solution,

$$z_1(t) = \gamma_1 \cos \beta(t - t_0) + \gamma_2 \sin \beta(t - t_0),$$

from which z_2 follows as $\beta^{-1}\dot{z}_1(t)$:

$$z_2(t) = \gamma_2 \cos \beta(t - t_0) - \gamma_1 \sin \beta(t - t_0).$$

Introducing initial conditions

$$z_1(t_0) = z_{10}, \qquad z_2(t_0) = z_{20},$$

we find

$$\begin{cases} z_1(t) = z_{10} \cos \beta(t - t_0) + z_{20} \sin \beta(t - t_0) \\ z_2(t) = z_{20} \cos \beta(t - t_0) - z_{10} \sin \beta(t - t_0) \end{cases}$$

or

$$\vec{z}(t) = \begin{bmatrix} c & s \\ -s & c \end{bmatrix} \vec{z}(t_0)$$

with obvious notation. The reader should check these results against the isocline and arrow method and convince himself that they are in perfect harmony.

(4)
$$\begin{bmatrix} \dot{z}_1 \\ \dot{z}_2 \end{bmatrix} = \begin{bmatrix} \alpha & \beta \\ -\beta & \alpha \end{bmatrix} \begin{bmatrix} z_1 \\ z_2 \end{bmatrix} \quad \text{or} \quad \begin{cases} \dot{z}_1 = \alpha z_1 + \beta z_2 \\ \dot{z}_2 = -\beta z_1 + \alpha z_2 \end{cases}.$$

Here we need to make a clever change of variables:

$$\vec{z}(t) = e^{\alpha t} \vec{w}(t), \qquad \vec{z}(t_0) = e^{\alpha t_0} \vec{w}(t_0).$$

This reduces our equation to a form we already know:

$$\begin{cases} \dot{w}_1 = \beta w_2 \\ \dot{w}_2 = -\beta w_1 \end{cases}.$$

Making the necessary substitution the reader will now easily find that

$$z(t) = e^{(t-t_0)\alpha} \begin{bmatrix} \cos \beta(t - t_0) & \sin \beta(t - t_0) \\ -\sin \beta(t - t_0) & \cos \beta(t - t_0) \end{bmatrix} \vec{z}(t_0).$$

Defining $r(t)$ as the distance between the origin and the running point $\vec{z}(t)$, the reader will also find $\langle r^2(t) = \vec{z}^T(t)\vec{z}(t)\rangle$:

$$r(t) = e^{(t-t_0)\alpha} r(t_0),$$

which shows that the point $\vec{z}(t)$ in the phase plane describes a spiral, inward as $t \uparrow \infty$ when α is negative, outward as $t \uparrow \infty$ when α is positive.

EXERCISES

1. An alternative way of handling (4) is to change to polar coordinates

$$\begin{cases} z_1(t) = r(t)\cos\varphi(t) \\ z_2(t) = r(t)\sin\varphi(t) \end{cases} \quad \text{and} \quad \begin{cases} z_1(t_0) = r(t_0)\cos\varphi(t_0) \\ z_2(t_0) = r(t_0)\sin\varphi(t_0) \end{cases}.$$

This approach leads to

$$\begin{cases} \varphi(t) = \varphi(t_0) - (t - t_0)\beta \\ r(t) = e^{(t-t_0)\alpha} r(t_0) \end{cases}.$$

2. Apply the isocline and arrow method (both for $\alpha > 0$ and for $\alpha < 0$; also for $\beta > 0$ and for $\beta < 0$) and demonstrate that its results are in perfect harmony with the above.

(2) (a)
$$\begin{bmatrix} \dot{z}_1 \\ \dot{z}_2 \end{bmatrix} = \begin{bmatrix} \lambda & 0 \\ 0 & \lambda \end{bmatrix}\begin{bmatrix} z_1 \\ z_2 \end{bmatrix} \quad \text{or} \quad \begin{cases} \dot{z}_1 = \lambda z_1 \\ \dot{z}_2 = \lambda z_2 \end{cases}.$$

The solutions follow immediately:

$$\begin{cases} z_1(t) = e^{(t-t_0)\lambda} z_1(t_0) \\ z_2(t) = e^{(t-t_0)\lambda} z_2(t_0) \end{cases}.$$

EXERCISES

3. Show that the point $\vec{z}(t)$ is in the same quadrant as $\vec{z}(t_0)$ for all t between $-\infty$ and $+\infty$.

4. Show that the orbits are straight half-lines, and that the direction of movement (away from or toward the origin as $t \uparrow \infty$) depends on the sign of λ.

5. Find the slope of the orbit at the point (z_1, z_2).

6. Show that in this case orbits and isoclines coincide.

(2) (b)
$$\begin{bmatrix} \dot{z}_1 \\ \dot{z}_2 \end{bmatrix} = \begin{bmatrix} \lambda & 1 \\ 0 & \lambda \end{bmatrix}\begin{bmatrix} z_1 \\ z_2 \end{bmatrix} \quad \text{or} \quad \begin{cases} \dot{z}_1 = \lambda z_1 + z_2 \\ \dot{z}_2 = \quad\quad \lambda z_2 \end{cases}.$$

EXERCISE

7. The isocline and arrow method is quite suggestive for this system. The horizontal axis is both orbit and isocline, but no other orbit coincides with any other isocline.

Sketch isoclines and orbits for this system. Distinguish between λ positive and λ negative.

The second equation of this system is easy to solve: $z_2(t) = e^{(t-t_0)\lambda} z_2(t_0)$. Plug this solution into the first equation, multiply the result by $e^{-\lambda t}$, and show that the derivative of $e^{-\lambda t} z_1(t)$ shall be equal to the derivative of $e^{-\lambda t_0} z_2(t_0) \cdot t$, from which result it easily follows that

$$\begin{cases} z_1(t) = e^{(t-t_0)\lambda} \langle z_{10} + z_{20} \cdot (t - t_0) \rangle \\ z_2(t) = e^{(t-t_0)\lambda} z_{20} \end{cases}.$$

EXERCISE

8. Analyze the orbits defined by this equation. First take *negative* λ and show that, for orbits with $(z_{10}, z_{20}) = \langle z_1(t_0), z_2(t_0) \rangle$ in the upper half-plane, $z_1(t)$ *reaches a maximum* at the point where the orbit intersects the line $\lambda z_1 + z_2 = 0$, which is the ($\dot{z}_1 = 0$) isocline (that makes sense!). How does this change either when (z_{10}, z_{20}) is in the lower half-plane or when λ is positive?

(1) $$\begin{bmatrix} \dot{z}_1 \\ \dot{z}_2 \end{bmatrix} = \begin{bmatrix} \lambda_1 & 0 \\ 0 & \lambda_2 \end{bmatrix} \begin{bmatrix} z_1 \\ z_2 \end{bmatrix} \quad \text{or} \quad \begin{cases} \dot{z}_1 = \lambda_1 z_1 \\ \dot{z}_2 = \lambda_2 z_2 \end{cases}.$$

Here we distinguish between the cases where λ_1 and λ_2 have the *same* sign, and where the two have *different* signs.

(a) $\lambda_1 < 0$ and $\lambda_2 < 0$. The solutions are

$$\begin{cases} z_1(t) = e^{(t-t_0)\lambda_1} z_1(t_0) \\ z_2(t) = e^{(t-t_0)\lambda_2} z_2(t_0) \end{cases}.$$

Again, the point $\vec{z}(t)$ is for all t in the same quadrant as $\vec{z}(t_0)$. The point $\vec{z}(t)$ will approach the origin as $t \uparrow \infty$. For all but two orbits (besides the origin itself) the asymptotic direction (as $t \uparrow \infty$) will be

$$\begin{cases} \text{the } z_1 \text{ axis iff } -|\lambda_2| < -|\lambda_1| < 0 \\ \text{the } z_2 \text{ axis iff } -|\lambda_1| < -|\lambda_2| < 0 \end{cases}.$$

EXERCISES

9. Find the equation of the orbits by eliminating t. Then express z_2 in terms of z_1 and show that the slope at the origin is given by

$$\begin{cases} \dfrac{dz_2}{dz_1} = 0, & \text{if } 0 < |\lambda_1| < |\lambda_2| \\[2mm] \dfrac{dz_1}{dz_2} = 0, & \text{if } 0 < |\lambda_2| < |\lambda_1|. \end{cases}$$

10. Identify the two orbits that are different. Hint: take $z_{10} = 0$, or $z_{20} = 0$.

(b) $\lambda_1 > 0$ and $\lambda_2 > 0$. The solutions are given by the same formulae, but now the point $\bar{z}(t)$ will go away from the origin as $t \uparrow \infty$, and approach the origin as $t \downarrow -\infty$. For all but two orbits (besides the origin itself) the asymptotic direction (as $t \downarrow -\infty$) will be

$$\begin{Bmatrix} \text{the } z_1 \text{ axis iff } 0 < \lambda_1 < \lambda_2 \\ \text{the } z_2 \text{ axis iff } 0 < \lambda_2 < \lambda_1 \end{Bmatrix}.$$

EXERCISE

11. Prove this and find the two exceptional orbits.

(c) $\lambda_1 < 0 < \lambda_2$. The solutions are given by the same formulae as in (a), but the result of the elimination of t is now

$$z_2^{|\lambda_1|} z_1^{|\lambda_2|} = z_{20}^{|\lambda_1|} z_{10}^{|\lambda_2|}$$

for all but four orbits (besides the origin itself).

EXERCISE

12. Explore these orbits; they look like hyperbolae, roughly speaking. Find the four exceptional orbits.

(d) $\lambda_2 < 0 < \lambda_1$. The reader will handle this case.

EXERCISE

13. The reader will put arrows on the diagrams of the orbits in cases (a), (b), (c), (d).

Check the following statement. In the canonical cases just discussed the origin is an *attractor* if the *real part* of *both eigenvalues* is *negative*; the origin is a *repulsor* if the *real part* of *both eigenvalues* is *positive*. The examples we have seen where both real parts are zero, showed orbits that neither approached the origin nor receded from it. If one eigenvalue is negative and the other positive, we have the peculiar arrangement of the saddle point: two orbits approach the origin, two orbits recede from it; the others first approach somewhat (if the initial point is located properly) and then recede.

Remark 3. The singular point is called an *improper node* if all orbits (with the exception at most of three) have the same asymptotic direction, either when $t \uparrow \infty$ or when $t \downarrow -\infty$. The singular point is called a *proper node* if the orbits are all straight lines with different directions. The singular point is called a *saddle point* when the two eigenvalues are real, one positive and one negative. The singular point is called a *spiral point* (or *vortex*, or *focus*) when the two eigenvalues are strictly complex (not pure imaginary). The

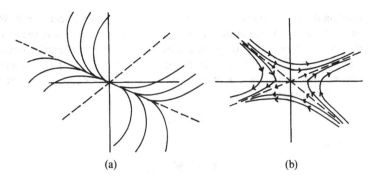

Figure 4.12. (a) Improper Node; (b) Saddle Point.

singular point is called a *center* if all orbits are closed curves around it. The singular point $\vec{0}$ is an *attractor* if, for all solutions $\vec{z}(t)$, $\lim_{t\uparrow+\infty}\vec{z}(t) = \vec{0}$, and a *repulsor* (or *repeller*) if the distance between it and $\vec{z}(t)$ increases as $t \uparrow +\infty$. In linear systems a repulsor becomes an attractor when time is reversed ($t = -\tau$). In order to avoid all ambiguity, we should point out that the asymptotic direction which is common to all (with the exception of at most three) orbits in the case of an *improper node* is the direction of these orbits as they *approach* the *singular point*. We are talking about the tangent line to these orbits at the singular point after we have "added" the singular point to each orbit. In the case of a *saddle point* for a linear system, the two lonely orbits tending to the singular point as $t \uparrow +\infty$ and the two lonely orbits tending to the singular point as $t \downarrow -\infty$ (going to infinity as $t \uparrow +\infty$) are called *separatrices*. The first two are referred to as the *incoming separatrices*, the latter two as the *outgoing separatrices*. The separatrices constitute the asymptotes of the other, hyperbola-like orbits.

Now we want to pick up the threads of the argument which we left when we introduced the six different classes of pairs of eigenvalues of the matrix A. We then discussed canonical representatives of the six classes of matrices A corresponding to these six classes of pairs of eigenvalues. Now we are ready to make the discussion completely general. We will use the same numbers, (1)–(6), to indicate the various cases.

(1) If the 2×2 matrix A has two *different, nonzero, real* eigenvalues, say λ_1 and λ_2, then we can construct a nonsingular matrix V such that

$$AV = V\Lambda \text{ or } V^{-1}AV = \Lambda,$$

where Λ is the diagonal matrix with elements λ_1 and λ_2, and V^{-1} plays the role of the matrix P quoted in the paragraph on the basic strategy following below (A2b).

EXERCISES

14. Since $\lambda_1 \neq 0$ and $\lambda_2 \neq 0$, the matrix A is nonsingular (why?).

Hint: Your answer depends on your criterion for a nonsingular matrix. A matrix

A is nonsingular iff *no nonnull vector* $\vec{v}$ exists with $A\vec{v} = \vec{0}$, or iff $\det A \neq 0$. With the earlier definition of eigenvalues as the roots of $\det(A - \lambda I) = 0$, the second criterion for A being nonsingular yields immediate results for our question (show!). Application of the first criterion needs the known result from linear algebra saying that for any given matrix A a nonnull vector $\vec{v}$ and a (real or complex) number λ can satisfy the equation

$$A\vec{v} = \lambda\vec{v}$$

if and only if

$$(A - \lambda I)\vec{v} = \vec{0},$$

which is *equivalent to*

$$\det(A - \lambda I) = 0;$$

this shows that the λ in $A\vec{v} = \lambda\vec{v}$ is an eigenvalue. (Be it known that the $\vec{v}$ in $A\vec{v} = \lambda\vec{v}$ is called an eigenvector!) Now note that

$$A\vec{v} = \vec{0} \text{ is equivalent to } A\vec{v} = 0 \cdot \vec{v},$$

which shows that the existence of a nonnull vector $\vec{v}$ with $A\vec{v} = 0$ is equivalent to the existence of an eigenvalue 0.

15. If $\vec{v}_1$ and $\vec{v}_2$ are both nonnull vectors, then show that

$$c_1\vec{v}_1 + c_2\vec{v}_2 = \vec{0}$$

implies that either c_1 and c_2 are both zero, or both nonzero. (c_1, c_2 are real or complex numbers; a null vector has all components zero; a nonnull vector has at least one nonzero component.)

For the further development we need the concept of linear (in)dependence of two vectors: two vectors are linearly *dependent* iff one is a scalar multiple of the other, $\vec{v}_2 = \gamma\vec{v}_1$ or $\vec{v}_1 = \delta\vec{v}_2$, which is equivalent to the definition that two vectors are linearly *dependent* iff a *nonnull* vector $\vec{c}$ (with components c_1 and c_2) exists such that

$$V\vec{c} = \vec{0} \text{ or } c_1\vec{v}_1 + c_2\vec{v}_2 = 0.$$

(According to Exercise 15 neither c_1 nor c_2 could be individually zero in this definition.) Obviously, the 2×2 matrix V built from the column vectors $\vec{v}_1$ and $\vec{v}_2$ is singular iff the vectors are dependent. Why? (See preceding exercises.)

EXERCISE

16. Now prove that if

$$\left\{ \begin{matrix} A\vec{v}_1 = \lambda_1\vec{v}_1 \\ A\vec{v}_2 = \lambda_2\vec{v}_2 \end{matrix} \right\}, \quad \vec{v}_1 \neq \vec{0}, \quad \vec{v}_2 \neq \vec{0},$$

then $\vec{v}_1$ and $\vec{v}_2$ are linearly independent if $\lambda_1 \neq \lambda_2$. *Hint:* Let $c_1\vec{v}_1 + c_2\vec{v}_2 = \vec{0}$.

Then the equality $\vec{0} = (A - \lambda_1 I)(c_1 \vec{v}_1 + c_2 \vec{v}_2) = c_2(\lambda_2 - \lambda_1)\vec{v}_2$ entails that $c_2 = 0$, hence that $c_1 = 0$ (why?).

So, whenever a matrix A has two *different* eigenvalues, say λ_1 and λ_2, then any one eigenvector corresponding to the first eigenvalue and any one eigenvector corresponding to the second eigenvalue are linearly independent. If a 2×2 matrix A has the maximum number (i.e., two) of different eigenvalues, then at least one eigenvector corresponds to each of these eigenvalues. Let $\vec{v}_1$ be an eigenvector for λ_1 and $\vec{v}_2$ for λ_2, then any other vector must be of the form $\gamma_1 \vec{v}_1 + \gamma_2 \vec{v}_2$. (Why?)

EXERCISES

17. After $\lambda_1 \neq 0$ and $\lambda_2 \neq 0$ have been found as the unequal roots of det $(A - \lambda I) = 0$, $\vec{v}_i$ is uniquely (except for a scalar coefficient) determined by

$$A\vec{v}_i = \lambda_i \vec{v}_i, \qquad i = 1, 2.$$

Prove! Also, the matrix

$$V = [\vec{v}_1 \quad \vec{v}_2]$$

is nonsingular. (Why?) As an exercise find the eigenvectors of

$$A' = \begin{bmatrix} 3 & 4 \\ 2 & 9 \end{bmatrix}, \qquad A'' = \begin{bmatrix} -1 & 3 \\ 2 & -2 \end{bmatrix}.$$

Also, for these two examples verify numerically the formula

$$V^{-1}AV = \Lambda,$$

quoted in the paragraph preceding Exercise 14. Also verify that scalar coefficients do not matter: the equality $V^{-1}AV = \Lambda$ is just as valid, and with precisely the same λ_1 and λ_2, when we replace $\vec{v}_1$ by $q_1 \vec{v}_1$ and $\vec{v}_2$ by $q_2 \vec{v}_2$.

18. Now execute the program as set forth at the beginning of this section. Transform the systems

$$\dot{\vec{x}} = A'\vec{x}, \qquad \dot{\vec{x}} = A''\vec{x},$$

where the single and double primes refer to the two matrices in Exercise 17, into systems

$$\dot{\vec{z}} = \Lambda'\vec{z}, \qquad \dot{\vec{z}} = \Lambda''\vec{z}$$

by means of the transformations

$$\vec{x} = V'\vec{z}, \qquad \vec{x} = V''\vec{z}$$

Find all kinds of asymptotic directions in the resulting $\vec{z}$ systems and, consequently, in the original $\vec{x}$ systems. Also write the solution functions both in $\vec{z}$ coordinates and in $\vec{x}$ coordinates.

The answers to Exercises 14–18 lead to the following *summary of case* (*1*). If the 2×2 matrix A has two *different, nonzero, real* eigenvalues λ_1

and λ_2, then λ_1 determines an eigenvector $\vec{v}_1$ and λ_2 determines an eigenvector $\vec{v}_2$, both essentially unique and such that the matrix

$$V = [\vec{v}_1 \ \vec{v}_2]$$

is nonsingular. The transformation

$$\vec{x} = V\vec{z}$$

transforms the system

$$\dot{\vec{x}} = A\vec{x}$$

into

$$\dot{\vec{z}} = V^{-1}AV\vec{z} = \Lambda\vec{z}.$$

The solutions of the z system are given by

$$\vec{z}(t) = e^{(t-t_0)\Lambda} \vec{z}_0,$$

with transparent notation. The solutions of the x system are given by

$$\vec{x}(t) = V\vec{z}(t) = Ve^{(t-t_0)\Lambda}\vec{z}_0 = Ve^{(t-t_0)\Lambda}V^{-1}\vec{x}_0.^6$$

As for the asymptotic directions, in the case of an improper node the preponderant *asymptotic direction* is that of the

$$\begin{cases} z_1 \text{ axis } (z_2 = 0), \text{ i.e., the vector } \vec{v}_1 \text{ iff } \lambda_2 < \lambda_1 < 0 \text{ or } 0 < \lambda_1 < \lambda_2, \\ z_2 \text{ axis } (z_1 = 0), \text{ i.e., the vector } \vec{v}_2 \text{ iff } \lambda_1 < \lambda_2 < 0 \text{ or } 0 < \lambda_2 < \lambda_1. \end{cases}$$

In the case of a *saddle point*, the "incoming separatrix" is carried by the z_1 axis (i.e., by the line through the singular point in the direction of the vector $\vec{v}_1$) iff $\lambda_1 < 0 < \lambda_2$, and by the z_2 axis (i.e., by the similar line parallel to $\vec{v}_2$) iff $\lambda_2 < 0 < \lambda_1$.

EXERCISE

19. Implement all details of the preceding summary and give a complete description of the solutions of

$$\dot{\vec{x}} = A'\vec{x} \quad \text{and} \quad \dot{\vec{x}} = A''\vec{x}$$

with A' and A'' as defined in Exercise 17.

(2) If the 2×2 matrix A has two eigenvalues that are *real* and *equal*, say λ_0, as well as *nonzero*, then there are two possibilities.

(a) *Two* linearly independent vectors $\vec{v}_1$ and $\vec{v}_2$ satisfy the equation $A\vec{v} = \lambda_0\vec{v}$ or $(A - \lambda_0 I)\vec{v} = \vec{0}$. In this case a transformation is not even

---

[6] Again the origin, the unique singular point of $\dot{\vec{x}} = A\vec{x}$, is an attractor iff both λ_1 and λ_2 are negative.

needed: linear algebra shows that now $(A - \lambda_0 I)$ must be of rank 0. This is possible only if every element of $(A - \lambda_0 I)$ is zero. So

$$A = \lambda_0 I;$$

the general case coincides here with the canonical case.

(b) Only *one* vector $\vec{v}_1$ (except for a scalar coefficient) satisfies the equation $A\vec{v} = \lambda_0 \vec{v}$ or $(A - \lambda_0 I)\vec{v} = \vec{0}$. In this case the reader will show (Exercise 21) that the can take any vector $\vec{w}$, not a multiple of $\vec{v}_1$, and that then a real number γ exists so that, say,

$$(A - \lambda_0 I)\vec{w} = \gamma\vec{v}_1 = \vec{u}.$$

Then

$$A[\vec{u} \quad \vec{w}] = [A\vec{u} \quad A\vec{w}] = [\lambda_0\vec{u} \quad \vec{u} + \lambda_0\vec{w}] = [\vec{u} \quad \vec{w}]\begin{bmatrix} \lambda_0 & 1 \\ 0 & \lambda_0 \end{bmatrix}.$$

Denoting $[\vec{u} \quad \vec{w}]$ by V and

$$\begin{bmatrix} \lambda_0 & 1 \\ 0 & \lambda_0 \end{bmatrix}$$

by Λ, we are back to

$$AV = V\Lambda.$$

The reader can complete the transformation of the present general case to the former special case (2) (b). The *asymptotic direction* of the orbits approaching the singular point is that of the z_1-axis, i.e. of the vector $\vec{v}_1$.

EXERCISES

20. Implement this procedure for $\dot{\vec{x}} = A\vec{x}$ with

$$A = \begin{bmatrix} -1 & 1 \\ -9 & 5 \end{bmatrix}.$$

21. In the development of point (2) (b), the following results for 2×2 matrices A were used.
    (α) If $\det(A - \lambda I) = 0$ has two equal roots λ_0, then every element of the matrix $(A - \lambda_0 I)^2$ is zero (a matter of patient, elementary algebra).
    (β) Defining $\vec{u} = (A - \lambda_0 I)\vec{w}$, show that $(A - \lambda_0 I)\vec{u} = \vec{0}$, which means that $\vec{u} = \gamma\vec{v}_1$. Why?
    (γ) $V = [\vec{u}\vec{w}]$ is nonsingular provided $\vec{w}$ is chosen not to be a multiple of $\vec{v}_1$. Prove.

(3), (4) If the 2×2 matrix A has two eigenvalues that are complex and different, say $\alpha + i\beta$ and $\alpha - i\beta$ with $\beta \neq 0$, and if $\vec{u}$ is the eigenvector corresponding to the eigenvalue $\alpha + i\beta$,

$$A\vec{u} = (\alpha + i\beta)\vec{u},$$

then the components of $\vec{u}$ obviously cannot be real or pure imaginary (why not?). So put

$$\vec{u} = \vec{v} + i\vec{w}, \text{ with } \vec{v} \neq \vec{0}, \vec{w} \neq \vec{0},$$

where the components of $\vec{v}$ and $\vec{w}$ are real. Taking the real and the imaginary part of the resulting equality,

$$A(\vec{v} + i\vec{w}) = (\alpha + i\beta)(\vec{v} + i\vec{w}),$$

we find

$$A\vec{v} = \alpha\vec{v} - \beta\vec{w}$$

$$A\vec{w} = \beta\vec{v} + \alpha\vec{w}.$$

EXERCISE

22. Prove that $\vec{v}$ and $\vec{w}$ are linearly independent. Because of the result of Exercise 15, we only need to prove that $c_1\vec{v} + c_2\vec{w} = \vec{0}$ entails that c_1 and c_2 cannot be both different from zero: the only remaining possibility is that both are zero, which proves our claim. Suppose c_1 and c_2 are both nonzero. Then

$$c_1\vec{v} = -c_2\vec{w}.$$

Show that the above equality $A(\vec{v} + i\vec{w}) = (\alpha + i\beta)(\vec{v} + i\vec{w})$ then yields

$$A\vec{w} = (\alpha + i\beta)\vec{w},$$

which contradicts $\beta \neq 0$. Why? So the assumption that $c_1 \neq 0$, $c_2 \neq 0$, leads to a contradiction. Hence $c_1 = 0 = c_2$; and $\vec{v}$ and $\vec{w}$ are linearly independent.

The pair of equations preceding Exercise 22 can be written as

$$AV = V\Lambda$$

where $V = [\vec{v} \ \ \vec{w}]$ is nonsingular and

$$\Lambda = \begin{bmatrix} \alpha & \beta \\ -\beta & \alpha \end{bmatrix}.$$

According to our usual method the solutions of

$$\dot{\vec{x}} = A\vec{x}$$

are of the form

$$\vec{x}(t) = V\vec{z}(t),$$

where

$$\vec{z}(t) = e^{(t-t_0)\alpha} \begin{bmatrix} c & s \\ -s & c \end{bmatrix} \vec{z}(t_0)$$

with $c = \cos \beta(t - t_0)$, $s = \sin \beta(t - t_0)$, $\vec{z}(t_0) = V^{-1}\vec{x}(t_0)$. Thus $\vec{z}(t)$ satisfies the equality

$$\vec{z}^T(t)\vec{z}(t) = e^{2(t-t_0)\alpha}\vec{z}^T(t_0)\vec{z}(t_0).$$

It follows that if $\alpha \gtreqless 0$, the point $\vec{z}(t)$, describing a solution curve, finds itself on

$$\left\{ \begin{array}{l} \text{gradually smaller} \\ \text{one and the same} \\ \text{gradually bigger} \end{array} \right\}$$

circle perimeter(s). The origin, a unique singular point for this system, is in these three respective cases

$$\left\{ \begin{array}{l} \text{attractor} \\ \text{center} \\ \text{repulsor} \end{array} \right\}.$$

Similarly, in terms of $\vec{x}(t)$,

$$\vec{x}^T(t)(VV^T)^{-1}\vec{x}(t) = e^{2(t-t_0)\alpha}\vec{x}_0^T(VV^T)^{-1}\vec{x}_0.$$

So, if $\alpha \gtreqless 0$, the point $\vec{x}(t)$, describing a solution curve, finds itself on

$$\left\{ \begin{array}{l} \text{gradually smaller} \\ \text{one and the same} \\ \text{gradually bigger} \end{array} \right\}$$

ellipse perimeter(s). Again the origin (singular point) is an attractor iff $\alpha < 0$.

(5) One eigenvalue zero. The equation for the eigenvalues, $\det(A - \lambda I) = 0$, can be written as $\lambda^2 - \lambda(a_{11} + a_{22}) + a_{11}a_{22} - a_{12}a_{21} = 0$. One root is zero iff $a_{11}a_{22} = a_{12}a_{21}$, which amounts to

(α) $a_{11}/a_{21} = a_{12}/a_{22} = p^{-1}$, say; putting $a_{11} = a$ and $a_{12} = b$, we find

$$A = \begin{bmatrix} a & b \\ pa & pb \end{bmatrix};$$

(β) $a_{12} = 0 = a_{22}$, special case of (α) (elaborate!);
(γ) $a_{22} = 0 = a_{21}$, special case of (α) (elaborate!);
(δ) other choices of zero elements reduce to (β) or (γ) by reassignment of subscripts.

Note that the other eigenvalue is nonzero iff in case (α) $a + pb \neq 0$, in cases (β) and (γ) $a_{11} \neq 0$.

EXERCISE

23. Since cases (β), (γ), (δ) are all special cases of (α), we need to study only (α). Prove that the nonzero eigenvalue is $a + pb$; its eigenvector has components 1 and p;

the other eigenvector has components $-b$ and a; these two eigenvectors are linearly independent; finally,

$$AV = V\Lambda$$

with A as defined under point (α) above, and with

$$V = \begin{bmatrix} 1 & -b \\ p & a \end{bmatrix}, \qquad \Lambda = \begin{bmatrix} a + pb & 0 \\ 0 & 0 \end{bmatrix}.$$

The results of Exercise 23 show how our general case (5) reduces to the canonical case of (5) discussed earlier, where

$$A = \begin{bmatrix} \lambda & 0 \\ 0 & 0 \end{bmatrix}.$$

No singular point is an *attractor* in this system!

(6) *Both* eigenvalues *zero.* In the matrix A quoted under the above point (α) in (5) we must now put $a + pb = 0$. (Why?) This reduces matrix A to the special form

$$A = \begin{bmatrix} -pb & b \\ -p^2b & pb \end{bmatrix}.$$

We have to distinguish two cases here.

(6) (a) $b = 0$. Then A is of the same form as the previously discussed special case (6) (a), all elements of A equal to zero.

(b) $b \neq 0$, p *arbitrary.* The reader will show that now

$$AV = V\Lambda,$$

with

$$A = \begin{bmatrix} -pb & b \\ -p^2b & pb \end{bmatrix}, \qquad V = \begin{bmatrix} 1 & 0 \\ p & b^{-1} \end{bmatrix}, \qquad \Lambda = \begin{bmatrix} 0 & 1 \\ 0 & 0 \end{bmatrix}.$$

Note that V is nonsingular. The reader will find all singular points and verify that none of them is an attractor.

Remark 4. This concerns finding the asymptotic directions for nodes, the directions for the separatrices for saddle points, and the absence of asymptotic directions for spiral points. In Exercises 9–11 of this section, in the discussion preceding Exercise 19, and in the last line before Exercise 20, we made observations regarding asymptotic directions of orbits in the neighborhood of an improper *node*: the preponderant asymptotic direction is given by that eigenvector of the system's matrix A which corresponds to the eigenvalue which is closer to zero, and the exceptional asymptotic direction is given by the eigenvector corresponding to the other eigenvalue. Similarly, in Exercise 12, in the latter part of Remark 3, and in the discussion preceding Exercise 19 we showed that the direction of the incoming separatrix around a *saddle point* is given by that eigenvector of the system's matrix A which corresponds to the negative eigenvalue, whereas the direction of the outgoing separatrix is given by the eigenvector corresponding to the positive eigenvalue. A fast method is available for obtaining the slopes of these two important directions, which, however, drops the distinction between the two. However, in many cases, when you construct a diagram of the phase portrait and sketch the two directions, this distinction is evident from the quick-and-dirty isocline-and-arrow method. Thus let k_1 and k_2 be the slopes of the (preponderant and the exceptional) asymptotic directions around an improper node, or let k_1 and k_2 be the slopes of the (incoming and outgoing) separatrices around a saddle point. Then k_1 and k_2 are the roots of the quadratic equation

$$a_{12}k^2 + (a_{11} - a_{22})k - a_{21} = 0,$$

where

$$\begin{bmatrix} a_{11} & a_{12} \\ a_{21} & a_{22} \end{bmatrix} = A$$

is the matrix of the system $\dot{\vec{x}} = A\vec{x}$. Note that no real roots exist for k when

$$(a_{11} - a_{22})^2 + 4a_{12}a_{21} < 0.$$

The reader will have no difficulty in showing that eigenvalues of A are nonreal under the same condition. So *spiral points* can be identified on the basis of nothing but the just-introduced *k-equation*. The distinction between a node and a saddle point follows geometrically, from the isocline-and-arrow method, or analytically, from the signs of the eigenvalues of the matrix A. The distinction between stable and unstable nodes or spiral points follows from the signs of the real parts of the eigenvalues of A. The distinction between stable and unstable nodes also follows from the arrow method, but not the distinction between stable and unstable spiral points.

EXERCISE

24. Let λ_i be an eigenvalue of the 2×2 matrix A, and $\vec{v}_i$ be the corresponding eigenvector, with the components v_{1i} and v_{2i} $(i = 1, 2)$. Then the reader will show that

$$k_i = \frac{v_{2i}}{v_{1i}} = \frac{\lambda_i - a_{11}}{a_{12}}, \qquad i = 1, 2$$

$$k_1 + k_2 = \frac{\lambda_1 + \lambda_2 - 2a_{11}}{a_{12}} = \frac{a_{22} - a_{11}}{a_{12}}$$

$$k_1 k_2 = \frac{-a_{21}}{a_{12}}$$

which directly shows that k_1 and k_2 are the roots of

$$a_{12}k^2 + (a_{11} - a_{22})k - a_{21} = 0.$$

Elaborate this proof!

Remark 5. What if in $\dot{\vec{x}} = A\vec{x}$ the vector $\vec{x}$ is an *n-vector* and the matrix A is an $n \times n$ matrix, $n > 2$? There is then a much greater variety of possibilities, more or less completely recorded only for $n = 3$.[7] One result that carries over rather straightforwardly is the one about stability: when all eigenvalues λ of the matrix A have *strictly negative* real parts, then all solution curves approach the singular point $\vec{0}$ as $t \uparrow +\infty$. When all $\text{Re}\,\lambda > 0$, then all solutions $\rightarrow \vec{0}$ as $t \downarrow -\infty$. Whenever some eigenvalues have positive real parts and others have negative real parts, the situation is as in the above saddle points: a great many trajectories approach $\vec{0}$ to a degree, and then take off for infinity. We will not go into the finer points of *n*-dimensional phase portraits.

A.4 Linearization

What is called linearization consists of the following method of investigating the phase portrait locally, i.e., in the neighborhood of any singular point. Given the *non*linear autonomous differential system

$$\dot{\vec{x}}(t) = \vec{f}(\vec{x}(t)) \tag{A3}$$

with a singular point $\vec{\xi}$,

$$\vec{f}(\vec{\xi}) = \vec{0},$$

$\vec{f}$ mapping *n*-vector space into *n*-vector space, perform the following steps.

(1) Transform $\vec{x}(t) = \vec{\xi} + \vec{y}(t)$:

$$\dot{\vec{y}}(t) = \vec{f}(\vec{\xi} + \vec{y}(t)). \tag{A4}$$

(2) Develop the second member of (A4) in a truncated Taylor series,

$$\vec{f}(\vec{\xi} + \vec{y}) = \vec{f}(\vec{\xi}) + D\vec{f}(\vec{\xi}) \cdot \vec{y} + o(\|\vec{y}\|),$$

where $D\vec{f}(^-)$ is the matrix with (i, j)-element $D_j f_i(^-)$, that is, the value of the partial derivative of the *i*th component of the vector $\vec{f}(\vec{x})$ with respect to the *j*th variable x_j, evaluated at $\vec{x} = \vec{\xi}$. Note that $\vec{f}(\vec{\xi}) = \vec{0}$.

(3) Study the linear system

$$\dot{\vec{y}}(t) = D\vec{f}(\vec{\xi})\,\vec{y}(t), \tag{A5}$$

especially the behavior of its solutions in the neighborhood of $\vec{y} = \vec{0}$.

(4) Assert that in a *neighborhood* of $\vec{\xi}$ the (asymptotic) behavior of the tra-

---

[7] See J. W. Reyn, "Classification and description of the singular points of a system of three differential equations," *Z. Angew. Math. Phys.* vol. 15, pp. 540–557, 1964.

jectories of $\dot{x} = \vec{f}(\vec{x})$ is "like" that of the trajectories of $\dot{\vec{y}} = D\vec{f}(\vec{\xi})\vec{y}$ in a neighborhood of $\vec{0}$.

Essentially, then, the linearization method substitutes the study of (one or more) linear systems for the study of a nonlinear system in the neighborhood of its (one or more) singular points. The local results are valid only under certain conditions (concerning the *eigenvalues of $D\vec{f}(\vec{\xi})$* as well as the nature of the correction term $o(\|\vec{y}\|)$; and the word "like" in step 4 has to be clarified and specified. The proofs concerning this method are too complicated for our present purposes. We will first give a few examples and counterexamples, and then list some of the theorems. For the routine applications of the linearization method one does not do much else than investigate the λ equation and the k equation connected with the matrix $D\vec{f}(\vec{\xi})$.

EXERCISES

1. The differential equation $\dot{x} = x(1 - x)$ has two singular points, $x = 0$ and $x = 1$. By the linearization method show that $x = 0$ is unstable and $x = 1$ is stable. *Hint:* Since this equation is one-dimensional, we can execute the whole program as follows. Find the Taylor series around $x = 0$, and the Taylor series around $x = 1$. Find the substitute linear differential equations in y:

$$\dot{y} = y \qquad\qquad \dot{y} = -y$$
$$\Downarrow \qquad\qquad\qquad \Downarrow$$
$$y(t) = e^{t-t_0}y_0 \qquad y(t) = e^{-(t-t_0)}y_0.$$

The conclusions re stability and instability follow.

 *Alternatively, $Df(\vec{\xi})$ is just a real number here instead of a matrix, or equivalently, $Df(\xi)$ is a 1×1 matrix; its eigenvalue equals $Df(\xi)$. For $f(x) = x - x^2$, find $Df(x)$, $Df(0)$, $Df(1)$ and show that your conclusions as based on these eigenvalues are the same as those following from the first approach, where you actually solved the substitute linear systems.

2. The system

$$\begin{cases} \dot{x}_1 = x_1(\alpha_1 - b_{11}\log x_1 - b_{12}\log x_2) \\ \dot{x}_2 = x_2(\alpha_2 - b_{21}\log x_1 - b_{22}\log x_2) \end{cases} \tag{A6}$$

has (among others) a singular point at (ξ_1, ξ_2) as determined by

$$\begin{cases} b_{11}\log \xi_1 + b_{12}\log \xi_2 = \alpha_1 \\ b_{21}\log \xi_1 + b_{22}\log \xi_2 = \alpha_2 \end{cases}.$$

Find $D\vec{f}(\vec{\xi})$, preferably without solving the equations for $\vec{\xi}$, and show that the corresponding λ-equation is

$$\lambda^2 + (b_{11} + b_{22})\lambda + (b_{11}b_{22} - b_{12}b_{21}) = 0.$$

Also make the substitution $\log x_i = y_i$ in (A6), and in the resulting equations for y_i make the substitution $y_i = \eta_i + z_i$, where $\eta_i = \log \xi_i$. The singular point $\vec{z} = \vec{0}$ corresponds to $\vec{x} = \vec{\xi}$. The differential equation for $\vec{z}(t)$ can be solved explicitly and the solutions for $\vec{x}(t)$ can be expressed in terms of the $\vec{z}$ solutions. The reader may check that $\bar{\xi}$ is stable iff $b_{11}b_{22} - b_{12}b_{21} > 0, b_{11} + b_{22} > 0$: a) directly from the explicit solutions, or b) from the λ-equation. The reader may also check that $\bar{\xi}$ is a stable singular point for the $\bar{x}$ equation iff $\bar{0}$ is a stable singular point for the $\bar{z}$ equation. Note that the amount of algebra needed to find the λ equation from $Df(\bar{\xi})$ is negligible relative to finding the explicit form of the x solutions. If the reader is a glutton for work, he may want to put $\bar{x}(t) = \bar{\xi} + \bar{e}(t)$, find the differential system for $\bar{e}(t)$, develop the necessary Taylor series, and find the linear parts in $e_1(t)$ and $e_2(t)$. The result should be easy to explain in the light of the above.

3. The system

$$\begin{cases} \dot{x}_1 = -\lambda_1 x_1 + x_2^2 \\ \dot{x}_2 = x_1^2 - \lambda_2 x_2 \end{cases} \tag{A7}$$

has two singular points, $(0, 0)$ and $((\lambda_1\lambda_2^2)^{1/3}, (\lambda_1^2\lambda_2)^{1/3})$. Analyze $Df(\bar{x})$ at both points. Find the eigenvalues and the slopes of the important directions. If $0 < \lambda_1 < \lambda_2$, then the x_1 axis is the preponderant asymptotic direction around the origin. Sketch some trajectories in that area, in detail (as if under a microscope).

4.
$$\left.\begin{array}{l} \dot{x}_1 = -x_1 - \dfrac{x_2}{\log\sqrt{x_1^2 + x_2^2}} \\[2ex] \dot{x}_2 = -x_2 + \dfrac{x_1}{\log\sqrt{x_1^2 + x_2^2}} \end{array}\right\}, \qquad \text{for } \bar{x} \neq \bar{0} \\[2ex] \dot{\bar{x}} = \bar{0}, \qquad\qquad\qquad\qquad \text{for } \bar{x} = \bar{0}. \tag{A8}$$

The solutions of this system can be constructed explicitly for $x_1^2 + x_2^2 < 1 - \delta$, where $0 < \delta < 1$, and they come out quite different from the solutions of the linearized system (Exercise 6 to follow)

$$\begin{cases} \dot{x}_1 = -x_1 \\ \dot{x}_2 = -x_2 \end{cases}. \tag{A8a}$$

Whereas the solutions of (A8a) are $\bar{x}(t) = e^{-(t-t_0)}\bar{x}_0$, with trajectories in the phase plane,

$$x_2(t)/x_1(t) = x_{20}/x_{10}$$

(straight lines radiating from the singular point at the origin), the solutions of (A8) are found after introduction of polar coordinates: $x_1(t) = r(t)\cos\varphi(t)$, $x_2(t) = r(t)\sin\varphi(t)$. Equations (A8) then reduce to

$$\begin{cases} \dot{r}(t) = -r(t) \\[1ex] \dot{\varphi}(t) = \dfrac{1}{\log r(t)} \end{cases} \tag{A8b}$$

with solutions defined for $t \geq t_0$ by

$$\begin{cases} r(t) = e^{-(t-t_0)}r_0 \\ \varphi(t) = \varphi(t_0) - \log(t - t_0 - \log r_0) + \log(-\log r_0) \end{cases} \tag{A9}$$

Note that we are studying (A8) only for $x_1^2 + x_2^2 < 1 - \delta$; so $t - t_0 - \log r_0 > t - t_0 \geq 0$, for all times later than t_0. The most obvious feature of these solutions is that they are *spirals*, winding around the origin, differing indeed from the straight lines of (A8a).

5. Although a great deal of difference lies between the straight-line solutions of (A8a) and the spiral solutions (see (A9)) of (A8), the two do agree in one important respect: if they start at a point in the interior of the unit circle about the origin, then they tend to the origin in the limit, as $t \uparrow +\infty$. Check this! Note that the λ equation for (A8a) has nonzero roots. The reason for the discrepancy between the phase-portraits of (A8) and of (A8a) is that the remainder terms, $x_i/\log r$, where $r = \sqrt{x_1^2 + x_2^2}$, do not tend to zero fast enough (see the relevant theorems below).

6. In Exercise 4 it was asserted that (A8a) is the linearized system of (A8). That looks very plausible indeed, since the terms $x_i/\log r$ are nonlinear and tend to zero faster than the linear terms. However, the description given of the linearization method in the beginning of Section 4 of this appendix requires that we determine the matrix $D\vec{f}(\vec{0})$ (since the singular point of (A8) is the origin, cf. Exercise 7). The reader will now actually compute the elements of the matrix $D\vec{f}(\vec{0})$. *Hint*: It is vastly more efficient to compute these partial derivatives at the origin directly from their definition, such as

$$\lim_{h \to 0} \frac{f_1(h, 0) - f_1(0, 0)}{h},$$

than from their general expressions for arbitrary x_1 and x_2.

7. Prove that the origin is the only singular point of the system defined by (A8). *Hint*: Assume it is not; then multiply the first equation by x_1, the second by x_2, and add. You find that the singular point must satisfy the equation $x_1^2 + x_2^2 = 0$.

Whereas the few preceding examples illustrate the fact that stability and instability are the same between a nonlinear system and its linearization, even in the face of marked differences between the phase portraits, provided the λ values have *nonzero* real parts, the following few examples will illustrate the fact that practically all bets are off if the λ values have *zero* real parts. In such cases the linearized system may, for instance, show a continuum of singular points in any neighborhood of the unique singular point of the nonlinear system, thereby disrupting any similarity in asymptotic behavior between the two systems.

EXERCISES

8. Study the system

$$\begin{cases} \dot{x}_1 = x_1^3 \\ \dot{x}_2 = -x_2 \end{cases} \tag{A10}$$

and its linearization re its singular point,

$$\begin{cases} \dot{x}_1 = 0 \\ \dot{x}_2 = -x_2 \end{cases}. \tag{A10a}$$

The phase portrait of this linear system is a collection of half-lines parallel to the x_2 axis. The phase portrait of the nonlinear system bears a strong resemblance to that of a linear system with a saddle point at the origin. The reader will fill in the details. *Hint:* The trajectories of (A10) have the equation

$$x_2 = e^{1/(2x_1^2)} e^{-1/(2x_{10}^2)} x_{20}.$$

Note that these trajectories have different horizontal asymptotes.

9. Study the system

$$\left\{ \begin{aligned} \dot{x}_1 &= -x_1^3 \\ \dot{x}_2 &= -x_2 \end{aligned} \right\}$$

(A11)

and its linearization re its singular point,

$$\left\{ \begin{aligned} \dot{x}_1 &= 0 \\ \dot{x}_2 &= -x_2 \end{aligned} \right\}.$$

(A11a)

This linearized system is the same as in the preceding question, but the behavior of the nonlinear system is vastly different. The origin is now asymptotically stable in the large (i.e., wherever the initial point $\vec{x}_0$ is, the corresponding solution will tend to the origin in the limit as $t \uparrow +\infty$), and looks pretty much like a stable node, with principal asymptotic direction that of the x_1 axis, and with the x_2 axis as carrier of two trajectories. *Hint:* The trajectories are now determined by

$$x_2 = e^{-1/(2x_1^2)} e^{+1/(2x_{10}^2)} x_{20}.$$

As $t \uparrow +\infty$, $x_2(t)/x_{20} \downarrow 0$ and $|x_1(t)| \downarrow 0$. Show that for every trajectory (except the two carried by the x_2 axis, and the origin itself):

$$\frac{x_2}{x_1} \downarrow 0 \quad \text{as} \quad |x_1| \downarrow 0,$$

which shows that all these trajectories have the x_1 axis as asymptotic tangent line. What happens as $|x_1| \uparrow +\infty$? Sketch the trajectories!

10. Study the system

$$\left\{ \begin{aligned} \dot{x}_1 &= x_1^2 \\ \dot{x}_2 &= -x_2 \end{aligned} \right\}.$$

(A12)

One half of the phase portrait looks like that of (A10), the other half like that of (A11). Elaborate!

11. Study the system

$$\left\{ \begin{aligned} \dot{x}_1 &= -x_2 + x_1(1 - r^2)r \\ \dot{x}_2 &= +x_1 + x_2(1 - r^2)r \end{aligned} \right\},$$

(A13)

where $r = \sqrt{x_1^2 + x_2^2} \geq 0$. Change to polar coordinates: $x_1 = r \cos \varphi$, $x_2 = r \sin \varphi$, and find

$$\left\{ \begin{aligned} \dot{r} &= (1 - r^2)r^2, \\ \dot{\varphi} &= 1, \end{aligned} \quad (r \geq 0) \right\}.$$

(A13a)

The first equation can be written as

$$\frac{\dot{r}}{r^2} + \frac{1}{2}\frac{\dot{r}}{1-r} + \frac{1}{2}\frac{\dot{r}}{1+r} = 1$$

which can be integrated to

$$e^{t-t_0} = e^{-(1/r)+(1/r_0)} \cdot \sqrt{\frac{1+r}{1+r_0}\cdot\frac{1-r_0}{1-r}}, \qquad r_0 > 0.$$

This equation shows (why?) that when $0 < r_0 < 1$, then $r = r(t)$ will for all $t > t_0$ remain in the open interval $]0, 1[$. For $0 < r < 1$ the second member of this equation is a monotone increasing function of r. So this equation does define r as a function of t. Prove that as $t \uparrow +\infty, r = r(t) \uparrow 1$. Noting that $\varphi(t) = t - t_0$, we find that the solutions of (A13) consist of outward spirals toward the unit circle (given $0 < r_0 < 1$): the origin is an *unstable spiral point*. The linearization of (A13),

$$\begin{cases} \dot{x}_1 = -x_2 \\ \dot{x}_2 = +x_1 \end{cases}, \tag{A13b}$$

has, however, a phase portrait consisting entirely of circles around the origin, which therefore is a *center* for (A13b).

Among the many theorems re linearization, which are discussed in great detail in Andronov *et al.* [4] as well as in E. A. Coddington and N. Levinson, [10, ch. 15],[8] we mention only a few. All refer to the situation in which the singular point under scrutiny is the origin (because of the transformation from (A3) to (A4) this does not hurt generality). All refer to the case in which the matrix $Df(0)$ is nonsingular, in fact to the case in which the eigenvalues of this matrix have *nonzero real parts*. Furthermore, certain restrictions need to be imposed on the nonlinear part of $\vec{f}(\vec{x})$, that is, on $\vec{f}(\vec{x}) - Df(0)\cdot\vec{x}$, even in the weaker theorem(s), viz., those on stability rather than on the shape of the phase portrait. First we will discuss (local) stability, then mode of approach to the singular point.

Theorem A1. *Consider the differential equation*

$$\dot{\vec{x}} = \vec{f}(\vec{x}). \tag{A14}$$

Let $\vec{f}(0) = \vec{0}$. *Let all eigenvalues of the matrix* $Df(0)$ *have negative real part. Let*

$$\vec{f}(\vec{x}) - Df(0)\cdot\vec{x} = o(\|\vec{x}\|). \tag{A15}$$

Then the origin is an attractor for the equation $\dot{\vec{x}} = \vec{f}(\vec{x})$. *(For an example, see Exercise 12 to follow.)*

Terminology. The meaning of (A15) is this:

---

[8] See also L. Cesari, *Asymptotic Behavior and Stability Problems in Ordinary Differential Equations*. New York: Springer, 1963, sec. 9.1.

$$\lim_{\vec{x} \to 0} \frac{\|\vec{f}(\vec{x}) - D\vec{f}(0) \cdot \vec{x}\|}{\|\vec{x}\|} = 0. \qquad (A15)$$

Here the vertical bars denote "norm of." The three most-used versions of norms will be

$$\|\vec{y}\| = \sqrt{y_1^2 + y_2^2}, \qquad \|\vec{y}\| = |y_1| + |y_2|, \qquad \|\vec{y}\| = \max(|y_1|, |y_2|).$$

The phrase, "the origin is an *attractor* for the equation $\dot{\vec{x}} = \vec{f}(\vec{x})$," needs to be defined more carefully for nonlinear equations than for linear ones. It is used here to mean the following. A real number $\varepsilon > 0$ exists such that each solution $\vec{x}(t)$ of our equation that at some time τ satisfies

$$\|\vec{x}(\tau)\| < \varepsilon,$$

exists for *all* $t > \tau$ and has the property that

$$\lim_{t \uparrow \infty} \|\vec{x}(t)\| = 0.$$

Remark 1. Note that $\|\vec{y}\| < \alpha$ has a slightly different meaning, varying with the definition of norm in use at the moment. The reader will not find it difficult to show that, according to the first definition,

$$\|\vec{y}\| < \alpha \text{ implies } |y_1| < \alpha \text{ and } |y_2| < \alpha;$$
$$|y_1| < \alpha/\sqrt{2} \text{ and } |y_2| < \alpha/\sqrt{2} \text{ imply } \|y\| < \alpha.$$

Similarly, according to the second definition,

$$\|\vec{y}\| < \alpha \text{ implies } |y_1| < \alpha \text{ and } |y_2| < \alpha;$$
$$|y_1| < \alpha/2 \text{ and } |y_2| < \alpha/2 \text{ imply } \|\vec{y}\| < \alpha.$$

Similarly, according to the third definition,

$$\|\vec{y}\| < \alpha \text{ implies } |y_1| < \alpha \text{ and } |y_2| < \alpha;$$
$$|y_1| < \alpha \text{ and } |y_2| < \alpha \text{ imply } \|\vec{y}\| < \alpha.$$

Consequently, according to any of those definitions,

$$\lim_{t \uparrow \infty} \|\vec{x}(t)\| = 0 \quad \text{iff} \quad \lim_{t \uparrow \infty} x_1(t) = 0 \text{ and } \lim_{t \uparrow \infty} x_2(t) = 0.$$

EXERCISE

12. Consider the equation

$$\begin{cases} \dot{x}_1 = a_{11}x_1 + a_{12}x_2 + b_{11}x_1^2 + 2b_{12}x_1x_2 + b_{22}x_2^2 \\ \dot{x}_2 = a_{21}x_1 + a_{22}x_2 + c_{11}x_1^2 + 2c_{12}x_1x_2 + c_{22}x_2^2 \end{cases}. \qquad (A16)$$

Prove that this equation satisfies (A15) no matter what definition of norm is used. *Hint:* Show that what you want to prove is equivalent to

$$\lim_{\vec{x} \to 0} \frac{b_{11}x_1^2 + 2b_{12}x_1x_2 + b_{22}x_2^2}{\sqrt{x_1^2 + x_1^2}} = 0,$$

and do the same with c instead of b; then switch to polar coordinates. Therefore, as soon as in (A16) the matrix A, with elements a_{ij}, has eigenvalues with negative real parts, the origin is an attractor.

Note that many of the examples in the main text of this module present such polynomials as occur in (A16). So the version of *Theorem A1* that is *used most often* is the version of Exercise 12: all you need to do with these polynomial models is to check the eigenvalues of the matrix of the linear part!

EXERCISE

13. Show that Theorem A1 also takes care of (A8) in Exercise 4. It proves that the origin is an attractor for equation (A8).

14. Theorem A1 can not take care of the differential equations discussed in Exercises 8–10. Why not?

Theorem A2. *Consider the differential equation*

$$\dot{\vec{x}} = \vec{f}(\vec{x}),$$

with $\vec{f}(\vec{0}) = \vec{0}$. *If the origin is a* spiral point *for the equation*

$$\dot{\vec{x}} = D\vec{f}(\vec{0}) \cdot \vec{x}$$

and if

$$\vec{f}(\vec{x}) - D\vec{f}(\vec{0}) \cdot \vec{x} = o(\|\vec{x}\|),$$

then the origin is also a spiral point for

$$\dot{\vec{x}} = \vec{f}(\vec{x}).$$

Terminology. The phase "the origin is a *spiral point* for the equation $\dot{\vec{x}} = \vec{f}(\vec{x})$" needs to be defined more carefully for nonlinear equations than for linear ones. It is used here to mean either one of two things: a *stable* spiral point or an *unstable* spiral point. The origin is a stable spiral point iff 1) the origin is an attractor (mind the role of $t \uparrow \infty$ in that definition), and 2) in polar coordinates the solutions

$$\begin{cases} x_1(t) = r(t)\cos\varphi(t) \\ x_2(t) = r(t)\sin\varphi(t) \end{cases}$$

have the properties that $r(t) \to 0$ as $t \uparrow \infty$ (which tells nothing but that the origin is an attractor) *and* $|\varphi(t)| \uparrow \infty$ (this is what makes $\vec{0}$ a spiral point). The definition of the origin being an unstable spiral point is obtained from that of a stable spiral point by time reversal: put $t = -T$ and write all definitions with T instead of t.

Remark 2. Theorem A2 is somewhat remarkable in that it makes a statement about the *mode of approach* of the solution curves to the singular point, not just about stability or instability, under a rather *weak condition*, viz.

$$\vec{f}(\vec{x}) - D\vec{f}(0) \cdot \vec{x} = o(\|\vec{x}\|).$$

The example discussed in Exercise 4 shows that this condition is not enough to keep a singular point a proper node under the transition from linearity to nonlinearity, but the spiral point property is apparently a bit sturdier. (For completeness' sake, we should mention that Coddington and Levinson [10, p. 378] point out that under this weak condition a spiral point may cease to be "proper" under the transition from linearity to nonlinearity, but we will not discuss this fine point.)

EXERCISE

15. The behavior of centers is quite the opposite from that of spiral points. If the origin is a center for

$$\dot{\vec{x}} = D\vec{f}(0) \cdot \vec{x}$$

then the origin may be a center, or a stable spiral point, or an unstable spiral point for

$$\dot{\vec{x}} = \vec{f}(\vec{x}),$$

even when the nonlinear part of $\vec{f}(\vec{x})$ satisfies more stringent conditions than (A15). Check this for the following three equations

$$\begin{cases} \dot{x}_1 = & x_2 + x_2 r \\ \dot{x}_2 = -x_1 & - x_1 r \end{cases}, \begin{cases} \dot{x}_1 = & x_2 - x_1 r \\ \dot{x}_2 = -x_1 & - x_2 r \end{cases}, \begin{cases} \dot{x}_1 = & x_2 + x_1 r \\ \dot{x}_2 = -x_1 & + x_2 r \end{cases}$$

where $r = \sqrt{x_1^2 + x_2^2}$. Another example of a nonlinear equation having a center at the same time as its linearization is given by the classical Volterra predator–prey model (see Section 2.1, Exercise 3).

Theorem A3. *Consider the differential equation ($\vec{x}$ being a 2-vector)*

$$\dot{\vec{x}} = \vec{f}(\vec{x}),$$

with $\vec{f}(0) = \vec{0}$. Let

$$\vec{f}(\vec{x}) - D\vec{f}(0) \cdot \vec{x} = o(\|\vec{x}\|).$$

Let the eigenvalues of $D\vec{f}(0)$ be real, strictly negative, and unequal, say $\lambda_2 < \lambda_1 < 0$. Then as $t \uparrow \infty$, every orbit of $\dot{\vec{x}} = \vec{f}(\vec{x})$, provided it starts close enough to 0, tends to the singular point $\vec{0}$ in one of four specific directions, an infinite number of orbits in the directions of $\vec{v}_1$ and $-\vec{v}_1$, and at least one orbit in each of the directions of $\vec{v}_2$ and $-\vec{v}_2$. Here $\vec{v}_1$ is the eigenvector of $D\vec{f}(0)$ corresponding to λ_1, and $\vec{v}_2$ is the eigenvector of $D\vec{f}(0)$ corresponding to λ_2.

Under stronger conditions re the nonlinear part of $\vec{f}(\vec{x})$, the local phase

portrait of our nonlinear equation is exactly like that of its linearization:
one orbit in the direction of $\vec{v}_2$, and *one* in the direction of $-\vec{v}_2$. An example
of such stronger conditions is the *continuity* of the *derivatives of* $\vec{f}(\vec{x})$ in a
neighborhood (nbhd) of the *singular point*:

$$D_j f_i(x_1, x_2) \text{ continuous in a nbhd of } \vec{0}.$$

Note that *polynomial* equations, such as those given by (A16) in Exercise 12,
satisfy these more stringent conditions: their local phase portrait is just
like that of their linearization.

Remark 3. If in *Theorem A3* the two strictly negative eigenvalues are allowed
to be equal, then Exercise 4 shows that the singular point $\vec{0}$ may well be a
spiral point for $\dot{\vec{x}} = \vec{f}(\vec{x})$. However, if $\vec{0}$ is a proper node for the linearization
of $\dot{\vec{x}} = \vec{f}(\vec{x})$ at $\vec{0}$, i.e., if $D\vec{f}(\vec{0})$ is a diagonal matrix with equal elements, and
if *in addition*

$$\vec{f}(\vec{x}) - D\vec{f}(\vec{0}) \cdot \vec{x} = o(\|\vec{x}\|^{1+\varepsilon}), \qquad \varepsilon > 0, \tag{A17}$$

then the singular point $\vec{0}$ will be a proper node for the nonlinear equation
$\dot{\vec{x}} = \vec{f}(\vec{x})$ as well. Note that condition (A17) imposes a stricter degree of
smallness on $\vec{f}(\vec{x}) - D\vec{f}(\vec{0}) \cdot \vec{x}$ than Theorem A3.

EXERCISE

16. Condition (A17) is satisfied, with $\varepsilon = \frac{1}{2}$, by (A16). Prove!

The last theorem we will quote concerns saddle points.

Theorem A4. *Consider the differential equation* ($\vec{x}$ *being a 2-vector*)

$$\dot{\vec{x}} = \vec{f}(\vec{x}),$$

with $\vec{f}(\vec{0}) = \vec{0}$. *Let* $D\vec{f}(\vec{0}) = A$ *have* two *unequal,* real *eigenvalues with*

$$\lambda_1 < 0 < \lambda_2,$$

and let the first-order partial derivatives of $\vec{f}(\vec{x})$ *exist and be continuous on a
neighborhood of the singular point* $\vec{0}$. *Then as* $t \uparrow \infty$, *exactly one orbit of*
$\dot{\vec{x}} = \vec{f}(\vec{x})$ *tends to the singular point* $\vec{0}$ *in the direction of* $\vec{v}_1$, *and another in the
direction of* $-\vec{v}_1$. *Again as* $t \downarrow -\infty$, *exactly one orbit of* $\dot{\vec{x}} = \vec{f}(\vec{x})$ *tends to the
singular point* $\vec{0}$ *in the direction of* $\vec{v}_2$, *and another in the direction of* $-\vec{v}_2$. *All
the other orbits eventually get away from* $\vec{0}$, *both as* $t \uparrow \infty$ *and as* $t \downarrow -\infty$.
*In other words, a saddle point remains a saddle point when we go from a
linear system to a nonlinear one under the above conditions, and the initial
directions of the separatrices are determined just as in the linear systems.*

Remark 4. All the above theorems and discussions were concerned with the
point $\vec{0}$ as a singular point of

$$\dot{\vec{x}} = \vec{f}(\vec{x}).$$

Now suppose $\vec{\xi}$ is a singular point of the same equation, i.e., $\vec{f}(\vec{\xi}) = \vec{0}$. Then put $\vec{x} = \vec{y} + \vec{\xi}$: it follows that, say,

$$\dot{\vec{y}} = \vec{f}(\vec{\xi} + \vec{y}) = \vec{g}(\vec{y}).$$

Consequently, $\vec{g}(\vec{0}) = \vec{f}(\vec{\xi})$ and $D\vec{g}(\vec{0}) = D\vec{f}(\vec{\xi})$. Thus the linearization method re the singular point $\vec{\xi}$ of $\dot{\vec{x}} = \vec{f}(\vec{x})$ amounts to the study of the matrix $D\vec{f}(\vec{\xi})$ instead of $D\vec{f}(\vec{0})$, and of the "nonlinear part" $\vec{f}(\vec{x}) - D\vec{f}(\vec{\xi}) \cdot (\vec{x} - \vec{\xi}) = \vec{g}(\vec{y}) - D\vec{g}(\vec{0}) \cdot \vec{y}$ instead of $\vec{f}(\vec{x}) - D\vec{f}(\vec{0}) \cdot \vec{x}$. Except for this modification, all theorems remain valid for the study of singular points $\vec{\xi}$.

Remark 5. The reader should go over all theorems and practice time-reversal, $t = -T$. This causes all eigenvalues to switch signs. Watch how this affects the conclusions.

EXAMPLE. Consider the equation

$$\begin{cases} \dot{x}_1 = x_1(\varepsilon_1 - \alpha_1 x_1 - \beta_1 x_2) \\ \dot{x}_2 = x_2(\varepsilon_2 + \alpha_2 x_1 - \beta_2 x_2) \end{cases}, \qquad \begin{cases} 0 < \varepsilon_2 \beta_1 < \varepsilon_1 \beta_2 \\ 0 < \alpha_i; 0 < \beta_i \end{cases}.$$

Singular points are $(0, 0)$, $(0, \varepsilon_2/\beta_2)$, $(\varepsilon_1/\alpha_1, 0)$, (ξ_1, ξ_2), where

$$\begin{cases} \varepsilon_1 - \alpha_1 \xi_1 - \beta_1 \xi_2 = 0 \\ \varepsilon_2 + \alpha_2 \xi_1 - \beta_2 \xi_2 = 0 \end{cases} \Rightarrow \xi_1 > 0 \text{ and } \xi_2 > 0.$$

Find $D\vec{f}(\vec{\xi})$ at each of these four singular points, check the nature of the relevant nonlinear parts, and determine the asymptotic directions or separatrices, as the case may be. The partial answer is that in the order given the above four singular points are an unstable node, a saddle point, a saddle point, and a stable node.

Appendix B: Bibliography

Section 1.3 presents a short list of journals in which ongoing research is published that should be of interest to the reader. Section 1.3 also gives a short list of fairly recent books in the general area of ecosystems. Most of the titles here, are listed simply to recognize the source of certain statements or ideas discussed in the text. Those are not at all crucial to the successful teaching of this module, and the instructor need not hunt for them unless the wish arises to expand upon certain topics. After each title one finds the section(s) of the module in which it is mentioned. A very few books are essential or very desirable to have around as a supplement to the written text. Most of these are available in fairly cheap paperbacks; they are indicated by the words *essential* or *very desirable*.

References

[1]   J. K. Aggarwal, *Notes on Nonlinear Systems*. New York: Van Nostrand, 1972, 214 pp.; in the paperback series "Notes on System Sciences." One of the titles mentioned at the end of Remark 5 in Section 2.1, it would be *very desirable* to have one of these around, and the present one is an inexpensive paperback.

[2]   W. C. Allee, A. E. Emerson, O. Park, T. Park, and K. P. Schmidt, *Principles of Animal Ecology*. Philadelphia: Saunders, 1949, 837 pp. See Sections 1.1 and 3. If the library on your campus has it, it is worthwhile for you and your students to have a good look at it, but don't have it ordered.

[3]   U.d'Ancona, *The Struggle for Existence*, A. Charles and R. F. L. Withers, Trs., vol. 6 of Bibliotheca Biotheoretica. Leiden: Brill, 1954, 274 pp. Available in hardcover and in paperback. See Sections 1.1, 1.2, 2.1 (Exercise 3), and 4. It is *very desirable*, in fact almost *essential*, to have this book available (for the instructor).

[4]   A. A. Andronov, E. A. Leontovich, I. I. Gordon, and A. G. Maier, *Qualitative Theory of Second-Order Dynamic Systems*. New York: Wiley, 1973, 524 pp. (Translated from a 1966 Russian edition.) One of the titles mentioned at the end of Remark 5 in Section 2.1, it would be *very desirable* to have one of these around. The present one is unusually detailed and exhaustive, but very expensive, and it does not discuss systems of dimension larger than two.

[5]   F. J. Ayala, "Competition, Coexistence, and Evolution," in *Essays in Evolution and Genetics in Honor of Th. Dobzhansky: A Supplement to Evolutionary Biology*, M. K. Hecht and W. C. Steere, Eds. New York: Appleton-Century-Crofts, 1970, pp. 121–158. See Section 3.3.

[6]   J. Balogh, Lebensgemeinschaften der Landtiere; ihre Erforschung unter besonderer Berücksichtigung der zoozönologischen Arbeitsmethoden; Budapest, Verlag der Ungarischen Akademie der Wissenschaften, and Berlin, Akademie-Verlag; 1958, 560 pp. See Section 1.1.

[7]   M. S. Bartlett, "Monte Carlo studies in ecology and epidemiology," in *Proc. 4th Berkeley Symp. on Mathematical Statistics and Probability*, vol. 4, J. Neyman, Ed. Berkeley, CA: Univ. of California Press, 1961, pp. 39–55. See Section 1.5.

[8]   M. Boudart, *Kinetics of Chemical Processes*. Englewood Cliffs, NJ: Prentice-Hall, 1968, 246 pp. See Section 2.1.

[9]   F. Brauer and J. A. Nohel, *The Qualitative Theory of Ordinary Differential Equations; An Introduction*. New York: Benjamin, 1969, 314 pp. One of the titles mentioned at the end of Remark 5 in Section 2.1, it would be *very desirable* to have one of these around. The present one is hardcover but not exceedingly expensive.

[10]   E. A. Coddington and N. Levinson, *Theory of Ordinary Differential Equations*. New York: McGraw-Hill, 1955, 429 pp. See Section A.4, Appendix A, before Theorem A1 and before Exercise 15.

[11]   W. A. Coppel, "A survey of quadratic systems," *J. Differential Equations*, vol. 2, pp. 293–304, 1966. See Section 4, Exercise 8.

[12]   H. Ellenberg, Ed., *Integrated Experimental Ecology; Methods and Results of Ecosystem Research in the German Solling Project*. New York: Springer, 1971, 214 pp. (of which pp. 1–15 carry an introductory survey by H. Ellenberg). See Section 1.1. The book is vol. 2 of the series, *Ecological Studies, Analysis and Synthesis*.

[13]   T. I. Êman, "O Nekotoryh Matematičeskih Modeliah Biogeocenozov," *Problemy Kibernetiki* (pod red. A. A. Liapunova) vol. 16, pp. 191–202, 1966, Moskva, Izd. Nauka. See Sections 2.2 and 4, (Exercise 7).

[14]   W. Feller, "Die Grundlagen der Volterraschen Theorie des Kampfes ums Dasein

in wahrscheinlichkeitstheoretischer Behandlung," *Acta Biotheoretica*, vol. 5, pp. 11–40. See Section 1.5. A famous paper, often quoted as starting the "stochastization" of deterministic models; not essential for the present purposes.

[15] *Feynman's Lectures in Physics*, vol. 1. Reading, MA: Addison-Wesley, 1963, 1965. See Section 1.5, point (γ). Sections 8-2, 8-3, and 9-5 of Feynman's book exemplify the classical argument for the derivative as a measure of speed or rate.

[16] S. E. Flanders and M. E. Badgley, "Prey–predator interactions in self-balanced laboratory populations, *Hilgardia*, vol. 35, pp. 145–183. See Section 2.2.

[17] G. F. Gause, *The Struggle for Existence*. New York: Dover, 1971, 163 pp. *Very desirable*. This paperback is well worth the price. The book gives a number of graphs representing data. See Sections 1.2, 1.5, 2.2, 3.3.

[18] ——, "Experimental demonstration of Volterra's periodic oscillations in the number of animals," *J. Experimental Biology*, vol. 12, pp. 44–48, 1935. See Section 1.2. This article has graphs of the same type as [17], but with experimentally controlled reproduction rates.

[19] M. E. Gilpin and F. J. Ayala, "Global models of growth and competition," *Proc. Nat. Acad. Sci. USA*, vol. 70, pp. 3590–3593, 1973. See Section 3.2, Exercise 1 and Section 3.3, Remark 1.

[20] M. E. Gilpin and K. E. Justice, "Reinterpretation of the invalidation of the principle of competitive exclusion, *Nature*, vol. 236, pp. 273–301, 1972. See Section 3.3, also Remark 1 therein.

[21] N. S. Goel, S. C. Maitra, and E. W. Montroll, *On the Volterra and Other Non-linear Models of Interacting Populations*. New York: Academic, 1971, 145 pp. (Reprinted from *Reviews of Modern Physics*, vol. 43, pp. 231–276, 1971.) See Sections 1.3, 2.1 (Remark 6), and 4. Too advanced; also contains errors.

[22] J. Gomatam, "A new model for interacting populations-I: Two-species systems," *Bulletin of Mathematical Biology*, vol. 36, pp. 347–353, 1974. See Section 2.2, equations (15) and (16).

[23] ——, "A new model for interacting populations-II: Principle of competitive exclusion," *Bulletin of Mathematical Biology*, vol. 36, (1974) pp. 355–364, 1974. See Sections 3.2 (Exercise 1) and 3.3.

[24] D. Greenspan, *Arithmetic Applied Mathematics*. Elsmford, NY: Pergamon, 1980, 172 pp. See Section 1.6, Remark 1. Available in hardcover and softcover.

[25] G. Hardin, "The competitive exclusion principle," *Science*, vol. 131, pp. 1292–1297, 1960. See Section 3.3.

[26] M. P. Hassell, *The Dynamics of Arthropod Predator–Prey Systems*. Princeton, NJ: Princeton Univ. Press, 1978, 237 pp. See Section 1.3.

[27] M. W. Hirsch and S. Smale, *Differential Equations, Dynamical Systems, and Linear Algebra*. New York: Academic, 1974, 358 pp. See Section 2.1, Discussion Question 3.

[28] C. S. Holling, "The functional response of invertebrate predators to prey density," *Memoirs Entomological Soc. of Canada*, vol. 48, pp. 1–86, 1966. See Section 2.2 (after Exercise 5). This paper could, together with [69], form a basis of a student project concerning some details of model building.

[29] C. S. Holling and S. Ewing, "Blind man's buff: Exploring the response space generated by realistic ecological simulation models," in *Statistical Ecology*, vol. 2, G. P. Patil *et al.*, Eds. University Park, PA: Pennsylvania State Univ. Press, 1971, pp. 207–233. See Section 2.2, Discussion Question 2.

[30] C. B. Huffaker, "Experimental studies on predation: Dispersion factors and predator-prey oscillations," *Hilgardia*, vol. 27, pp. 343–383, 1958. Reprinted in *Readings in Population and Community Ecology*, W. E. Hazen, Ed. Philadelphia, PA: Saunders, 1964, pp. 164–204. See Sections 1.5 (first paragraph), 2.2 (first paragraph), and 2.3 (Remark 2). Huffaker describes extensive experiments,

highlighting certain tensions between reality and certain models discussed in our chapter. Hazen's book of readings has more papers of interest; it would be *desirable* to have this paperback available. Huffaker's paper is also quoted by Leigh [38].

[31] W. Hurewicz, *Lectures on Ordinary Differential Equations*. Cambridge, MA: M.I.T. Press, 1964, 122 pp. (paperback). One of the titles mentioned at the end of Remark 5 in Section 2.1, it would be *very desirable* to have one of these around, and the present one is an inexpensive paperback (beautiful, but a bit more abstract than Aggarwal).

[32] D. L. Iglehart, "Multivariate competition processes," *Ann. Math. Stat.*, vol. 35, pp. 350–361, 1964; also see D. L. Iglehart, "Reversible competition processes," *Z.f. Wahrscheinlichkeitstheorie und verwandte Gebiete*, vol. 2, pp. 314–331, 1964. See Section 1.5 (second paragraph). The work on competition processes is not really in the stage of biological applicability yet.

[33] G. J. Jacobs, Ed., *Proceedings of a Conference on Theoretical Biology* (conference organized by the Amer. Inst. of Biol. Sci. under the sponsorship of NASA, Princeton, NJ, November 1963). Scientific and Technical Information Division of NASA (Number NASA SP-104), 1966, 188 pp. See end of Section 2.1.

[34] S. Kakutani and L. Markus, "On the non-linear difference–differential equation $y'(t) = [A - By(t - \tau)] \ y(t)$," in *Contributions to the Theory of Nonlinear Oscillations*, vol. 4, S. Lefschetz, Ed. Princeton, NJ: Princeton Univ. Press, 1958. (This is *Ann. of Math. Studies*, vol. 41.) See Section 1.5, Discussion Question 5.

[35] E. H. Kerner, *Gibbs Ensemble: Biological Ensemble; the Application of Statistical Mechanics to Ecological, Neural, and Biological Networks*. New York: Gordon and Breach, 1972, 167 pp. See Section 2.1, Remark 6. This book consists of four reprinted articles with a lengthy (66 pp.) and far from flawless introduction; the book will be too advanced for most of our readers.

[36] A. N. Kolmogorov, "Kačestvennoe izučenie matematičeskih modelei dinamiki populíacii" (Qualitative investigation of mathematical models of population dynamics), *Problemy Kibernetiki*, vol. 25, pp. 101–106, 1972. See Section 2.2, after Exercise 2. All that is needed for the questions on those pages is spelled out, so the original reference is not needed for teaching this material.

[37] L. Lapidus and J. H. Seinfeld, *Numerical Solution of Ordinary Differential Equations*. New York: Academic, 1971, 299 pp. See Section 1.6, Exercise 3 (f).

[38] E. G. Leigh, Jr., "The ecological role of Volterra's equations," in *Lectures on Mathematics in the Life Sciences*, vol. 1, *Proc. Symp. on Mathematical Biology— December 1966*. Providence, RI: American Mathematical Society, 1968, 117 pp. See Section 1.4, last paragraph. The tables on pages 58–60 of that paper are of interest. However, upon comparing the numbers in these tables with the graphs from which E. G. Leigh took them, it becomes apparent that the accuracy of the process was low. So the reader would do better to look at these graphs and obtain these numbers, if he wants them. The graphs are to be found in Huffaker [30, figure 18], and in MacLulich [48, figures 16 and 17, pp. 109 and 110].

[39] ——, *Adaptation and Diversity; Natural History and the Mathematics of Evolution*, San Francisco, CA: Freeman, Cooper and Company, 1971, 288 pp. See Section 2.3, Remark 2. Its Figure 7-5, is the same as [60, fig. 1]. What the figure does should rather be done by the students themselves: take a graph from Huffaker [30] and from these data construct the size of the horizontal and the vertical arrows and their resultants. Thus one obtains a phase portrait.

[40] P. H. Leslie, "A stochastic model for studying the properties of certain biological systems by numerical methods," *Biometrika*, vol. 45, pp. 16–31, 1958. See Sections 1.6 (Discussion Question 1) and 2.2 (paragraph preceding Exercise 4 and in Discussion Question 5). See remark re Leslie and Gower [42].

[41] ——, "A stochastic model for two competing species of Tribolium and its application to some experimental data, *Biometrika*, vol. 49, pp. 1–25, 1962. See Section 1.5, second paragraph. See remark re Leslie and Gower [42].

[42] P. H. Leslie and J. C. Gower, "The properties of a stochastic model for the predator-prey type of interaction between two species," *Biometrika*, vol. 47, pp. 219–234, 1960. See Section 1.5, second paragraph. The above two papers by Leslie and the present one are typical for a number of publications in that time from the Bureau of Animal Population in Oxford.

[43] T. -Y. Li and J. A. Yorke, "Period three implies chaos," *Amer. Math. Monthly*, vol. 82, pp. 985–992, 1975. See Section 1.6, end of first paragraph.

[44] A. J. Lotka, "Studies on the mode of growth of material aggregates," *American J. Science*, 4th ser., vol. 24 (whole number 174), pp. 199–216, 1907, with an addendum on 375–376. See Section 1.2 (second paragraph).

[45] ——, *Elements of Physical Biology*, Baltimore, MD: Williams and Wilkins, 1925. Reprinted as *Elements of Mathematical Biology*. New York: Dover, 1956, 465 pp. See Sections 1.2 (second paragraph), and 2.1 (first paragraph). Somewhat desirable, available as an inexpensive paperback.

[46] R. H. MacArthur and J. H. Connell, *The Biology of Populations*, New York: Wiley, 1966, 200 pp. See Section 2.2, first paragraph. Of this book, chapter 6 is closest to our present concerns.

[47] R. H. MacArthur, *Geographical Ecology; Patterns in the Distribution of Species*, New York: Harper and Row, 1972, 269 pp. See Section 1.3.

[48] D. A. MacLulich, *Fluctuations in the Numbers of the Varying Hare (Lepus americanus)*, Biological Series, University of Toronto Studies, no. 43. Toronto, ON, Canada: Univ. of Toronto Press, 1973, 136 pp. See remarks regarding Leigh [38].

[49] M. Mamdani, *The Myth of Population Control; Family, Caste, and Class in an Indian Village*, New York: Monthly Review Press, 1972, 173 pp. See Appendix C, remarks made regarding Discussion Question 1 in Section 1.5. This book gives a detailed discussion of the cultural and economic barriers against birth control in a typical Indian village.

[50] R. M. May, *Stability and Complexity in Model Ecosystems*, Princeton, NJ: Princeton Univ. Press, 1973, 235 pp. See Sections 1.3, 2.2 (paragraph preceding Discussion Question 6), and 3.1. Section 1.3 gives a short description of the book. It is *very desirable* for the instructor to have it around.

[51] ——, "On the relationships among various types of population models," *The American Naturalist*, vol. 107, pp. 46–57, 1973. See Section 1.6 (end of first paragraph).

[52] J. M. Smith, *Mathematical Ideas in Biology*, New York: Cambridge Univ. Press, 1968, 152 pp. See Section 1.3, where a short characterization is given.

[53] ——, *Models in Ecology*, New York: Cambridge Univ. Press, 1974, 146 pp. See Section 1.3, where a short characterization is given.

[54] D. B. Mertz, "The Tribolium model and the mathematics of populations growth," *Annual Review of Ecology and Systematics*, vol. 3, pp. 51–78, 1972. See Sections 1.3, 1.5 (end of second paragraph), and 3.2 (Remark 1). If this volume is in the campus library, it is quite worthwhile to take a good look at this article.

[55] J. Neyman, T. Park, and E. L. Scott, "Struggle for existence; the Tribolium model; Biological and statistical aspects," in *Proc. 3rd Berkeley Symp. on Mathematical Statistics and Probability*, vol. 4, *Contributions to Biology and Problems of Health*, Berkeley, CA: Univ. of California Press, 1956, pp. 41–79. See Sections 1.5 (end of second paragraph) and 3.2 (Remark 1). Emphasis is on how the stochastic model is different from the deterministic model, and how it is similar to it.

[56] R. Pearl and L. J. Reed, "On the rate of growth of the population of the United States since 1790 and its mathematical representation," *Proc. of the National*

Academy of Sciences, vol. 6, pp. 275–288, 1920. See Section 1.5, Discussion Question 4.

[57] I. A. Poletaev, "O mathmatičeskih modeliah elementarnyh processov v biogeocenozah," *Problemy Kibernetiki* (pod red. A. A. Liapunova), vol. 16, str. 171–190, 1966, Izd. Nauka, Moskva. See Sections 2.2 (paragraph after Discussion Question 5) and 4 (Exercise 7).

[58] *Problemy Kibernetiki*, an ongoing serial publication, A. A. Liapunov, Ed., published in Moscow by Nauka, on any subject related to cybernetical problems. Volume 25 (1972), is especially heavy on population dynamics. It may be available in translation. See Section 2.2, paragraph preceding Discussion Question 6.

[59] G. E. Reuter, "Competition processes," in *Proc. 4th Berkeley Symp. on Mathematical Statistics and Probability*, vol. 2, *Probability Theory*. Berkeley, CA: Univ. of California Press, 1961, pp. 421–430. See Section 1.5, second paragraph. The work on competition processes is not really in the stage of biological applicability yet.

[60] M. L. Rosenzweig, "Why the prey curve has a hump," *The American Naturalist*, vol. 103, pp. 81–87, 1969. See Section 2.3, Remark 2.

[61] T. Royama, "A comparative study of models for predation and parasitism," *Researches on Population Ecology*, supplement 1, September 1971. Kyoto, Japan: Society of Population Ecology, c/o Entomological Laboratory, Kyoto University, 91 pp. See Section 2.2, paragraph preceding Discussion Question 6. Theoretically oriented, this would be useful for a far more detailed course.

[62] F. M. Stewart and B. R. Levin, "Partitioning of resources and the outcome of interspecific competition: A model and some general considerations," *The American Naturalist*, vol. 107, pp. 171–198, 1973. See Section 3.3, second paragraph.

[63] A. Tansley, "The use and abuse of vegetational concepts and terms," *Ecology*, vol. 16, pp. 284–307, 1935. See Section 1.1.

[64] C. P. Tsokos and S. W. Hinkley, "A stochastic bivariate ecology model for competing species," *Mathematical Biosciences*, vol. 16, pp. 191–208, 1973. See Section 1.5, second paragraph.

[65] M. B. Usher and M. H. Williamson, eds., *Ecological Stability*, London: Chapman and Hall; New York: Wiley, 1974, 196 pp. See Section 1.3.

[66] H. R. van der Vaart, "A comparative investigation of certain difference equations and related differential equations: Implications for model-building," *Bulletin of Mathematical Biology*, vol. 35, pp. 195–211, 1973. See Section 1.6. Essential if Section 1.6 is used for a student project.

[67] V. Volterra, "Variazioni e fluttuazioni del numero d'individui in specie animali conviventi," Atti della R. Accademia Nazionale dei Lincei, Anno 324; Serie sesta, *Memorie Della Classe di Scienze Fisiche, Matematiche e Naturali*, vol. 2, pp. 31–113, 1927. See Sections 1.2 and 2.1 (Remark 1). This title is almost the same as the title of the article published by the *R. Comitato Talassografico Italiano* (see Section 1.2). There are no observational data in the present title, only mathematical theory.

[68] ——, *Theory of Functionals and of Integral and Integro-Differential Equations*, Blackie and Sons, 1929. (New York: Dover, 1959, [39] + *xiv* + 226 pp.) See Section 1.2, first paragraph. The separately numbered pages, [5]–[39], contain a good biography, written by E. Whittaker. See especially pp. [19]–[25], [32]–[33], and [36]–[39].

[69] K. E. F. Watt, "A mathematical model for the effect of densities of attacked and attacking species on the number attacked," *The Canadian Entomologist*, vol. 91, pp. 129–144, 1959. See Section 2.2, paragraph preceding Discussion Question 6. See remark regarding [28].

[70] ——, *Ecology and Resource Management: A Qualitative Approach*. New York:

McGraw-Hill, 1968, 450 pp. See Section 2.2, paragraph preceding Discussion Question 6.

[71] M. Williamson, "The Analysis of Biological Populations," London: Arnold; and New York: Crane and Russak, 1972, 180 pp. See Section 1.3, where a short characterization is given.

Appendix C: Suggestions and Solutions

Some of the exercises, and especially the discussion questions, could puzzle the instructor or class as to what kind of answer should be expected. We hope that the following remarks about some of them may alleviate such confusion. These should be particularly helpful to persons with scant experience in applications of mathematics to biology.

Section 1.5

Discussion Question 1. In human populations, for instance, behavioral and cultural patterns established during an era of relatively low population density and primitive medical knowledge tend to change more slowly than might be desirable for increased population density. So family size or, equivalently, the percentage-wise rate of increase is not really determined by today's population density, but by that of a century ago, say. For example, see the difficulties encountered by family planning or population control in India, as discussed by Mamdani [49]. On a different time scale, long gestation periods introduce delays in the conversion of food into increases in population numbers. Students or instructors, especially those with a biological background, might come up with more examples.

Discussion Question 2. Answers: $\varphi(x, y)$ and $\psi(x, y)$, any pair of functions independent of h.

Exercise 2. Any of the following methods will be fine (it would be useful to show more than one). (1) Substitute (5d) into (5c); this also decides the question of existence of a solution. (2) Divide both members of (5c) by x^2 and change variables according to

$$y(t) = \frac{1}{x(t)};$$

this results in a linear equation in $y(t)$. (3) Multiply both members of (5c) by $K/[x(K - x)]$; the use of the method of partial fractions will then yield the differential equation

$$\frac{\dot{x}(\square)}{x(\square)} + \frac{\dot{x}(\square)}{K - x(\square)} = \gamma K;$$

now integrate with respect to $\square$ from t_0 to t. The third method is the most delicate one:

$$\int_{t_0}^{t} \frac{\dot{x}(\square)}{x(\square)} d\square = \log\left|\frac{x(t)}{x_0}\right|,$$

and one has to worry about $x(t)$ not taking the value zero, so that $x(t)/x_0$ will have a constant sign and the absolute value bars can be deleted.

Exercise 3. We recommend that the students draw more than one graph: two or three in the strip $0 < x < K$, one or two in the halfplanes $x > K$ and $x < 0$.

Discussion Question 3. Experience shows that some readers have a quick understanding of this question, others wrestle with it. At a more intuitive level, the point is that it is *not* true that every quadruple of values (t_0, x_0, γ, K) with $0 < \gamma$, $0 < K$, $0 < x_0 < K$, determines a different function of the form (5d). At a formal level the question can be rephrased as follows. Show that a one-to-one correspondence does *not* exist between the points of four-dimensional (t_0, x_0, γ, k)-space (with $0 < \gamma$, $0 < K$, $0 < x_0 < K$) and the collection of all logistic curves of the form (5d). Rather, a one-to-one correspondence exists between the points of three-dimensional (A, B, C)-space (with $0 < A, 0 < B, 0 < C$) and the collection of all logistic curves, as can be seen by rewriting (5d) as

$$x(t) = \frac{A}{1 + Be^{-Ct}}.$$

Specifically, the individual values of x_0 and t_0 do not matter: the only thing that counts is the value of

$$\frac{K - x_0}{x_0} e^{+rt_0}.$$

The question is important in view of statistical estimation of parameters: (t_0, x_0) is not identifiable.

Discussion Question 4. Re the question at the very end. Verhulst said that his agricultural argument does lead to an expression for $f(x)$ of the given form, but it does not really. According to the verbal argument given, the population grows purely exponentially until the level $x = b$ is reached (at time t_b, say). For $x > b$ the differential equation model is of the form

$$\frac{\dot{x}}{x} = (r - m \cdot (x - b)) = r + mb - mx$$

$$= m(K - x),$$

with $mK = r + mb$, and $x(t_b) = b$. The curve that answers Verhulst's description consists, therefore, of two parts, each part described by a different formula.

Discussion Question 5. The rationale for the equation displayed here is as follows. Think of a human population in which things like family size are decided on the basis of traditional attitudes (cf. remarks on Discussion Question 1, Section 1.5). Then $\tau \sim 100$ years, say: the factor in the formula that is supposed to represent increased procreational caution, viz. $(K - x)$, should be evaluated 100 years before t; this is the factor that should reflect attitudes about family size, and these attitudes were formed under the influence of the population size of τ years ago. On the other hand, the number of families now is more or less proportional to the population size now, or, at least, to the population size of a much shorter time ago than the above-postulated period of adjustment of attitudes to population size. The same equation is proposed with essentially the same argument (though less elaborate) by Kakutani and Markus [34]. Of course, in a population in which family size would be determined less by tradition than by the experiences and feelings of the parents during their childhood, and in which the bulk of people are having children during the same relatively short age span, a more logical model would be

$$\dot{x}(t) = (r/K) \cdot x(t - \tau) \cdot [K - x(t - \tau)],$$

with a time lag of $\tau = 20$ or 25 years. As for the construction of the graphs of the solutions of the equations

$$\dot{x}(t) = (r/K) \cdot x(t) \cdot [K - x(t - \tau)] \qquad \text{(a)}$$

and

$$\dot{x}(t) = (r/K) \cdot x(t - \tau) \cdot [K - x(t - \tau)], \qquad \text{(b)}$$

it will become clear (as soon as you try to do it) that the knowledge of $x(t_0)$ is now not enough to get started: $\dot{x}(t_0)$ cannot be computed from $x(t_0)$, not for equation (a), and not for equation (b). One needs to know the function $x(\ )$ over the time interval from $t_0 - \tau$ to t_0: an *arc instead of a point*. Suppose this initial arc represents a monotone increasing function of t, then the solution of equation (a) will, at any level x up to K, be steeper than any logistic with the same γ and K. Suppose this initial arc represents a piece of a regular logistic with the same γ and K, then the solution of equation (b) will be obtained by translating a suitable logistic (with that γ and K) upwards over the distance $x(t_0) - x(t_0 - \tau)$. Finally, going back to equation (a), suppose that $x(t') = K$; then $x(t' - \tau) < K$ and $\dot{x}(t') > 0$. So the population size will increase beyond K, and $\dot{x}(\ )$ will be zero only at $t' + \tau$. Thereafter $\dot{x}(\ ) < 0$ for a while. Pursuing this argument, one can make the oscillations of $x(t)$ around K as shown by Kakutani and Markus [34], very plausible indeed. Similar argument for (b).

Section 2.1

Exercise 1. Choose β_1 and β_2 such that $p\beta_2 = q\beta_1$.

Exercise 2. See sections A.1 and A.2 in Appendix A.

Exercise 4. The intention of this question should be clear by comparison with Exercise 1. The point is that no scale change of the form $x = \beta_1 x_1$, $y = \beta_2 x_2$ will be able to turn the matrix

$$\left\{ \begin{matrix} \delta & -p \\ +q & -\zeta \end{matrix} \right\}$$

into a skew-symmetric one. The reason for this is that a skew-symmetric matrix has diagonal elements equal to *zero*, and neither $-\delta\beta_1$ nor $-\zeta\beta_2$ will ever be zero, since δ and ζ are given as positive numbers, and $\beta_i = 0$ would make the change meaningless.

Exercise 5. See Sections A.1 and A.2 in Appendix A.

Exercise 6. See Section A.4 of Appendix A, especially the final example in that section. One should not find any contradictions, but some of the things conjectured from the arrow method should now become more precise and certain.

Discussion Question 1. There are too many nonzero coefficients in (10). So we can*not* now get rid of all the unwanted terms and thus separate variables.

Discussion Question 2. Looking at (10) we can say that the ratio δ/γ_1 indicates how much worse the presence of one prey individual makes the environment for the prey species, whereas the ratio q/γ_2 indicates how much better the presence of one prey individual makes the environment for the predator. The model yields coexistence of predator and prey iff the percentage deterioration for the prey is less than the percentage improvement for the predator. In the opposite case the advantage for the predator to have the prey around is apparently not enough to keep the predator in business. Now this sounds as if it would make the biologist moderately happy. The only question the biologist could raise to is: Why does ζ not play a role in the decision re coexistence of the two species? It does to some extent: it helps determine the size of the predator population at equilibrium. Other than that I do not see a ready answer to this remark, and it is a bit odd for the crowding effect in the *predator* not to be terribly important in the question of coexistence, while the crowding effect in the *prey* is that important.

Another possible question would be, Why should q be considered relative to γ_2? Well, γ_2 describes how much the predator needs just to stay in business.

Discussion Question 3. The locus of all points with $\dot{x} = 0$ should be a horizontal line through the singular point. The locus of all points with $\dot{y} = 0$ should be .. ? .. (see Eq. (7); and neither is the case in this diagram.

Section 2.2

Exercise 1. Any trajectory that crosses that portion of the isocline, reaches its left-most point there, at that crossing point. Thereafter, the danger for the prey to decrease more has passed. So if that isocline keeps far enough away from the y axis, the prey will not become extinct.

Exercise 2. In a manner somewhat similar to Exercise 1, the prey cannot $\uparrow +\infty$.

Exercise 3. The one term which makes (10) different from (12) is obviously $y \cdot (\ldots - \zeta y)$. It contradicts Kolmogorov's assumption that the predators act independently of each other (see point (1) in the latter half of this exercise).

Discussion Question 1. If the equation $K_2(x) = 0$ has any roots, then the horizontal isocline is the union of the x axis ($y = 0$) and any vertical line $x = \xi$, where ξ is a root of $K_2(x) = 0$. Also any singular point must belong to the horizontal isocline. All of Kolmogorov's sketches portray only one singular point outside the coordinate axes. So the only spot on any trajectory (outside the x axis) where that trajectory can have a horizontal tangent line, must be on the vertical line through that lonely singular point. Most of Kolmogorov's sketches lack this property.

Discussion Question 2. The y axis belongs to the vertical isocline iff $L(0) = 0$.

Discussion Question 3. $K_1(x)$ is the relative rate of increase of the prey in the absence of the predator. The assumption that it is monotone decreasing represents the crowding effect and is therefore not unreasonable (except perhaps for extremely small values of x); whether $K_1(x)$ should be negative for large enough x is something else. The assumptions re $K_2(x)$ and $L(x)$ are in line with our earlier discussions, except maybe for $L(0) > 0$; this inequality means that a prey population of size zero keeps decreasing as long as some predators are left, which sounds odd (whoever saw a population of size less than zero?). See the last sentence of Discussion Question 3 in Section 2.2. The equation of the vertical isocline is

$$y = \frac{K_1(x)}{L(x)} \cdot x.$$

From the definition of $K_1(\ )$ and $L(\ )$, these functions clearly have some positive value for each value of x less than the root of $K_1(x) = 0$. So for *each value* of x less than that root a value of y (viz., $x \cdot K_1(x)/L(x)$) exists such that the trajectory through (x, y) has a *vertical* tangent line at (x, y). Looking at Figure 4.5, one sees that several of the diagrams do not show this property (and are, hence, erroneous). Several other difficulties can be found with these diagrams. The author of this module does not see, for instance, how the singular points can possibly be located as in diagram 2: the singular point $(A, 0)$ must be on the vertical isocline, so $K_1(A) \cdot A - L(A) \cdot 0 = K_1(A) \cdot A = 0$; therefore $K_1(A) = 0$, so $K_1(x) < 0$ for $x > A$. The singular point (B, C) must also be on the vertical isocline, so $K_1(B) \cdot B - L(B) \cdot C = 0$. However, for $B > A$ and $C > 0$ it is clear that $K_1(B) \cdot B - L(B) \cdot C < 0$. These remarks should give a good idea of what all can be uncovered with respect to these diagrams, and we will not spoil your fun by spelling it all out. Note that for some of the questions you need to use the linearization method as discussed in Section A.4 of Appendix A.

Exercise 4. On the y axis the system is not defined. Therefore, although the trajectories in the neighborhood of the origin behave as if the origin were a saddle point, we cannot apply the customary criteria for saddle points. Let $\vec{p} = (p_1, p_2)$ be the singular point in the interior of the first quadrant. (Prove such a singular point exists!) Then show that

$$Df(\vec{p}) = \begin{bmatrix} -a_1 p_1 & -b_1 p_1 \\ +a_2 p_2^2 p_1^{-2} & -a_2 p_2 p_1^{-1} \end{bmatrix}.$$

Therefore, the product of the two eigenvalues is positive, and their sum is negative. Hence the eigenvalues have negative real parts. (Prove!) The singular point $\vec{p}$ is, therefore, either a stable node or a stable spiral point, and the behavior of this model is not all that much different from that of (10), nor all that much of an improvement.

Section 2.3

Exercise 1. The four answers are, respectively, 0, 0, positive, negative.

Exercise 2. They consist of at least one saddle point and one stable or unstable spiral point.

Discussion Question 1. At any point on the vertical isocline $\psi(x, y)$ (cf. (17)) is nonzero (unless that point is also on the horizontal isocline), that is, $\psi(x, y)$ is either positive or negative. Because of the continuity of $\psi(x, y)$ it will have the same sign at points off the isocline as at points on the isocline, provided they are close enough. "Close enough" here means "at the same side" of the horizontal isocline, because $\psi(x, y)$ will not be able to change sign without hitting zero; and $\psi(x, y)$ can hit zero only on the horizontal isocline. (Why?) Finally, when $\psi(x, y) > 0$, then $\dot{y} > 0$ and the vertical arrow points upwards; when $\psi(x, y) < 0$, then $\dot{y} < 0$ and the vertical arrow points downwards. The same applies to horizontal arrows. This should enable the reader to explain all the arrows in Figure 4.9.

Discussion Question 2. The two possibilities depicted in the two diagrams on the left of Figure 4.9 seem to allow populations to explode all the way to infinity. This would be biologically unacceptable: even insect pests eventually come down.

Section 3.2

Exercise 1. The trick is in getting the isoclines to be convex graphs; y a convex function of x, or x a convex function of y for both the horizontal and the vertical isoclines.

PART II

BIOMEDICINE: EPIDEMICS, GENETICS, AND BIOENGINEERING

CHAPTER 5

Malaria: Models of the Population Dynamics of the Malaria Parasite

Helen Marcus–Roberts* and Fred S. Roberts**

1. Introduction

Malaria is a tropical disease which at times has seriously depleted the populations of whole nations. The disease is still an important health problem in many parts of Africa, the Mideast, and Asia. In this chapter, we present a series of mathematical models attempting to describe the development of the disease through its various stages in an infected human or other mammal.

We shall start with a very simple model, confront its predictions with data, and add a series of increasingly more complex assumptions. Finally, after constructing a fourth model, we shall see the need to introduce an element of uncertainty into our modeling, and we shall present a second series of four models, analogous to the first four, but assuming that certain processes are governed by laws of chance.

Even the most complicated of our models are not capable of giving an adequate description of what happens in malaria. But they should give the reader a feeling for what additional complications would have to be added to obtain a realistic model.

In the next section, we discuss briefly the course of the malarial infection, as background for the models which follow.

* Department of Mathematics and Computer Science, Montclair State College, Upper Montclair, NJ 07043.
** Department of Mathematics, Rutgers University, New Brunswick, NJ 08903.

2. Malaria

Humans or animals contract malaria through the bite of a mosquito which is carrying malaria parasites (*Plasmodia*). These parasites first enter cells of the liver, and there begin to multiply rapidly. When enough parasites are present, the liver cells burst, and the parasites are released into the blood stream, each finding a red blood cell (rbc) which it will parasitize (infect). The parasites entering a given rbc will reproduce within that cell up to a characteristic range, at which point that cell will burst, releasing more parasites into the blood stream, who in turn attach themselves to new rbc's. The bursting of rbc's and release of malaria parasites happens with great regularity, every 48 or 72 hours, depending on the species. The bursting of the cells produces a form of protein shock, which leads to the sudden onset of high fever and chills characteristic of the disease.

3. The First Model

Since the bursting of rbc's and the release of malaria parasites into the blood stream occur with such great regularity, to speak of *time periods* or *generations* makes sense. Thus the *0th generation* is the first set of parasites which enter red blood cells. The *first generation* is the set of parasites which are produced by the bursting of these cells and which enter more rbc's. These in turn reproduce, producing the second generation of parasites. And so on.

Let Z_n be the number of parasitized rbc's at the nth generation. Let us assume for simplicity that in each parasitized rbc, the same number k of malaria parasites are produced. The number k will of course depend on the species of parasite, but it is certainly greater than one.

What does this simple model predict? If there are Z_n parasitized rbc's at the nth generation, and each produces k new parasites, then at the $(n + 1)$st generation, there are exactly kZ_n parasitized rbc's. Hence

$$Z_{n+1} = kZ_n.$$

Thus it is easy to show that

$$Z_n = k^n Z_0,$$

where Z_0 is the number of malaria parasites released from the liver cells. Since k is greater than one, the model therefore predicts that the number of parasitized rbc's grows exponentially. (Compare the graph of $Z_n = Z_0 k^n$ to that of $y = ak^x$.) Is that what happens in malaria? The second column of Table 1 lists the number of parasitized rbc's out of 10^6 rbc's sampled every 48 hours during the course of a typical malaria infection. (The data are from Hawking (personal communication.)) Figure 5.1 plots the data. Clearly, the number Z_n does not continue to grow every period; rather the number Z_n

Table 1. Number of Parasitized Red
Blood Cells out of 10^6 Sampled at
48-hour Intervals[†]

Date	Time	Number of Parasitized rbc's	rk	r if $k = 10$
10/24	22:15	5600	0.218	0.022
10/26	22:30	1220	1.09	0.109
10/28	22:00	1330	0.902	0.090
10/30	22:30	1200	1.3	0.13
11/1	22:30	1560	0.923	0.092
11/3	22:30	1440	1.389	0.139
11/5	22:30	2000	0.685	0.069
11/7	23:00	1370	0.118	0.012
11/9	23:15	161		

[†] Data from Hawking (personal communication).

grows, then drops, then grows, then drops, and so on. We shall have to
modify our model. (Figure 5.2 shows more detailed data.)

4. The Second Model: Survival Proportions

One of the simplifications in our first model was that we assumed that all
the parasites released into the blood stream survive. This is not a reasonable
assumption biologically. Suppose for simplicity that a fixed proportion r of
the released parasites survive and enter new rbc's. What does the introduction
of survival proportions do to our model? From the initial Z_0 parasitized
rbc's, kZ_0 parasites are released, and a fraction r of these survive. Thus

$$Z_1 = r(kZ_0) = (rk)Z_0.$$

Similarly,

$$Z_{n+1} = (rk)Z_n$$

and so

$$Z_n = (rk)^n Z_0.$$

If $rk > 1$, this model predicts that the number of parasites at the nth generation grows exponentially. If $rk < 1$, the model predicts that the number of
parasites at the nth generation decreases exponentially to 0. If $rk = 1$, the
model predicts that the number of parasites at the nth generation is constant
over n. None of these predictions account for fluctuations like those seen
in Figure 5.1. We shall once again have to modify our model.

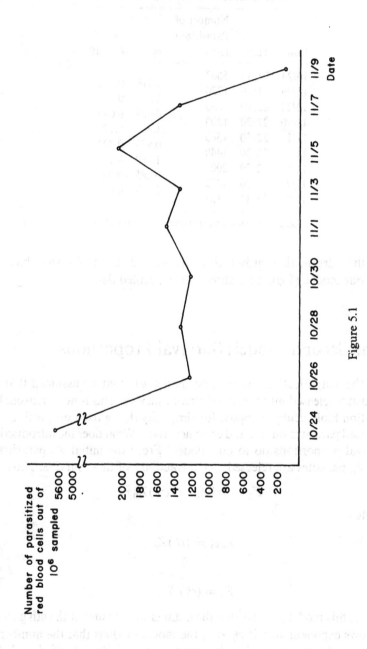

Figure 5.1

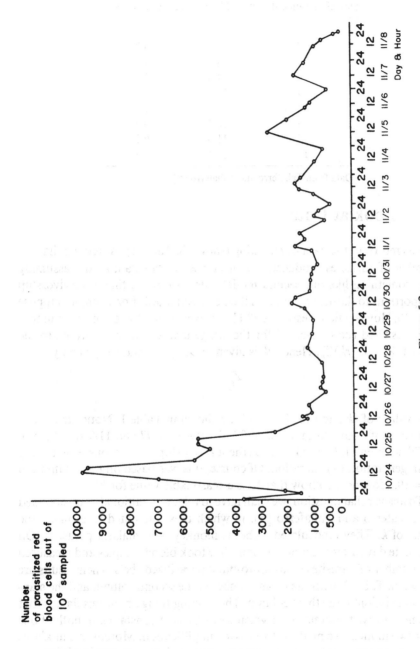

Figure 5.2

Table 2. Number of Parasites in an
About-to-Burst Parasitized Red Blood Cell[†]

Day after Innoculation	Mean	Standard Deviation
3	17.4	0.2
5	8.9	0.2
7	11.8	0.2
9	10.7	0.3
11	11.2	0.3
13	10.7	0.2
15	11.3	0.2
17	12.1	0.3

[†] Data from Taliaferro and Taliaferro [5].

5. A Look at Data

Let us return to the data of Hawking (shown in Table 1). Assuming that the number of parasites produced in a given rbc is a constant k, and assuming that something like our second model holds, we can estimate survivorship proportions to the next generation if we can estimate k. For example, suppose $k = 10$. How would we estimate r? The answer is that if Z_n counts the number of parasitized rbc's observed for the nth generation, then according to the model, Z_{n+1} is $(rk)Z_n$. Hence rk is given by Z_{n+1}/Z_n, and r is given by

$$\frac{Z_{n+1}}{kZ_n}.$$

The values of rk and of r if $k = 10$ are shown in Table 1. Notice that these estimates of r vary from a low of 0.012 between 11/7 and 11/9 to a high of 0.139 between 11/3 and 11/5. Thus the survivorship proportions seem to vary from generation to generation. Of course, this was based on the assumption $k = 10$. How do we know that 10 is a reasonable value for k?

To answer that question, we shall have to refer to additional data, obtained by Taliaferro and Taliaferro [5], in which they attempted to estimate the value of k. They inoculated a rhesus monkey with malaria parasites. On alternate days after the innoculation, they took blood samples and measured the number of parasites in about-to-burst parasitized rbc's. Their results are shown in Table 2, with the mean number in the second column and the standard deviation in the third column. The striking thing about this data is that k is not always the same. Thus when we assumed a constant k in both of our first two models, we made a strong oversimplification. Moreover, our above calculation *suggests* that assuming a constant r also is an oversimplification. This is only suggestive, since the calculations were done under the assumption of fixed k.

In any case, it looks as though we shall have to modify our models to allow both k and r to vary. Rather than introduce both of these complications at once, we shall introduce them one at a time.

6. The Third Model: Varying Survival Proportions

Let us start by assuming that the number k of offspring in each generation is fixed, but that the proportion of these that will survive varies. In particular, let us assume that this survival proportion depends only on the generation n. We will have to be a little careful about our definition of generation. Let Z_0 count the number of rbc's which are initially parasitized. Let Z_{1M} be the number of malaria parasites released from these rbc's. According to our model,

$$Z_{1M} = kZ_0.$$

Of these Z_{1M} parasites, a certain proportion r_1 survive to enter rbc's, with r_1 dependent only on the conditions at this time. Let Z_1 count this number, the number of parasitized rbc's in the *first* generation. Therefore,

$$Z_1 = r_1 Z_{1M}$$
$$= (r_1 k)Z_0.$$

Similarly, the parasitized rbc's of the first generation burst and release Z_{2M} parasites. Of these, a certain proportion r_2 survive to enter rbc's, with r_2 dependent only on the conditions at the time. Let Z_2 count this number, the number of parasitized rbc's in the *second* generation.

Similarly, we define Z_n, Z_{nM}, and r_n for every n. The definitions of these symbols should be clear. Our model says that

$$Z_{(n+1)M} = kZ_n \tag{1}$$

and that

$$Z_n = r_n Z_{nM}. \tag{2}$$

Putting Equations (1) and (2) together, we obtain

$$Z_{n+1} = (r_{n+1}k)Z_n. \tag{3}$$

Hence it is easy to show that

$$Z_n = r_1 r_2 \cdots r_n k^n Z_0. \tag{4}$$

It might help at this point to give a concrete example. Suppose $Z_0 = 1000$, $k = 10$, and r_n alternates between 0.6 and 0.01, starting with $r_1 = 0.6$. Then we calculate Z_n and Z_{nM} for various n in Table 3, and we plot Z_n and Z_{nM} in Figure 5.3. Notice the fluctuations which our new model already predicts.

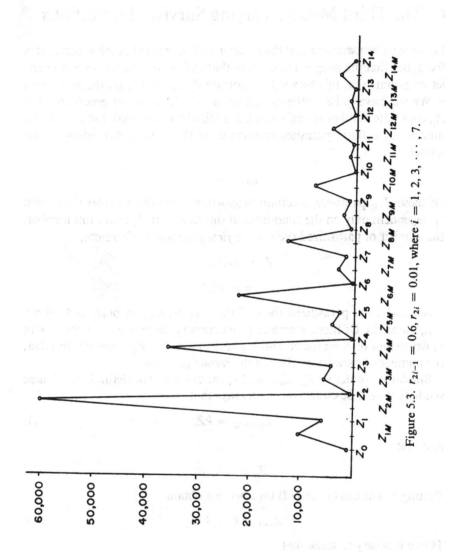

Figure 5.3. $r_{2i-1} = 0.6$, $r_{2i} = 0.01$, where $i = 1, 2, 3, \ldots, 7$.

Table 3. Values of Z_n and Z_{nM} Calculated Using Third Model if $Z_0 = 1000$, $k = 10$, and r_n Alternates between 0.6 and 0.01.

n	Z_n	$Z_{(n+1)M}$	r_{n+1}
0	1000	10,000	0.6
1	6000	60,000	0.01
2	600	6,000	0.6
3	3600	36,000	0.01
4	360	3,600	0.6
5	2160	21,600	0.01
6	216	2,160	0.6
7	1296	12,960	0.01
8	129.6	1,296	0.6
9	777.6	7,776	0.01
10	77.76	777.6	0.6
11	466.56	4,665.6	0.01
12	46.66	466.6	0.6
13	279.936	2,799.36	0.01
14	27.994		

7. The Fourth Model: Varying Reproduction Numbers

Introducing variations in the reproduction numbers k into our third model is easy. We simply modify Equation (1) in such a way that k can change from generation to generation. In particular, (1) is replaced by

$$Z_{(n+1)M} = k_n Z_n. \tag{5}$$

Equation (2) stays the same. Equation (3) becomes

$$Z_{n+1} = (r_{n+1} k_n) Z_n. \tag{6}$$

In fact, even (5) is rather simplified, because evidence suggests that reproduction rates of parasites vary from rbc to rbc. Thus it would be more realistic to speak of each individual parasite (in an rbc) as having characteristic numbers of offspring or a characteristic reproduction rate. This gets fairly complicated unless we look at it probabilistically. That is the attack of the next set of models. The reader who wishes to skip the remaining sections should realize that the models presented so far are highly oversimplified. Some additional oversimplifications are described in Section 12, and that section should be read.

8. First Probabilistic Model

To see how the process we have been studying can be treated probabilistically, let us start with a very simple situation, the situation which again disregards the fact that some parasites do not survive.

Let us assume that a given malaria parasite, having entered an rbc, gives rise to a number of offspring, with exactly k offspring occurring with probability p_k, $k = 0, 1, 2, \cdots$. We also assume that the parasites in different rbc's reproduce independently, but with the same probabilities governing the number of offspring. Let generations be defined as before. Let $X_{n,j}$ be the number of parasite offspring produced in the jth parasitized rbc of the nth generation. Thus, if Z_n counts the number of parasitized rbc's in the nth generation, we have

$$Z_{n+1} = X_{n,1} + X_{n,2} + \cdots + X_{n,Z_n} = \sum_{j=1}^{Z_n} X_{n,j}. \tag{7}$$

Thus Z_{n+1} is the sum of a random number Z_n of independent, identically distributed random variables. The model we have defined is called a *branching process*. The reader who is not familiar with the notion of branching process and its many applications may want to consult such references as Karlin and Taylor [3], Cox and Miller [1], or Harris [2].

Predictions from this branching process model can be obtained using probability generating functions (pgf's). We assume that the reader is familiar with the notion of a pgf. For a brief discussion, see Marcus–Roberts [4] or Karlin and Taylor [3]. Among the properties of pgf's we will use are the following: if $g(s)$ is the pgf of a random variable X, then

$$g(1) = 1 \tag{8}$$

$$E(X) = g'(1) \tag{9}$$

$$\text{Var}(X) = g''(1) + g'(1) - [g'(1)]^2. \tag{10}$$

Let $f(s)$ be the pgf of each of the independent identically distributed random variables $X_{n,1}, X_{n,2}, \cdots, X_{n,Z_n}$. Thus

$$f(s) = \sum_{k=0}^{\infty} p_k s^k.$$

Let $f_n(s)$ be the pgf of the distribution of Z_n.

Assuming $Z_0 = 1$ for the sake of discussion, we have

$$f_1(s) = f(s), \tag{11}$$

since the number in the first generation is the number of parasite offspring of the single 0th generation parasite. In general, by properties of generating functions

$$f_{n+1}(s) = f_n(f(s)), \qquad n = 1, 2, \cdots. \tag{12}$$

(See Karlin and Taylor [3, pp. 394–395] for a derivation.)

We would like to calculate the expected number of parasitized rbc's in the nth generation $E(Z_n)$. By Eq. (9), this is given by $f_n'(1)$. We differentiate Eq. (12) and set $s = 1$, obtaining

$$f_{n+1}'(1) = f_n'[f(1)]f'(1)$$
$$= f_n'(1)f'(1),$$

since $f(1) = 1$ by (8). Similarly, we obtain

$$f_{n+1}'(1) = [f_{n-1}'(1)f'(1)]f'(1)$$
$$= f_{n-1}'(1)[f'(1)]^2.$$

By induction,

$$f_{n+1}'(1) = f_1'(1)[f'(1)]^n.$$

Since $f_1'(1) = f'(1)$, we obtain

$$f_{n+1}'(1) = [f'(1)]^{n+1}$$

or

$$f_n'(1) = [f'(1)]^n.$$

Now $f'(1) = f_1'(1) = E(Z_1)$. Letting $E(Z_1) = \mu$, we have

$$E(Z_n) = \mu^n.$$

It is natural to assume that $\mu > 1$. Thus our model has predicted that the expected number of parasitized rbc's in the nth generation grows exponentially. This is similar to the prediction in our first model. If $\mu < 1$, the prediction is that this expected number declines exponentially to 0. This prediction is similar to a prediction of our second model. Neither prediction matches the behavior of the population of parasitized rbc's in malaria, since we have seen that this population can fluctuate rather wildly.

It should be emphasized that this model and the remaining probabilistic ones give more information than simply the expected value of Z_n. The variance can also be calculated, and it gives some idea of possible deviations. The variance is calculated as follows (the reader is asked to provide some of the details in Exercise 13):

$$f_{n+1}''(1) = f_n''(1)[f'(1)]^2 + f_n'(1)f''(1).$$

Now by Eq. (10),

$$f''(1) = \sigma^2 - \mu + \mu^2,$$

where $\sigma^2 = \text{Var}(Z_1)$. Thus

$$f_{n+1}''(1) = \mu^2 f_n''(1) + (\sigma^2 - \mu + \mu^2)\mu^n.$$

We can now easily show by induction that

$$f_n''(1) = (\sigma^2 - \mu + \mu^2)[\mu^{2n-2} + \mu^{2n-3} + \cdots + \mu^{n-1}].$$

Hence Eq. (10) implies

$$\text{Var}(Z_n) = (\sigma^2 - \mu + \mu^2)[\mu^{2n-2} + \mu^{2n-3} + \cdots + \mu^{n-1}] + \mu^n - (\mu^n)^2$$
$$= \sigma^2[\mu^{2n-2} + \mu^{2n-3} + \cdots + \mu^{n-1}].$$

If $\mu \neq 1$, we obtain

$$\text{Var}(Z_n) = \sigma^2 \mu^{n-1} \frac{\mu^n - 1}{\mu - 1}.$$

If $\mu = 1$, we have

$$\text{Var}(Z_n) = n\sigma^2.$$

Summarizing,

$$\text{Var}\, Z_n = \begin{cases} \sigma^2 \mu^{n-1} \dfrac{\mu^n - 1}{\mu - 1}, & \text{if } \mu \neq 1 \\[2mm] n\sigma^2, & \text{if } \mu = 1. \end{cases}$$

9. Second Probabilistic Model: Survival Probabilities

Let us vary the previous model to introduce the fact that some parasites do not survive. We assume again for simplicity that $Z_0 = 1$. All parasites released into the blood stream upon bursting have a fixed probability r of surviving to enter an rbc. The formula (7) no longer applies, but we can still speak of the random variables $X_{n,j}$ and of the generating functions $f(s)$ and $f_n(s)$. We have

$$f_1(s) = f(s),$$

as before. As we ask the reader to verify in Exercise 17,

$$f_{n+1}(s) = f_n[rf(s) + t], \tag{13}$$

where

$$t = 1 - r.$$

As before, $E(Z_n)$ is given by $f_n'(1)$, which is calculated as follows.

$$f_{n+1}'(1) = f_n'[rf(1) + t]rf'(1)$$
$$= f_n'[r + t]rf'(1)$$
$$= f_n'(1)rf'(1).$$

By induction,

$$f_{n+1}'(1) = f_1'(1)[rf'(1)]^n$$

$$= f'(1)[rf'(1)]^n$$
$$= r^n[f'(1)]^{n+1},$$

or

$$f'_{n+1}(1) = r^n\mu^{n+1},$$

or

$$E(Z_n) = f'_n(1) = r^{n-1}\mu^n = \frac{1}{r}[r\mu]^n,$$

where

$$\mu = E(Z_1).$$

We leave calculation of the variance as an exercise (Exercise 14).

This model has a prediction analogous to that of the first probabilistic model except that whether or not the expected number of parasitized rbc's in the nth generation grows exponentially or declines exponentially depends now on the product $r\mu$ rather than on the number μ. This model is also completely analogous to our second deterministic model, where the prediction was that $Z_n = (rk)^n Z_0$. (The slight difference is that we relate $E(Z_n)$ to $E(Z_1)$ rather than to Z_0.)

10. Third Probabilistic Model: Varying Survival Probabilities

If the survival probability becomes a function of the generation, and is denoted r_n, then it is easy to modify the computations of the previous section. The basic equation

$$f_1(s) = f(s)$$

still holds, and Eq. (13) becomes

$$f_{n+1}(s) = f_n[r_n f(s) + t_n], \tag{14}$$

where $t_n = 1 - r_n$. Calculation of $E(Z_n)$ and $Var(Z_n)$ is left as an exercise (Exercise 15).

11. Fourth Probabilistic Model: Varying Reproduction Probabilities

Analogous to our fourth deterministic model, where we let the number of parasite offspring k_n produced in the nth generation vary with n, we shall discuss in this section what happens if the probability that a given parasite has k offspring varies with the generation n. We shall omit the problem of survivorship, asking the reader to introduce this complication as an exercise. In this case, we let $g_n(s)$ be the pgf of the number of offspring produced by an individual of the $(n-1)$st generation. Then we have

$$f_1(s) = g_1(s) \tag{15}$$

and

$$f_{n+1}(s) = f_n[g_{n+1}(s)]. \tag{16}$$

Thus

$$f'_{n+1}(1) = f'_n[g_{n+1}(1)]g'_{n+1}(1)$$
$$= f'_n(1)g'_{n+1}(1)$$

because $g_{n+1}(1) = 1$, which is true for any pgf. Thus, by induction,

$$f'_n(1) = f'_1(1)g'_2(1)g'_3(1) \cdots g'_n(1)$$
$$= g'_1(1)g'_2(1)g'_3(1) \cdots g'_n(1).$$

If $\mu_i = g'_i(1) =$ expected number of parasite offspring from the $(i-1)$st generation, then

$$E(Z_n) = \mu_1\mu_2 \cdots \mu_n.$$

The reader should compare this result to that of the fourth deterministic model (cf. Exercise 6).

12. Discussion

We have presented four deterministic models for the population dynamics of the malaria parasite in a mammalian host, and four corresponding probabilistic models. Even the fourth model of each kind is almost certainly much too simple to adequately account for these population dynamics. In particular, the following complications are not accounted for:

(1) some of the parasites which have entered rbc's do not survive to have offspring;
(2) several infections may start at different times, meaning that several of these periodic processes may be going on at the same time, with a delay factor;
(3) the reproduction of malaria parasites really starts in the liver;
(4) the time of release into the blood stream of parasites from the liver varies;
(5) some of the offspring from the malaria parasites within a parasitized rbc

do not, in turn, enter new rbc's, or die off, but instead become sperms and eggs which are ingested by mosquitoes biting an infected mammal. (These, in turn, become the source of the malaria infection when the mosquito bites a new subject.)

These complications can be accounted for by various modifications of the branching process, but we shall not discuss how to do so here. However, we do consider some of them in the exercises.

Exercises

1. In the first model, plot Z_n versus n for $n = 0, 1, 2, \cdots, 10$ if $Z_0 = 1$ and
   (a) $k = 2$,
   (b) $k = 4$,
   (c) $k = 8$.
   Discuss the effect of a doubling in k.

2. In the first model, assume for the sake of discussion that k can be less than 1, and plot Z_n versus n for $n = 0, 1, 2, \cdots, 10$ if $Z_0 = 1000$ and
   (a) $k = 1/2$,
   (b) $k = 1/4$.
   Discuss the difference in predictions between $k > 1$ and $k < 1$.

3. In the second model, plot Z_n versus n for $n = 0, 1, 2, \cdots, 10$ if $Z_0 = 1$ and
   (a) $k = 10$ and $r = 0.5$,
   (b) $k = 10$ and $r = 0.001$.
   Discuss the differences between the two cases.

4. In the third model, tabulate and then graph Z_n versus n for $n = 0, 1, 2, \cdots, 15$ in the following cases.
   (a) $Z_0 = 1000$, $k = 10$, r_n alternates between 0.6 and 0.5, with $r_1 = 0.6$.
   (b) $Z_0 = 1000$, $k = 10$, r_n alternates between 0.6 and 0.05, with $r_1 = 0.6$.
   (c) $Z_0 = 1$ billion, $k = 10$, r_n alternates between 0.08 and 0.05, with $r_1 = 0.08$.
   (d) $Z_0 = 1000$, $k = 10$, r_n going from 0.6 to 0.01 to 0.4 and then repeating, with $r_1 = 0.6$.

5. Suppose the quantities r and k are both allowed to vary, as in the fourth model.
   (a) If Z_{n+1} is observed to be greater than Z_n, what does this imply about the value of $r_{n+1}k_n$?
   (b) What if Z_{n+1} is observed to be less than Z_n?
   (c) The next-to-last column of Table 1 can be used as an estimate of $r_{n+1}k_n$. Use these estimates to predict whether or not Z_{n+1} will be greater than Z_n. Check against the data in the table or against the diagram of Figure 5.2.

6. In the fourth model, derive an equation for Z_n in terms of Z_1.

7. In the fourth model, plot Z_n versus n for parameters r_n and k_n of your choice. Observe how the behavior of the population variable Z_n varies (increases, decreases, blows up, dies out, etc.) with different choices of these parameters.

8. In the third model, derive a formula for Z_{nM} in terms of Z_0.

9. One of the simplifications in our models is that we do not consider the possibility of secondary malaria infections begining at later times. Suppose a second infection starts one generation later than the first infection. Suppose we are in the situation of our second model. The first infection proceeds with each parasite producing $k = k^{(1)}$ new parasites and with a proportion $r = r^{(1)}$ of these surviving. The second infection proceeds with perhaps different parameters $k = k^{(2)}$ and $r = r^{(2)}$.
   (a) Find an equation for Z_{n+1} in terms of Z_n.
   (b) Derive a formula for Z_n in terms of Z_0.
   (c) Discuss the qualitative nature of the graphs of Z_n versus n for all possible combinations of parameters.
   (d) Whenever a model is proposed, one wants to know if the parameters needed to make predictions can be estimated from data. Could we estimate the parameters $k^{(1)}$, $k^{(2)}$, $r^{(1)}$, and $r^{(2)}$? Discuss the possible difficulties in this.

10. Another simplification in our models of malaria is that some of the offspring from the malaria parasites within a parasitized rbc do not in turn enter new rbc's, but instead become sperms and eggs which are ingested by mosquitoes biting an infected mammal. Discuss how we might bring this phenomenon into our first four models.

11. Suppose $p_k = b(k; n, p)$, the probability of k successes in n Bernoulli trials if p is the probability of a success.
   (a) Find $E(Z_n)$ in the first probabilistic model.
   (b) Find Var (Z_n) in the first probabilistic model.
   (c) Find $E(Z_n)$ in the second probabilistic model.

12. Repeat Exercise 11 if $p_k = e^{\lambda}(\lambda^k/k!)$, $k = 0, 1, \cdots$ (p_k is Poisson).

13. In the first probabilistic model,
   (a) verify that $f_{n+1}''(1) = f_n''(1)[f'(1)]^2 + f_n'(1)f''(1)$;
   (b) verify that $f_n''(1) = (\sigma^2 - \mu + \mu^2)[\mu^{2n-2} + \mu^{2n-3} + \cdots + \mu^{n-1}]$;
   (c) verify that

   $$\text{Var}(Z_n) = (\sigma^2 - \mu + \mu^2)(\mu^{2n-2} + \mu^{2n-3} + \cdots + \mu^{n-1}) + \mu^n - (\mu^n)^2; \qquad (17)$$

   (d) verify that if $\mu \neq 1$, the right-hand side of Eq. (17) equals

   $$\sigma^2 \mu^{n-1}\left(\frac{\mu^n - 1}{\mu - 1}\right);$$

   (e) verify that if $\mu = 1$, the right-hand side of (17) equals $n\sigma^2$.

14. For the second probabilistic model,
   (a) derive a formula for Var (Z_n);
   (b) calculate Var (Z_n) in the binomial case (Exercise 11);
   (c) calculate Var (Z_n) in the Poisson case (Exercise 12).

15. For the third probabilistic model,
   (a) derive a formula for $E(Z_n)$;
   (b) derive a formula for Var (Z_n);
   (c) calculate $E(Z_n)$ in the binomial case (Exercise 11);
   (d) calculate $E(Z_n)$ in the Poisson case (Exercise 12);
   (e) calculate Var (Z_n) in the binomial case;
   (f) calculate Var (Z_n) in the Poisson case.

16. In the fourth probabilistic model, find an expression which gives $\text{Var}(Z_{n+1})$ in terms of $\text{Var}(Z_n)$.

17. Derive Eq. (13). Hint: Since survival is binomial, one can show that the generating function for the number of surviving offspring is $rf(s) + t$.

References

[1] D. R. Cox and H. D. Miller, *The Theory of Stochastic Processes*. New York: Wiley, 1965.

[2] T. E. Harris, *The Theory of Branching Processes*. Berlin: Springer, 1963.

[3] S. Karlin and H. Taylor, *A First Course in Stochastic Processes*. New York: Academic Press, 1975.

[4] H. Marcus–Roberts, "A comparison of some deterministic and stochastic models of population growth," this volume, chapter 3.

[5] W. H. Taliaferro and L. G. Taliaferro, "Asexual reproduction of *Plasmodium Cynomolgi* in rhesus monkeys," *J. Infectious Diseases*, vol. 80, pp. 78–104, 1947.

Notes for the Instructor

Prerequisites. This chapter presents a series of eight models of the population dynamics of the malaria parasite in a mammalian host. The first four of these are increasingly complex deterministic models, and these form a self-contained unit. The last four of these are probabilistic analogues of the deterministic ones.

The first part requires some knowledge of sequences and the concept of exponential growth (the graph of the function $f(x) = ak^x$). The second part requires knowledge of probability generating functions. For the second part, some previous exposure to branching processes is recommended, though not required. This chapter can easily be combined with a standard treatment of branching processes and their applications.

The first part is appropriate for a finite math course or math for liberal arts course in which the notion of sequence and the graph $y = ak^x$ have been discussed, or a finite math course with a prerequisite of one semester of calculus. The second part is appropriate for a probability course. Together, both parts are appropriate for a modeling course.

Time. The first part should take less than an hour to present or can be given as a reading assignment. The whole chapter should take from two to three hours, depending on the details the instructor wishes to add about the branching processes.

CHAPTER 6

MacDonald's Work on Helminth Infections

Donald Ludwig* and Benjamin D. Haytock**

1. Introduction

Parasitic infections are among the most important world health problems. Malaria leads the list, followed by schistosomiasis and other helminth infections. These diseases are endemic in most of the tropical and subtropical areas of the world, and their effect can be so severe as to make certain areas nearly uninhabitable. Although large scale efforts have been made to control schistosomiasis, the long-term effects of these efforts have been disappointing. The reasons for this lack of success and suggestions for improved control measures are given by George MacDonald [3].[1]

MacDonald's results are derived with the aid of a mathematical model which describes the complicated interaction between parasitic worms, human hosts, and secondary hosts (snails). The conclusions MacDonald draws from his analysis of the model are given in [3, pp. 501–502]. Basically, he concludes that a control effort will have little effect unless it is extremely intensive. Once control efforsts reach a certain level, that is, once a "break point" is reached, then the level of infection will decline sharply, and the disease may be eradicated within a few years. However, before the break point is reached, only a small effect will be observed.

The sharpness of the decline in the parasite population at the break point is due to a peculiar feature of helminth infections: in order for the parasites to reproduce, male and female worms must be paired within the body of a

* Department of Mathematics, University of British Columbia, Vancouver, BC, Canada V6T 1W5.

** Department of Mathematics, Allegheny College, Meadville, PA 16335.

[1] A copy of this article, reproduced with permission, appears at the end of this chapter.

human host. As the mean number of worms per hums per human declines, there is also a decline in the probability that a given female will be able to find a male with whom to mate. Therefore once low average numbers of worms per human are reached, a sharp decline in the parasite population will be observed.

Although MacDonald argues eloquently on the need for a mathematical model and the relevance of its conclusions, he does not supply all of the equations which he used in deriving his results. Also, he failed to utilize the fact that certain of his results can be given explicitly in terms of Bessel functions. The following discussion is intended as an introduction to the mathematical features of MacDonald's model and its solution. It is provided to make the paper more accessible to those with a mathematical background.

2. The Schistosomiasis Model

Schistosomes have a complicated life history. Male and female worms must mate within a human host. Thereafter, the female deposits eggs, some of which leave the host in the feces. Other eggs may be trapped in various organs of the body, and these cause the symptoms of the disease. If an egg comes into contact with fresh water, a larva called a miricidium hatches. In order to continue the cycle, the miricidium must penetrate the body of a snail. Once a snail is so infected, a large number of larvae called circariae are produced by asexual means. Each circaria swims freely. It seeks to penetrate the skirt of a human in order to complete the cycle.

The main quantities of interest are the mean number of worms infecting each human (denoted by m) and the number of infected snails (denoted by I). We first consider the variation of I with time. If we assume that the relative death rate of infected snails is a constant, which we denote by δ, and that the rate at which snails are infected is proportional to the number of healthy snails, then I will satisfy an equation of the form

$$\frac{dI}{dt} = -\delta I + C(m)(S - I). \tag{1}$$

Here S denotes the total number of snails, and $C(m)$ is the infection rate. This infection rate depends upon the mean number of paired worms per human $P(m)$, since the number of eggs produced (and hence the number of miricidia) is proportional to $P(m)$. Therefore, we may write

$$C(m) = P(m)B, \tag{2}$$

where B is a factor which is independent of m. For simplicity, it is also assumed that S is constant.

A similar argument leads to an equation for the rate of change of m. We may write

$$\frac{dm}{dt} = -rm + A\frac{I}{S}. \tag{3}$$

Here r denotes the death rate for worms inside a human host, and A is a factor which takes into account the number of circariae produced per infected snail.

The basic equations which govern the course of the infection are (1) and (3). In order to simplify their analysis, we observe that m changes very slowly since the life span of a worm inside a human is on the order of three years. Therefore, we first think of $C(m)$ as constant in Eq. (1). Let I^* denote the point where $dI/dt = 0$; thus

$$I^* = \frac{C}{C + \delta}S. \tag{4}$$

If $I < I^*$, then $dI/dt > 0$, and I will increase. Likewise, I will decrease if $I > I^*$. We conclude that $I \to I^*$ as $t \to \infty$. This fact can also be verified from the exact solution of (1). MacDonald assumed that if m varies slowly as a function of t, I should be close to I^* (this assumption is discussed in the appendix). Therefore, to a good approximation, we may replace (1) by

$$\frac{I}{S} \cong \frac{I^*}{S} = \frac{BP(m)}{BP(m) + \delta}. \tag{5}$$

This relation is the same as expression (12) of MacDonald's paper (identify δ with his $-\log P$ and $P(m)$ with his $m\alpha$).

After substitution (5) into (3), we obtain

$$\frac{dm}{dt} = -rm + \frac{ABP(m)}{BP(m) + \delta}. \tag{6}$$

3. The Poisson Probability Distribution

In order to proceed further we must obtain an expression for $P(m)$, and in order to do this we must know something about the probability distribution for the worms. We shall think of the population as being one large "region" in space and make the following assumptions about the distribution of worms within this region.

(1) The number of worms in a region is independent of the number of worms in any nonoverlapping region.
(2) The probability distribution for the number of worms in any region is the same as that for any other region of the same size. The size of a region is an appropriate measure of its length, area or volume depending upon the physical nature of the region. We suppose that size is measured by one real variable.

(3) If the size of a region is small, then the probability of exactly one worm in that region is approximately proportional to the size of the region.

(4) If the size of a region is small, then the probability of more than one worm in that region is negligeable in comparison to the probability of one worm.

Let $p_n(t)$ denote the probability of n worms in a region of size t. Assumption, 2 makes this notation meaningful. Assumptions 3 and 4 may now be stated more precisely as follows.[2]

3: $p_1(h) = \lambda h + o(h)$, for some $\lambda > 0$,

4: $\sum_{k=2}^{\infty} p_k(h) = o(h)$.

The function $p_0(t)$ can easily be determined. We proceed in the following way. From the relationship

$$p_0(t + h) = p_0(t)p_0(h),$$

which follows from assumption 1, and

$$p_0(h) = 1 - \lambda h + o(h),$$

which follows from assumption 4 and the definition of a probability distribution, we obtain

$$\frac{p_0(t + h) - p_0(t)}{h} = \frac{-\lambda h p_0(t) + o(h)}{h}$$

and hence, taking the limit as $h \to 0$,

$$p_0'(t) = -\lambda p_0(t). \tag{7}$$

Since a worm occupies a finite amount of physical space the probability of one or more worms being in a region of size zero is zero. Therefore, $p_0(0)$ must be one, and it follows that

$$p_0(t) = e^{-\lambda t}.$$

We can determine $p_n(t)$ in much the same way. Using the assumptions as we did above, we obtain

$$p_n(t + h) = p_n(t)p_0(h) + p_{n-1}(t)p_1(h) + p_{n-2}(t)p_2(h) + \cdots + p_0(t)p_n(h)$$

$$= p_n(t)p_0(h) + p_{n-1}(t)p_1(h) + o(h)$$

and consequently

$$p_n'(t) = \lim_{h \to 0} \frac{p_n(t + h) - p_n(t)}{h} = \lim_{h \to 0} \frac{-\lambda h p_n(t) + \lambda h p_{n-1}(t) + o(h)}{h}$$

$$= -\lambda p_n(t) + \lambda p_{n-1}(t), \qquad n = 1, 2, \cdots. \tag{8}$$

[2] $o(h)$ denotes a term $t(h)$ satisfying $\lim_{h \to 0} t(h)/h = 0$.

The differential equations (8) can be solved successivley (along with the conditions $p_n(0) = 0$ for $n \geq 1$) to get

$$p_n(t) = e^{-\lambda t}\frac{(\lambda t)^n}{n!}, \qquad n = 1, 2, 3, \cdots. \tag{9}$$

EXERCISES

1. Justify each of the steps in the derivation of Eqs. (7) and (8) and verify that formula (9) actually provides the solution.

2. Show that $\Sigma_{n=0}^{\infty} p_n(t) = 1$. Why is this to be expected?

If we choose our unit of size in such a way that the average human being has size 1 and let p_n denote the probability of a given person carrying n worms, it follows that $p_n = p_n(1) = e^{-\lambda}\lambda^n/n!$. This probability distribution is known as the Poisson distribution.

3. Show that if $p_n = e^{-\lambda}\lambda^n/n!$, then the expected number of worms per person is λ.

4. Calculation of $P(m)$

If m is the expected number of parasites harbored by a given human, we shall assume that the expected numbers of male and female parasites are each $m/2$. Moreover, we shall assume that the numbers of male and female parasites are independent random variables each with a Poisson distribution. Therefore,

$$\Pr[p \text{ males}] = e^{-m/2}\frac{1}{p!}\left(\frac{m}{2}\right)^p, \tag{10}$$

$$\Pr[q \text{ females}] = e^{-m/2}\frac{1}{q!}\left(\frac{m}{2}\right)^q, \tag{11}$$

$$\Pr[p \text{ males and } q \text{ females}] = e^{-m}\frac{1}{p!q!}\left(\frac{m}{2}\right)^{p+q}. \tag{12}$$

For simplicity, we shall assume that pairs are formed whenever possible; i.e., if there are p males and q females present, the number of pairs is given by $\min(p, q)$. Therefore, the number of paired parasites is given by 2 $\min(p, q)$. Hence from (12) we conclude that

$$P(m) = \sum_{p=0}^{\infty}\sum_{q=0}^{\infty} 2 \min(p, q)e^{-m}\frac{1}{p!q!}\left(\frac{m}{2}\right)^{p+q}. \tag{13}$$

From (13), it is already apparent that

$$P(m) \sim \frac{m^2}{2} \text{ for small values of } m, \tag{13'}$$

since the only term which is not of higher degree corresponds to $p = 1$, $q = 1$. For large values of m, one could approximate the Poisson distribution by a normal distribution and show that $P(m)$ is approximately equal to m. Instead of elaborating upon these remarks, we shall evaluate the sum (13) in terms of known functions. The following calculation is based upon Leyton [2] and Nåsell and Hirsch [4].

The expression (13) will be evaluated by summing the doubly infinite matrix along diagonals $p = q + l$, with l fixed. If the matrix is denoted (a_{pq}), then the diagonals are shown in the matrix below

$$
\begin{array}{c}
\begin{array}{cccc}
l = 0 \qquad\qquad\qquad l = -1 \;\; l = -2 \\
\end{array}\\
\begin{array}{ll}
l = 1 \!-\!\!\!\! &
\begin{bmatrix}
a_{11} & a_{12} & a_{13} & a_{14} & \cdots \\
a_{21} & a_{22} & a_{23} & a_{24} & \cdots \\
a_{31} & a_{32} & a_{33} & a_{34} & \cdots \\
a_{41} & a_{42} & a_{43} & a_{44} & \cdots \\
\vdots & \vdots & \vdots & \vdots &
\end{bmatrix}
\end{array}
\end{array}
$$

As a preparation, we first sum the original distribution (12) along diagonals. If $l > 0$, we define

$$
I_l(m) = \sum_{q=0}^{\infty} \frac{1}{q!(q + l)!} \left(\frac{m}{2}\right)^{q+q+l}. \tag{14}
$$

It turns out that $I_l(m)$ is a modified Bessel function (see Abromowitz and Stegun [1, p. 375]). This is a considerable advantage, since these functions have been studied and tabulated. In view of the symmetry of the distribution, we set $I_{-l} = I_l$. By summing over all of the diagonals, we obtain the identity (see [1, p. 376, eq. 9.6.37])

$$
e^{-m} \sum_{l=-\infty}^{\infty} I_l(m) = 1. \tag{15}
$$

This expresses the fact (which can be verified by summing (12) in the usual way) that the probabilities of all of the possibilities add up to 1.

Let A_l denote a diagonal sum corresponding to (13); if $l \geq 0$

$$
A_l = \sum_{q=0}^{\infty} \frac{q}{q!(q + l)!} \left(\frac{m}{2}\right)^{2q+l}. \tag{16}
$$

We set $A_{-l} = A_l$, in view of the symmetry in (13). It follows from (13) and (16) that

$$
P(m) = 2e^{-m} \sum_{l=-\infty}^{\infty} A_l. \tag{17}
$$

On the other hand a comparison of (14) and (16) shows that if $l \geq 0$, then

$$
A_l = \frac{m}{2} I_{l+1}(m). \tag{18}
$$

Therefore (17) can be rewritten as

$$P(m) = me^{-m}\left(\sum_{l=1}^{\infty} I_l + \sum_{l=2}^{\infty} I_l\right). \tag{19}$$

The identity (15) then implies that

$$P(m) = m[1 - e^{m}(I_0(m) + I_1(m))]. \tag{20}$$

The factor within the brackets gives the proportion of paired parasites. MacDonald denotes this quantity by α and has tabulated it in the second column of Table II, page 192. The asymptotic expansion of [1, p. 377, eq. 9.7.1] shows that if m is large, then

$$\frac{P(m)}{m} \cong 1 - \left[\frac{2}{\pi m}\right]^{1/2}. \tag{21}$$

This approximation yields $P(m)/m \cong 0.748$ for $m = 10$. It is even more accurate for larger values of m. For small values of m the table shows that indeed $P(m)/m$ is close to $m/2$.

EXERCISE

4. Verify the computations in Eqs. (14)–(20).

5. Analysis of Equation (6)

We begin by looking for equilibrium solutions, i.e., those for which $dm/dt \equiv 0$. Using the notation $\alpha(m)$ for $P(m)/m$ (MacDonald's α) and setting $dm/dt = 0$ in (6) we obtain

$$-rm + \frac{ABm\alpha(m)}{Bm\alpha(m) + \delta} = 0. \tag{22}$$

Clearly, $m \equiv 0$ is one solution. To find the others it is helpful to rewrite (22) in the form

$$\alpha(m) = \frac{r\delta}{AB - mBr}. \tag{23}$$

The graph for $y = \alpha(m)$ can be constructed from the graphs of $e^{-m}I_0(m)$ and $e^{-m}I_1(m)$ found in [1, p. 375]. It follows from (13′) that the slope of this graph at the origin is $1/2$, and it follows from (21) that the graph is asymptotic to the line $y = 1$. The graph of $y = r\delta/(AB - mBr)$ is a branch of a hyperbola, and the solutions of (23) correspond to the points of intersection shown in Figure 6.1.

Notice that for the particular choices of the parameters A, B, r, δ corresponding to the graphs shown in Figure 6.1 there are two positive roots of

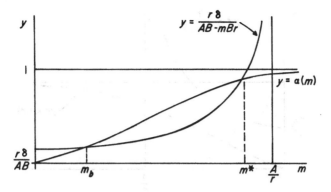

Figure 6.1

(22), denoted by m^* and m_b. Thus we find three equilibrium solutions of (6),

$$m \equiv 0$$

$$m \equiv m_b$$

$$m \equiv m^*.$$

Rewriting (6) in the form

$$\frac{dm}{dt} = \left(\frac{m}{mB\alpha + \delta}\right)\left(AB - mBr\right)\left(\alpha - \frac{r\delta}{AB - mBr}\right),$$

it is clear that if $m > m^*$, then $dm/dt < 0$; and if $m_b < m < m^*$, then $dm/dt > 0$. Thus m^* is stable, and if m is any solution of (6) with $m > m_b$, then $m(t) \to m^*$ as $t \to \infty$. If $0 < m < m_b$, then $dm/dt < 0$ and $m \to 0$. The number m_b is the number called the break point. If a treatment program succeeds in bring m below m_b, then the infection will die out. If not, the level of infection will again rise to m^*.

A comprehensive program aimed at controlling or eradicating the infection will affect all of the parameters A, B, r, and δ as well as m. The relationship of the points m_b and m^* to A, B, r and δ lies at the heart of MacDonald's paper. A qualitative feeling for these relationships can be obtained from Figure 6.2.

Sanitation improvements have the effect of decreasing B. This in turn has the effect of shifting the hyperbola upward which leads to a shift of m_b to the right. The vertical asymptote at A/r is unaffected by B and consequently large changes in B lead to relatively small changes in m^*. A concentrated program of medical treatment has several effects, one of which is to reduce m and the second of which is an increase in r, the death rate of worms. The vertical asymptote is shifted to the left, the intercept $r\delta/AB$ is raised, and the effect is to decrease m^* and increase m_b. A campaign to kill snails has a similar effect since A is decreased and δ increased.

The ideal situation is to modify the parameters in such a way that the

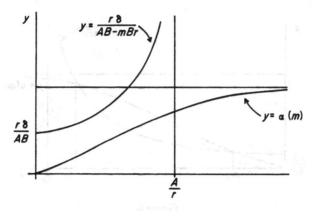

Figure 6.2

hyperbola does not intersect $\alpha(m)$ at all (Figure 6.2). In this case, the only stable solution is $m \equiv 0$, and every solution will die out.

With this introduction, the reader is urged to turn to MacDonald's original work. A more elaborate and complete mathematical treatment of this problem is contained in Nåsell and Hirsch [4].

Appendix: An Alternate Model

In deriving Eq. (6), which is the basis of his model, MacDonald made the assumption that since m varies slowly with respect to time, I will remain near an equilibrium value I^* (see pages 193–194 in MacDonald's paper or page 180 of this introduction). The assumption seems somewhat dubious, however, when one considers that killing snails is one of the major methods of control. One might therefore expect Eqs. (1) and (3) to provide a more realistic model. In what follows, we will sketch a phase portrait for the system of Eqs. (1), (3). We will see that from a qualitative point of view we can draw conclusions similar to MacDonald's but that the interdependence of m and I will become more apparent.

The equations under consideration are

$$\frac{dI}{dt} = -\delta I + BP(m)(S - I) \tag{1}$$

$$\frac{dm}{dt} = -rm + \frac{A}{S}I. \tag{3}$$

We begin by observing that $dI/dt = 0$ whenever $\delta I = BP(m)(S - 1)$ or when $I = BP(m)S/(BP(m) + \delta)$. This curve, labeled c, is sketched in Figure 6.3. Since $P(m) \sim m$ for large values of m, c will be asymptotic to the line $I = S$. For small values of m, c behaves like the parabola $I = m^2 s/2\delta$. Above c, dI/dt is negative and below c, dI/dt is positive.

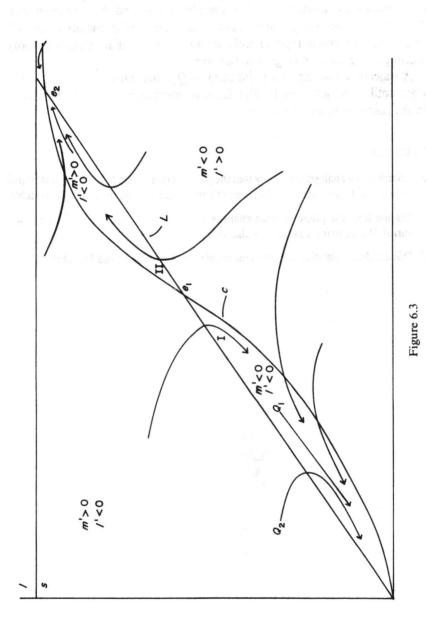

Figure 6.3

Similarly, $dm/dt = 0$ when $I = (S/A)\,rm$. This line is labled L. Above L, dm/dt is positive, and below L, dm/dt is negative. The three points of intersection 0, e_1, and e_2 are the equilibrium solutions.

Now consider a trajectory starting at a point Q_1 inside region I. Such a curve must move toward the origin since both dI/dt and dm/dt are negative. Furthermore, such a trajectory cannot cross either line L or the curve c (why?) and so must remain in region I and continue in to 0. Similarly, any trajectory starting in region II must go into the point e_2.

A trajectory starting at a point such as Q_2 must move down and to the right until it crosses L (vertically). Once it enters region I it must behave as in the case above, and go into 0.

EXERCISES

5. Complete the analysis, and show that the phase portrait must look like that sketched in Figure 6.3. Show that 0 and e_2 are both asymptotically stable while e_1 is unstable.

6. Discuss how the phase portrait changes as the parameters A, B, r, δ, and S are varied. Recall that a change in S also affects A.

7. Discuss the similarities and differences between these results and MacDonald's.

Appendix: Reprint of MacDonald's Article

TRANSACTIONS OF THE ROYAL SOCIETY OF
TROPICAL MEDICINE AND HYGIENE.
Vol. 59. No. 5. September, 1965.

THE DYNAMICS OF HELMINTH INFECTIONS, WITH SPECIAL REFERENCE TO SCHISTOSOMES

BY

GEORGE MACDONALD

Director, Ross Institute of Tropical Hygiene; Professor of Tropical Hygiene, London School of Hygiene and Tropical Medicine

All medically significant helminths are bisexual, differing in this way from almost all other types of infecting agents. Whereas bacterial, virus and protozoal infections may multiply with relative ease from small origins, owing to the absence of immunity against them, and find growth restricted when they become common, the helminth inevitably to some extent experiences the reverse, the probability of the two sexes meeting being less when they are rare than when they are common, with consequent restriction of multiplication from a small start. Though this must modify to some degree the dynamics of infection with helminths—and there are many comments to this effect in the literature—the exact nature of the modification does not appear to have been explored. The primary object of this paper is to do so.

However, this is not the only point of principle on which helminth infections differ from others. The reaction of immunity to many of them is low; superinfection is not only possible, but the general rule; multiple infections occur in considerable numbers and the infectivity of the host to others is related to the order of multiple infections carried, and consequently varies greatly from host to host and from time to time. The unit of infectivity is, in fact, the number of parasites harboured, whereas in most other infections it is the number of infected hosts. This again must have an important effect on the dynamics of infection and also does not appear to have been adequately explored.

Other characteristics to be taken into account are that most helminths do not complete multiplication within the vertebrate host, and require an alternative environment. When this is a living alternative host such as a snail or mosquito, superinfection may be possible but is necessarily limited if only by the relative size of the two organisms, with the result that infectivity of the alternative host cannot for long remain proportional to the number of infections which it has received. Its status as regards infectivity resembles that of the vertebrate host of bacterial and similar infections, an infective unit rather than the carrier of an almost infinitely variable number of discrete infections.

The implications of these characteristics and their working are too complicated to follow by direct reasoning or to infer from field observation without a preliminary hypothesis as a background on which to work. The most effective way of studying them is through creation of a model by strict definition of these characteristics, their interpretation into a form which can be manipulated mathematically, analysis of the manner in which the different characteristics influence dynamic happenings, and study of the effect of changes in them on the total volume of transmission.   Such a model does not primarily depend on a quantitative knowledge of these characteristics, but rather on their nature, and, by indicating which are the most significant, it may be a sound guide to the general policies of both research and operational prevention.

Important contributions to the dynamics of schistosome infections have been made by HAIRSTON (1962) and WHO (1965), though without reference to the sexual feature on which attention is here concentrated.

The model should incorporate all the factors known to have a significant influence on the nature of transmission, despite the resultant complication.   Indeed, the advantage of a model is that it enables one to study the whole structure, made up of a number of complicated parts, in a manner which could not be otherwise understood.   The model here presented includes two different aspects of probability theory: the consequences of random distribution of invading larvae between people, and the probable numbers of pairs resulting from invasion by different numbers.   These are both basically simple but, when brought together, form series which cannot be handled by ordinary analytical methods.   After considerable preliminary exploration, it was decided that only a computer technique could solve them.   After the necessary re-writing, all the various series except those presented in Table I have been worked on the Atlas computer of the University of London Institute of Computer Science.   The results are expressed for the most part as a series of graphs in the text, and the main expressions, together with the principles of their development, are set out in an Appendix.   Abbreviated tabular statements are given of 3 sets of figures which it is thought may be of general use as working tools for research, but the many other sets of figures involved are not otherwise reproduced.*

The model is presented in two sections.   The first is a basic statement of the relationship between the number of invading organisms and the probability of pairing, for both a given number of invading organisms per individual and for a random distribution within a population of a given mean number of infections.   The second part incorporates this basic material in a general model of a schistosome infection, studying particularly the happenings following the first introduction of infection to a community, the influence of different factors on its increase and ultimate level, together with the relative efficacy of different means of prevention.

The probability of pairing

It is here assumed that the probabilities of invasion by male and female larvae are equal, though the actual distribution of the two sexes is determined by chance; that a pairing, once it has occurred, is permanent—as is thought to represent happenings in the schistosomes.

Probability for known numbers

Clearly invasion by a single larva cannot result in pairing.   Invasion by two may be in the form of two male, one of each sex, or two female, with the respective probability of 1/4, 2/4 and 1/4, giving a 0·5 probability of pairing.   The probability is the same for the next odd number, 3, but increases to 0·625 for 4 and 5, and again increases for subsequent sets of even and odd numbers.   The justification for this is set out in the Appendix, together with general expressions from which the probable proportion of any given number of invading larvae which are paired can be calculated.   The results

---

* The author can supply a tabular statement of the figures on which any of the graphs are based, or a fuller statement of Table II, if a research worker requires them.

of some of these calculations are set out in Table I in sufficient detail for graphic representation and interpolation, it being remembered that the figures are not properly represented by a true curve, but by a histogram proceeding by stages from even number to even number, though this may not be significant with high numbers where there is little change from one to another.

TABLE I. The probability of pairing for known numbers of worms in the host. The probabilities for odd numbers are the same as for the immediately preceding even number.

Number	Probability
1	0
2	0·5
4	0·625
6	0·687
8	0·726
10	0·754
12	0·774
14	0·790
16	0·804
18	0·816
20	0·825
30	0·855
40	0·875
60	0·897
80	0·911
100	0·921
400	0·960
1,000	0·975

Probability for randomly distributed numbers

It is most unlikely that in any given group or community all individuals would be invaded by the same number of larvae, the best representation being that the proportion receiving 0, 1, 2, 3, etc., varies with the ordinary laws of chance, represented for small numbers by the Poisson series. Under this random condition it may well occur that some receive 2 or more even when the mean number is considerably less, and some amount of pairing may therefore occur. Exploration of the combination of these two probabilities is therefore essential, and the conclusions apply whether the host is regarded as a single entity within which a male and female parasite will inevitably meet, or as a compartmentalized structure within which pairing only occurs if male and female enter the same compartment. Exploration of this aspect is particularly important because the special features of bisexual infections are thought to occur mainly when the invading numbers are small.

A general expression for this relationship is given in the Appendix. Calculation of actual values in a dynamic series cannot be done by analytical means, and is excessively laborious by desk calculation mechanisms, but constitutes a simple exercise for the computer. Table II sets out the probable proportion of all worms in a host community which are paired for given mean numbers per community member, for a series of means up to 10·0. After this it is justifiable to use the values given in Table I because the two then, to all intents and purposes, merge with each other. This element of the proportion of randomly distributed worms which are paired enters into all the various dynamic equations used in the later model.

TABLE II. The probabilities, for a random distribution of a mean load of worms throughout a host community, of worms being paired, and of hosts harbouring paired worms or worms whether paired or not.

Mean Load	Probable proportions of worms paired	Probable proportions of hosts with	
		Paired worms	Worms, whether paired or not
0·1	0·048	0·0024	0·095
0·2	0·091	0·0091	0·181
0·3	0·130	0·0194	0·259
0·4	0·166	0·0329	0·330
0·5	0·199	0·0489	0·393
0·6	0·229	0·0671	0·451
0·7	0·256	0·0721	0·503
0·8	0·281	0·109	0·551
0·9	0·305	0·131	0·593
1·0	0·326	0·155	0·632
1·2	0·365	0·204	0·699
1·4	0·398	0·253	0·753
1·6	0·428	0·303	0·798
1·8	0·453	0·352	0·835
2·0	0·476	0·400	0·865
3·0	0·560	0·604	0·950
4·0	0·614	0·748	0·982
5·0	0·652	0·843	0·993
6·0	0·681	0·903	0·998
7·0	0·704	0·941	0·999
8·0	0·722	0·964	} > 0·999
9·0	0·738	0·978	
10·0	0·751	0·987	

Probable proportion of hosts with paired worms

Though it is the proportion of paired worms which constitutes the significant dynamic factor, the common epidemiological measures are in terms of people who are infected or, more properly, the proportion of people with paired worms. The two are not the same inasmuch as a host enters the class of having paired worms as soon as it harbours a single pair, though there may be several unpaired specimens present. The probability of having one or more pairs when infection is randomly distributed involves another combination of the Poisson series with a binomial expression, which is also set out in the Appendix and requires computer calculation. Relevant values of this series, which again may be useful as a working tool, are set out in the second column of Table II, in column 3 of which they are contrasted with the probable proportion of people carrying one or more worms, whether paired or not, from which it will be seen that there is a substantial difference between the two proportions when the level of infection is low.

The schistosomiasis model

Basic assumptions

The adequacy of representation of an infection by a model turns principally on the basic assumptions built into it, and their accuracy in qualitative representation of transmission. If they are sound, the model can give a qualitative picture of transmission with the relative significance of different factors, and of modification of these factors, even though their quantitative values may be almost unknown. Such a qualitative model will show which factors are most important and therefore most merit quantitative measurement, and thereby ultimately lead to a fully quantitative model. The one here presented aspires to the first, qualitative, form.

It concerns a bisexual helminth: infection occurs through invasion by larvae randomly distributed, with equal probability of male and female larvae, through the members of a host community in an ecological complex. The worms are considered as monogamous, a single union taking place. They are long-lived and the female lays continuously throughout life, the eggs being passed out in urine or stool. In numerical working, a mean life of 3 years and a mean daily egg-laying of 1,000 eggs has been attributed to them (cf. HAIRSTON, 1962), but even very substantial modification of these values would make no difference to the points of principle which are subsequently elaborated on the basis of the working.

The daily number of eggs reaching the water within any given ecological complex turns on two sets of variables: firstly on the host population within the complex, its mean worm load, the proportion of worms which are paired and the daily egg output per fertilized worm; and secondly on the proportion of these eggs which are carried directly or indirectly into the water. The first group is a function of the prevalence of infection, and the second a function of environment and sanitary habit which are subject to considerable modification. This last is referred to henceforth as the "contamination factor".

The probability of a miracidium coming into contact with a snail depends principally on the numbers of the latter, being naturally lower when they are sparse, though account must be taken of the fact that the number of miracidia per snail may then be increased, since penetration of a snail removes a miracidium from circulation and therefore to some degree protects others.

The next group of factors involved are those which control multiplication within the snail host; principally the number of susceptible snails within the ecological complex, their length of life, the daily cercarial output from an infected snail and its duration. The significantly variable factor among these is the number of susceptible snails, and the whole group of factors is subsequently referred to as the "snail factor". No account is taken in the model of the mortality experienced by snails as a result of infection, a considerable study of the influence which such mortality would have resulting in the conclusion that it would be quantitative only and would not interfere in any way with the principle of dynamics or the qualitative findings which are developed in this paper. The well accepted possibility of multiple infections in the snail has also been ignored. There have been many demonstrations of this happening, though all of those known to the writer concern multiple infections due to virtually simultaneous penetration of two or more miracidia, and there is some doubt as to whether superinfection can occur on top of an already well developed infection. However, the important point in considering dynamics is that cercarial production is not quantitatively related to the number of invading miracidia. PESIGAN et al. (1958) found a reduction of output with multiple infections and, though there is no evidence that this is generally true, or that there is not some increase with double or treble infections, the dynamic picture depends on whether or not a direct quantitative relationship can be almost indefinitely maintained over a long series of superinfections, and this is certainly not the case.

The next group of factors concerns the probability of a cercaria finding a suitable host, in which there are two constituents: a biological constant representing the efficiency of the cercaria in this respect, and a variable, the number and extent of contacts with water by potential hosts. The picture incorporated in the model is of variable number of contacts of a standard mean extent, and it is referred to as the "exposure factor" which can be modified at will. Since the biological factor is presumably a constant its actual value has no influence on the principle of happenings, though it has been necessary to attribute a value to it for numerical working and one has been selected which seems to accord realistically with natural happenings.

Within the vertebrate host, incomparably the most important factor in modifying principle is the probability of male and female worms mating, which is handled on the lines already explained. A second important characteristic is the longevity of the worm which is naturally determined and is normally regarded as a constant, but which can be modified by systematic case-finding and treatment mechanisms aiming at periodically detecting and treating a large proportion of positive cases. Since this may be a significant item in control or eradication programmes, the length of life of the worm is treated as a variable, and referred to as the "longevity factor".

No account is taken here of two factors which may be thought to be relevant: the extent to which the volume of the host limits the probability of male and female larvae meeting, and the way in which immunity may interfere with the process. It is almost certainly true that the very large extent of the vascular system limits the probability of male and female meeting, and that it would be more correct to regard the body as consisting of a number of compartments of limited size, mating taking place if male and female found themselves in the same compartment. The effect this would have on the dynamics of infection has been explored, and it would certainly have a very large quantitative effect in that the probability of mating for given numbers of larvae would be greatly reduced, but the general form of happenings would not be in any way altered. It is mainly for this reason that the model is presented purely as a qualitative one, dealing with terms of principles and not with actual numbers of parasites harboured.

The uncertainty about the scale on which this isolation occurs could probably be removed if it were possible to relate the number of eggs in the excreta to the worm load carried even in a few cases—a subject on which the literature is silent. If this gap in knowledge could be filled, it would probably be possible to convert the present qualitative model into one which was largely quantitative and, particularly, to relate the conclusions about "break points" to actual infection rates measured by traditional means, and thus to give precision to the science of prevention. The part played by immunity in restricting transmission has the same entirely quantitative consequence. It is probable that people are susceptible only to a finite number of infections, becoming ultimately resistant to others, but this number is certainly large. Though allowance could readily be made for it, its influence on dynamics is probably so much smaller than that of isolation by volume, discussed above, that it does not justify inclusion until that subject can be clarified.

The model based on these characteristics has certain features which can be deduced in a general manner by inspection but it is only by actual calculation by computer that they can be confirmed and precision given to them. The findings described henceforward are, therefore, all based on a series of computer programmes in which different values have been given to the main factors, contamination, snails, exposure, and longevity in the vertebrate host. Programmes were run first to identify the probable course of events following original introduction of the infection into an ecological complex, which has been visualized as a village community with its neighbouring water holes or pools, which members of the community enter from time to time for their domestic purposes. After gaining a picture of happenings following introduction leading to an equilibrium level in the population, a number of programmes have been run representing efforts at control.   For this a single set of parameters, previously tested in the introduction phase and thought by their consequences to be realistic, have been accepted as the standard and control has been represented by reduction of the value of one or other of the parameters to a stated fraction of the original, the general principles being to test the effects of equivalent reduction in each.

During this working, it has been shown both by deduction and calculation that the level of prevalence in the community is subject to both lower and upper limiting values which are analagous to the critical level of the transmission and the equilibrium level in other infections, though there are certain important differences from them.   The characteristics of the lower limit have such an important bearing on the policy of control that it is here distinguished by a different name, the "break point", the significance of which should be apparent from findings noted in a later section.

The break point

A normal infection by an asexual parasite may be introduced to a community by a minimal amount of infectivity, typically by a single introduced case, and it may then find its optimum opportunity for multiplication which, when represented on log-metric or "ratio" paper, is likely to take the form of curve B in Fig. 1.   The question of whether it multiplies and at what rate depends exclusively on characteristics of the environment, which determine the degree of effective contact between the primary case and susceptibles.

By contrast the establishment of a bisexual infection in a community depends both on environmental factors determining the degree of contact, and also on the quantity of infection introduced.   A potential introduction may be on a sufficiently small scale to make it unlikely that it will produce enough multiple infections in recipients to ensure continuation of the chain of transmission, for which it is necessary to postulate the introduction of a notable number of fertile worms, whether in one or several hosts.   For any given environment there is a critical number of worms; the presence of more will lead to multiplication till equilibrium is reached, and of less to progressive diminution.   This is represented in terms of the mean worm load for the community concerned and is termed the "break point," the significance of this term being that this number of worms is not only critical in preventing or allowing introduction of the infection but also, as will be shown later, in causing an abrupt break between maintained transmission and eradication when control measures are introduced.   It is determined almost equally by the four factors of contamination, snails, exposure, and longevity, so that introduction and maintenance are relatively easy when these are high but may demand quite massive invasion for establishment of the chain of transmission when they are low.   It follows that introduction to a previously uninfected area by a single traveller would be improbable, though the risk of introduction by groups of people from an infected place would be considerably greater, and there is ample evidence in the history of both schistosomiasis and filariasis to support this.

Introduction of infection

If the scale of introduction is slightly above the break point, multiplication at first occurs at a substantially slower rate than would be expected with an asexual infection,

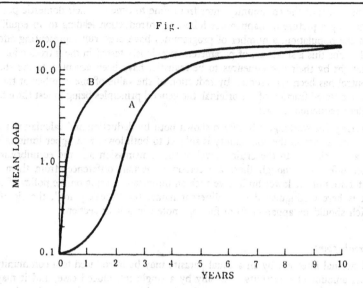

FIG. 1. Curves on log/metric or ratio paper showing A, the expected
course of happenings following introduction of a sexual helminth infection
as described in the text, contrasted with B, the expected course of a
hypothetical asexual parasite, otherwise identical, to show the modification of principle determined by the sexual feature.

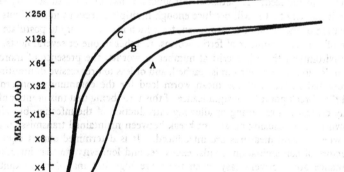

FIG. 2. The "standard" introduction, A, and the curves expected
following doubling the contamination factor, B, and either the exposure
or snail factor, C.

but gradually accelerates as the mean load increases until after a considerable lapse of time, which in the examples worked is 2 or more years, it reaches the same rate of development as would otherwise occur.

When the mean load is low the infection meets a considerable obstruction to multiplication and it is then unstable; if conditions are unchanged it is liable to multiply considerably, but some quite small change might result in reversal and disappearance. When, however, the infection has become common it achieves stability, a substantial change being then needed to modify the equilibrium level in any significant manner.

The contrast between the asexual and bisexual types of curve is shown in curves A and B of Fig. 1, from which it will be seen that, following this original sharp discrepancy between them, there is a rise to the same plateau of equilibrium.

Fig. 2 shows the effect of modification of the contamination factor and of the exposure or snail factors on introduction of infection. Increase in either of them lowers the break point so that introduction would have been effective with a smaller invading group. In both cases the time factor of multiplication is substantially altered so that the rapid increase occurs very much earlier, though the general shape of the curve with the initial period of relatively slow development remains. Both rise to a plateau. In the case of increased contamination, this is virtually identical with the original whereas with increased exposure, and also with a greater number of snails, the resultant plateau is at a mean load which is increased almost proportionately to the increase in exposure or snails.

Heavy contamination of the water, though it makes introduction of the infection easier, appears to have virtually no effect on the ultimate level of endemicity attained, which is almost exclusively dependent on the numbers of snails, the frequency of entry to water and the longevity of the worm. Further aspects of this characteristic will be discussed in relation to control where it has most significant implications for policy. The explanation is that whatever the degree of contamination of water, the mean load ultimately rises in most circumstances, to a level where miracidia are much more numerous than are susceptible snails, so that even quite considerable modification in their number within a very wide range produces an insignificant change in ultimate numbers of infective snails.

After running a number of programmes, a set of parameters has been arbitarily selected as the standard for subsequent testing of the effects of control by alteration of their value. The standard curve is that for bisexual infections, in curve A of Fig. 1. Among its assumptions other than those already stated, are contamination equivalent to 1,000th part of the total excreta of the population reaching the water and a snail density of 5 per linear metre of water bank. No specific figure has been given for the number of water entries per person per day, but the total exposure factor previously described, which includes a still unmeasured biological constant, has been adjusted to produce what is thought to be a realistic result. The value used is $0 \cdot 02$, which would mean that, with an average of one entry daily per person, scanning one square metre of water, the probability of the individual cercaria within that square metre successfully penetrating would be $0 \cdot 02$, though the actual values used are quite immaterial to the present context.

Representation of control

The effect of modifying any of the factors involved is two-fold: to change the level at which equilibrium is established, and also to change the level of the break point in this set of circumstances. In this context the break point represents a mean load below which the infection is unable to maintain itself. If it is passed, diminution is not only progressive but accelerating.

B*

A first set of programme runs shows the effect of reducing transmission factors to a degree which does not cause the equilibrium level to sink below the break point, and they are illustrated in Fig. 3. In this group of programmes 4 types of control scheme have been tested, superficially of the same degree in that, in each, one of the relevant factors was decreased to the same degree, here one fifth of its original level, and the consequences tested over a period of 10 years.

Improvement of sanitation is represented as a decrease of the amount of contamination of water, so that one 5,000th of the excreta reaches water. The consequential reduction of mean load in the population, shown in curve A of Fig. 3, is so small as to be quite invisible in the graph, and is in fact less than 1%. Despite this reduction to a level of contamination which represents quite good sanitation, the number of miracidia in the water remains higher than the number of snails, and the chain continues almost unabated.

The effects of reduction of snail factor and of the exposure factor, shown in curve B, are so nearly identical that they are represented here by a single line which ultimately descends to about a fifth of its original level. The slope of descent is extremely slow and more than 10 years elapse before the new, lower equilibrium level is established.

Treatment is considered as a continuous campaign of diagnosis and treatment which results in the examination of every individual once a year, followed by effective treatment of the positives. This is looked on as reducing the expectation of life of the average worm from about 3 years to about 6 months, the average time elapsing between infection and subsequent treatment, but to allow for imperfections in the programme the

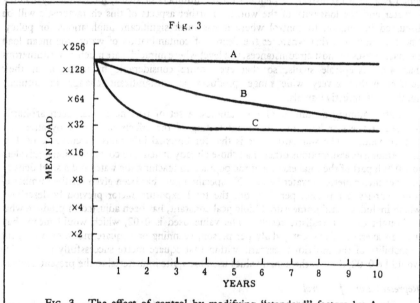

FIG. 3. The effect of control by modifying "standard" factors by A, reducing the contamination factor to 1/5th; B, reducing either snails or exposure to 1/5th; and C, reducing the mean longevity of the worm by systematic treatment campaigns to 1/5th.

actual reduction claimed has been only to one fifth of the original figure. This produces a fall in the mean load, shown in curve C, to a new equilibrium level which is almost identical with that obtained by long-continued control of snails or exposure, but the new level is much more rapidly attained, almost complete results being visible between 2 and 3 years after the start. A side issue of the programme demonstrates, however, that this treatment has no "public health significance" in the form of reducing the inoculation rate for the general population and thus lessening the risk to those who do not themselves undergo treatment, this rate showing only a small decline to 83% of its original level during this programme. The explanation of this relative lack of effect lies in the form that protection of the general population would take—reduction of contamination—in itself a relatively ineffective measure. Treatment carried out to an extent which does not approach eradication of the infection is, therefore, of great value to the recipients but is of little value to others. The only method of limited control which has any public health significance within this definition is the control of the snail factor.

These schemes were ineffective for eradication in that they never led to the equilibrium level approaching the break point. A following series of programmes attempts to enhance them until the break point is passed. For this purpose the programme of treatment illustrated in Fig. 3 was taken as a basis, but since it was thought to be impractical to attempt to improve any programme of treatment beyond the standard here

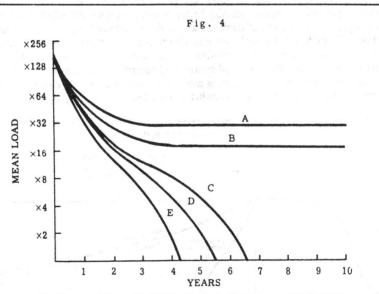

FIG. 4. The break point. The "standard" has been modified in A by reduction of the longevity of the worm through treatment to 1/5th. To this has been added decrease of exposure, or of snails, to give a total reduction of transmission factors to $1/8 \cdot 75$ in B, 1/10 in C, $1/11 \cdot 25$ in D and 1/15 in E. No significance is attached to the actual numerical values of these reductions, but great significance is attached to the slight relative difference between B and C and the consequences of this small difference.

described, enhancement of effect was produced by super-added reduction of the exposure factor, though the influence of super-added snail control would have been the same. The concept of reduction was that the longevity of the worm already having been reduced to 1/5, a further reduction of exposure to, for instance, one half reduced the total factors to 1/10 of the original level. On this basis an attempt was made to bracket the break point. Fig. 4 shows the results. Curve A is the same as that for treatment in Fig. 3. B shows super-added control to reduce the factors to 1/8·75 of their original value, and this also fails to reach the break point and establishes a new equilibrium at a somewhat lower point. C shows the effect of reducing the total to 1/10 of the original, a very small increment on the efficiency of the previous programme which does, however, pass the point, undergo an inflection and thereafter decrease at a rapidly accelerating rate. D and E show the effect of reduction of the total to 1/11·25 and 1/15 of the original level, with results which are exactly the same in principle as the third curve, though somewhat altered in time scale. This inflection occurs when the mean load is approximately 0·8, which, it will be seen by comparison with Table II, would correspond to an infection rate in the community of roughly 10%, but no great attention is paid to this quantitative inference. The significant point is that a sufficiently intense programme can be expected to pass a break point and thereafter increase rapidly in efficiency and lead to eradication, while one which falls short of the required degree of intensity, even by only a small measure, will have no hope of ever attaining anything other than a reduction of general prevalence.

A following set of programmes illustrated in Fig. 5 completes these observations by testing over a long period, 20 years, the effects of equal reduction in contamination, snails, exposure, and worm longevity by treatment, supported by reduction of exposure, to a degree at which some of them at least would be expected to produce ultimate eradication. The effect of reduced contamination to one 15,000th of excreta reaching water, which represents a very high standard of sanitation, is virtually negligible over the entire period. The effects of snail control and control of exposure in the form of entry to water are virtually identical during most of the period of fall, though during the later stages control of exposure is somewhat more effective, resulting in a slightly earlier

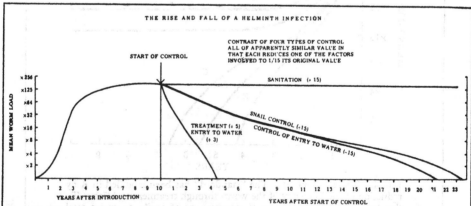

FIG. 5. The rise and fall of a helminth infection. Happenings after introduction above the break point, followed by application of 4 apparently equivalent control programmes: reduction of contamination; reduction of snails; reduction of exposure; and treatment with complementary lessening of exposure or of snails.

disappearance of the infection.   Ultimate disappearance following either of these methods is delayed for over 20 years, throughout all of which effective measures would have to be carried out, and even improvement to a level approaching perfection would only slightly reduce the time involved, to 14 or 15 years, owing to the long mean length of life postulated for the worms, 3 years.   By contrast, the combination of systematic treatment with either reduction of exposure or snail control produces a rapid result, the final effects of which are visible between 4 and 5 years after the start.

This Figure is introduced by the reproduction of the standard entry previously described, and since it is thought to epitomize the whole story, it can be described as the rise and fall of a helminth infection.

Discussion

"The inescapable conclusion from these experiments is that the sanitation produced no measurable effect on infection with the four species of worm parasite (one *S. mansoni*) under study."   These words were used by SCOTT and BARLOW (1938) in a classical study, and the conclusion that it could have no effect is equally inescapable from the present study.   No significant effect, that is, on reduction of the worm load in the community; so that, as a prime measure of control it is virtually useless, because an absolute standard of sanitation can never be achieved in any community.   It follows also that once the infection is established it could be maintained by minute amounts of contamination, the amounts conveyed from slightly fouled clothing being sufficient to keep up transmission.   This is not to say, however, that it is without value in all circumstances.   The standard of sanitation has as large an influence as any of the other factors on determining the break point; a good standard therefore both lessens the probability of introduction and increases the probability of success of other measures, which with this help may reach the break point.   However, the common supposition that "sanitation diseases" are best controlled by provision of latrines finds very little support in these programmes.

A very much more effective aspect of sanitation is reduction of the frequency of contact with possibly contaminated water, chiefly by provision of safe water supplies which makes frequent resort to natural water unnecessary.   Allowance has only been made in the model for actual reduction of exposure to infection, but it is highly probable that reduction of entry would also greatly lessen contamination of the water itself and would thus contribute further to the raising of the break point, if not to the original rate of fall, and therefore to the likelihood of ultimate eradication.   However, the results of reduction of exposure or reduction of snails are so slow as to be almost despairing, both in the model and in experience, and the inclusion of the most effective possible case-finding and treatment mechanisms would be essential to any scheme which hoped for visible success in forseeable time.

It seems, however, that such treatment as is now conceivable could rarely, if practised alone as a control measure, lead to eradication, so that a combination of methods is essential.

A very strong implication of the break point is that campaigns should be very intensive.   Concentrated effort with a full treatment campaign supported by snail control and provision of safe water supplies is likely to be effective, and could be carried out in relatively limited areas because the risks of early re-introduction are relatively low.   On the other hand, diffuse activities with local imperfections in them, or reliance on a single method of control as has, up till now, been the common practice, are very unlikely to produce more than amelioration without prospect of eradication.   When these points are taken together with observations by many past observers, and recently by FORSYTH and BRADLEY (in press) and FORSYTH and MACDONALD (1965), that infection is often of a focal character, there would seem often to be great advantages in a control programme which concentrated effort on the identification of foci.

The model deprecates the "public health value" of treatment, unless the treatment is systematic, regular, and supplemented by other intensive measures with the object of passing the break point and going on to eradication, in which case it has paramount value by introducing an acceptable time scale. The greatest weakness of present programmes lies in the field of therapy, and is largely due to the inadequacy and toxicity of drugs now available. Probably the most significant research contribution which could be made to control mechanisms would be the development of schistosomicidal drugs without these defects.

The presentation has treated the host as an entity within which any male and female worm would probably meet, whereas it is highly probable that a better representation would be as a number of compartments, with the probability of pairing dependent on meeting within a compartment. The uncertainty in this could be removed if, within any ecological complex, it was possible to estimate both the proportion of people with paired worms (the "infection rate") and the mean worm load. A first step in this direction would be to relate worm load to egg output in a few individual cases. All studies of the quantitative aspects of transmission are valuable, but study of this point would perhaps be the most productive step towards gaining a full quantitative appreciation of transmission. This would not be expected to alter the picture here put forward, but should make it possible to estimate the actual degree of improvement of the environment and thoroughness of treatment programmes needed to achieve eradication.

Although the model has been developed with special reference to schistosomiasis, it has some general implications which are applicable to all helminth infections. Of the two aspects of sanitation, reduction of dissemination of contaminated material and reduction of exposure to the medium which may be contaminated, the latter is incomparably the most important. Safe water supplies are more important than latrines, as are shoes in the prevention of ancylostomiasis, and sanitation policy should be reorientated in this way. To be effective, a control programme should be intensive, if necessary limited to a small area, but employing within it all available means of control. Such a programme might have prospects of complete success, and the safeguarding of any area or community which has been cleared may not present great problems.

Appendix

Probability of pairing, for known numbers

If the probabilities of invasion by male and female larvae are equal and mutually exclusive, and the total number invading is an even number n, then the probability of a larva being unmatched by one of the opposite sex is:—

$$\frac{n!}{\left(\frac{n}{2}!\right)^2 2^n} \qquad [1]$$

and the probability of being matched, or pairing, is therefore :—

$$1 - \frac{n!}{\left(\frac{n}{2}!\right)^2 2^n} \qquad [2]$$

The most effective confirmation of this is by taking the binomial expansion of $(a + b)^n$ for any value of n and checking the total number of pairs of a and b which can be made as a proportion of the total numbers in the expression.

The probability for an odd number is identical with that for the preceding even number.

These expressions hold good for any value of n, and can be worked with relative ease when this value is low, but become cumbersome for high values. Fortunately it is then possible to use a simplified expression which is based on the substitution of Stirling's approximation to the factorial for $n!$ in [2], which then approximates:—

$$1 - 0 \cdot 7979 n^{-0 \cdot 5} \qquad [3]$$

It becomes legitimate to use this approximation in the present context when n exceeds 10, at which point the error is less than $0 \cdot 5\%$ and rapidly decreases thereafter.

Table I is based on expression [2] for values up to 10, and [3] thereafter.

Probability of pairing, for random distribution of a known mean

If a known number of larvae are distributed within a finite community on a random basis, so that the mean number per individual is m, then the proportion of the community receiving 0, 1, 2, 3 etc. is given by successive elements of the Poisson series:—

$$e^{-m} \left\{ 1 + m + \frac{m^2}{2!} + \frac{m^3}{3!} + \ldots \ldots \ldots \frac{m^n}{n!} \right\} \qquad [4]$$

and the proportion of larvae in hosts with 0, 1, 2, 3, etc. is given by successive elements of:—

$$\frac{e^{-m}}{m} \left\{ 0 + m + \frac{2m^2}{2!} + \frac{3m^3}{3!} + \ldots \ldots \ldots \frac{m^n}{(n-1)!} \right\} \qquad [5]$$

The probable proportion of larvae which are unpaired is found by multiplying successive pairs (even and odd) of items of [5] by the relevant value of [1] to give an expression in the form:—

$$\frac{e^{-m}}{m} \left\{ \left(0 + m \right) 1 + \left(\frac{m^2}{1} + \frac{m^3}{2!} \right) \left(\frac{2!}{1.1.2^2} \right) + \left(\frac{m^4}{3!} + \frac{m^5}{4!} \right) \left(\frac{4!}{2!2!2^4} \right) + \right.$$
$$\left. \ldots \ldots \left(\frac{m^n}{(n-1)!} + \frac{m^{n+1}}{n!} \right) \left(\frac{n!}{\left(\frac{n}{2}! \right)^2 2^n} \right) \right\} \qquad [6]$$

which, after slight simplification, gives the proportion paired as:—

$$1 - e^{-m} \left\{ 1 + \left(\frac{m}{1} + \frac{m^2}{2!} \right) \left(\frac{2!}{1.1.2^2} \right) + \left(\frac{m^3}{3!} + \frac{m^4}{4!} \right) \left(\frac{4!}{2!2!2^4} \right) + \ldots \ldots \right.$$
$$\left. \ldots \ldots \left(\frac{m^n}{n!} + \frac{m^{n+1}}{(n+1)!} \right) \left(\frac{n!}{\left(\frac{n}{2}! \right)^2 2^n} \right) \right\} \qquad [7]$$

Expression [7] gives the probable proportion of worms paired for any mean number per person randomly distributed, for the range of means suitably represented by the Poisson series. For present purposes this has been taken as a mean of up to 10, when the Poisson series is merging into a normal distribution. For higher values expression [3] has been used, it having been shown by calculation that the two then merge within fully acceptable limits of error.

Random distribution is taken as characteristic of the infections studied, and consequently expressions [7] or [3], whichever is appropriate according to the value of m, enter into all dynamic expressions. Series [7] cannot be estimated analytically, and is excessively cumbersome for serial working by desk methods, and its invariable presence as a constituent of dynamic expressions is the principal bar to their ready appraisal or calculation. For this reason it has been adapted to the computer with an automatic switch from [7] to [3] at a mean of 10, both as a main programme which forms the basis of column 1 of Table II, and as a subroutine incorporated in other later expressions.

The proportion of hosts with paired worms

For any known number, n, of male and female larvae or worms, the sexes being randomly allocated, the probability that they will all be of one sex is:

$$2^{(1-n)} \tag{8}$$

and the consequent probability of one or more pairs being present is:—

$$1 - 2^{(1-n)} \tag{9}$$

As in the previous case, when larvae are randomly distributed throughout the population and it is desired to know the probable proportion of the population with or without any paired worms, it is necessary to combine expression [8] with the Poisson series, [4], producing the following probable proportion of the population with one or more pairs:—

$$1 - e^{-m} \left\{ 1 + m + \frac{m^2}{2!2} + \frac{m^3}{3!2^2} + \cdots\cdots \frac{m^n}{n!2^{n-1}} \right\} \tag{10}$$

which is the basis of column 2 of Table II. Column 3 is directly derived from the Poisson series.

The schistosomiasis model

The course of infection is considered in an ecological complex with an evenly distributed population numbering P, with regular habits, entering water on an average E times daily each. A certain proportion, c, of the eggs they pass reach water. Host snails exist in the water at a density of S per linear metre of bank, the total length of water in the complex being L. The chance of a miracidium which is in the water reaching and penetrating a snail is:—

$$(1 - e^{-0.15}) \tag{11}$$

a probability which is reasonably supported by the critical examination of miracidial behaviour by CHERNIN and DONOVAN (1962).

Transmission can, then, be represented in 4 stages: the inoculation rate to which snails are subject; multiplication of the larvae within those snails which become infected; the consequent inoculation rate to which man is subject; and the growth of infection in man.

The inoculation rate of snails depends on: the number of people in the complex, their mean worm load and the proportion of these which are fertile; the proportion of eggs passed which reach water; the chance which the average miracidium has of coming into effective contact with a snail ; and the number of snails among which these miracidia are distributed.

Among these the mean worm load and the proportion paired are variables within any one programme, and so must be given separate expression, in the form $m\alpha$, in which α is the function of m given in [7]. The remaining factors are parameters which normally remain constant throughout any one programme though the size of the population, the proportion of eggs reaching water and the number of snails can all be modified between programmes. These factors come together in the form of a simple product and so can for simplicity be identified by a single symbol, but for further simplification it is justifiable and convenient to include another factor, the probability of an infected snail living till cercariae develop, within this product, which is then referred to as B, and the total inoculation rate as $Bm\alpha$.

The infection rate in snails can then be represented in a very similar manner to the infection rate of mosquitoes with malarial sporozoites. If p is the probability of a snail surviving through one day, it is:—

$$\frac{Bm\alpha}{Bm\alpha - \log_e p} \qquad [12]$$

Multiplication within infected snails depends, apart from their infection rate, on the number of snails, the mean daily cercarial output of an infected snail and the time for which they live in an infective state. The infection rate and the time for which they remain infective have already been accounted for in [12], which leaves only the number of snails and the cercarial output. This probability of multiplication is, however, followed by one of certain decrease, related to the frequency of human contact with water and the biological efficiency of cercariae in attaching themselves and penetrating. There are no internally variable factors in this group which, however, includes the parameters, fixed within any one programme, of snail density and frequency of human entry into water. The combined probabilities again constitute a simple product which is henceforth represented by A, which can be adjusted by modification of the two parameters mentioned.

The inoculation rate, h, to which man is subject is then:—

$$h = \frac{ABm\alpha}{Bm\alpha - \log_e p} \qquad [13]$$

Superinfection is the rule, and in a simple model making no allowance for migration of hosts, the same basic derivative which has previously been applied to superinfection in malaria (MACDONALD, 1957) can be applied:—

$$\frac{dm}{dt} = h - rm \qquad [14]$$

$$= \frac{ABm\alpha}{Bm\alpha - \log_e p} - rm \qquad [15]$$

However, unlike the malaria case, this derivative remains unchanged whatever the relative values of h and r, and represents the change in the mean worm load within unit time.

Inspection suggests that the integral of this would have an upper limit, L_m, and a lower point of inflexion when the sign of the derivative would inevitably change. The difficult character of α makes precise calculation of the limit and inflexion point impossible, though the following approximate values are indicated. For the upper limit:—

$$L_m \simeq \frac{A}{r} - \frac{(-\log_e p)}{B} \qquad [16]$$

and the point of inflexion is passed when:—

$$\alpha \simeq \frac{r(-\log_e p)}{AB} \qquad [17]$$

Though exact justification of these by analytical means is not feasible, calculation of a considerable number of programmes with a wide range of parameters shows without doubt that the limit and inflexion point exist, with values about those given in [16] and [17], which can therefore be taken as applicable when precision is not needed.

The inflexion point is the "break point" described in the text. It will be noted from [17] that it depends equally on 4 factors, including B. The amount of faecal contamination of water forms a constituent of this, and this is the justification for the statement that, although sanitation has little influence on equilibrium, it materially affects the break point and so supports other control measures.

Acknowledgements

Grateful acknowledgement is made to the University for the facility of using the Atlas computer of the University of London Institute of Computer Science, and to Mrs. Ian McBean for so capably undertaking novel types of secretarial assistance.

REFERENCES

FORSYTH, D. M. & BRADLEY, D. J. *Bull. World Hlth. Org. In press.*
——— & MACDONALD, G. (1965). *Trans. R. Soc. trop. Med. Hyg.*, 59, 171.
HAIRSTON, NELSON G. (1962). CIBA Foundation Symposium on Bilharziasis, p. 36.
MACDONALD, G. (1957). *The Epidemiology and Control of Malaria.* London: Oxford University Press.
PESIGAN, T. P. et al. (1958). *Bull. World Hlth. Org.*, 18, 481.
SCOTT, J. A. & BARLOW, C. H. (1938). *Amer. J. Hyg.*, 27, 619.
WHO Expert Committee on Bilharziasis, 3rd Report (1965). *World Hlth. Org. Tech. Rep. Ser.*, No. 299.

References

[1] M. Abromowitz and I. A. Stegun, *Handbook of Mathematical Functions*. New York: Dover, 1958.

[2] M. K. Leyton, "Stochastic models in populations of helminthic parasites in the definitive host. II. Sexual mating functions," *Math. Biosci*, vol. 3, pp. 413–419, 1968.

[3] G. MacDonald, "The dynamic of helminth infections, with special reference to schistosomes," *Trans. Roy. Soc. Trop. Med. and Hyg.*, vol. 59, no. 5, 1965.

[4] I. Nåsell and W. M. Hirsch, "A mathematical model of some helminth infections," *Com. Pure Appl. Math.*, vol. 25, pp. 459–478, 1972.

CHAPTER 7

A Model for the Spread of Gonorrhea

Martin Braun*

Gonorrhea ranks first today among reportable communicable diseases in the United States. There are more reported cases of gonorrhea every year than the combined totals for syphilis, measles, mumps, and infectious hepatitis. Public health officials estimate that more than 2,500,000 Americans contract gonorrhea every year. This painful and dangerous disease, which is caused by the gonococcus bacterium, is spread from person to person by sexual contact. A few days after the infection there is usually itching and burning of the genital area, particularly while urinating. About the same time a discharge develops which males will notice but which females may not notice. Infected women may have no easily recognizable symptoms, even while the disease does substantial internal damage. Gonorrhea can only be cured by antibiotics (usually penicillin). However, treatment must be given early if the disease is to be stopped from doing serious damage to the body. If untreated, gonorrhea can result in blindness, sterility, arthritis, heart failure, and ultimately death.

In this section we construct a mathematical model of the spread of gonorrhea. Our work is greatly simplified by the fact that the incubation period of gonorrhea is very short (3–7 days) compared to the often quite long period of active infectiousness. Thus we will assume in our model that an individual becomes infective immediately after contracting gonorrhea. In addition, gonorrhea does not confer even partial immunity to those individuals who have recovered from it. Immediately after recovery, an individual is again susceptible. Thus we can split the sexually active and promiscuous portion of the population into two groups, susceptibles and infectives. Let $c_1(t)$ be the total number of promiscuous males, $c_2(t)$ the total number of promis-

* Department of Mathematics, Queens College, Flushing, NY 11367.

cuous females, $x(t)$ the total number of infective males and $y(t)$ the total number of infective females, at time t. Then the total numbers of susceptible males and susceptible females are $c_1(t) - x(t)$ and $c_2(t) - y(t)$, respectively. The spread of gonorrhea is presumed to be governed by the following rules:

(1) Male infectives are cured at a rate a_1 proportional to their total number, and female infectives are cured at a rate a_2 proportional to their total number. The constant a_1 is larger than a_2 since infective males quickly develop painful symptoms and therefore seek prompt medical attention. Female infectives, on the other hand, are usually asymptomatic, and therefore are infectious for much longer periods of time.
(2) New infectives are added to the male population at a rate b_1 proportional to the total number of male susceptibles and female infectives. Similarly, new infectives are added to the female population at a rate b_2 proportional to the total number of female susceptibles and male infectives.
(3) The total numbers of promiscuous males and promiscuous females remain at constant levels c_1 and c_2, respectively.

It follows immediately from rules 1–3 that

$$\frac{dx}{dt} = -a_1 x + b_1(c_1 - x)y$$
$$\frac{dy}{dt} = -a_2 y + b_2(c_2 - y)x. \tag{1}$$

Remark. The system of equations (1) treats only those cases of gonorrhea which arise from heterosexual contacts; the case of homosexual contacts (assuming no interaction between heterosexuals and homosexuals) is treated in Exercises 5 and 6. Now, the number of cases of gonorrhea which arise from homosexual encounters is a very small percentage of the total number of incidents of gonorrhea. Surprisingly, this situation is reversed in the case of syphilis. Indeed, more than 90% of all cases of syphilis reported in the state of Rhode Island during 1973 resulted from homosexual encounters. (This statistic is not as startling as it first appears. Within 10–90 days after being infected with syphilis, an individual usually develops a chancre sore at the spot where the germs entered the body. A homosexual who contracts syphilis as a result of anal intercourse with an infective will develop a chancre sore on his rectum. This individual, naturally, will be reluctant to seek medical attention, since he will then have to reveal his identity as a homosexual. Moreover, he feels no sense of urgency, since the chancre sore is usually painless and disappears after several days. With gonorrhea, on the other hand, the symptoms are so painful and unmistakable that a homosexual will seek prompt medical attention. Moreover, he need not reveal his identity as a homosexual since the symptoms of gonorrhea appear in the genital area.)

Our first step in analyzing the system of differential equations (1) is to show that they are plausible. Specifically, we must show that $x(t)$ and $y(t)$ can never become negative and can never exceed c_1 and c_2, respectively. This is the content of Lemmas 1 and 2.

Lemma 1. *If $x(t_0)$ and $y(t_0)$ are positive, then $x(t)$ and $y(t)$ are positive for all $t \geq t_0$.*

Lemma 2. *If $x(t_0)$ is less than c_1 and $y(t_0)$ is less than c_2, then $x(t)$ is less than c_1 and $y(t)$ is less than c_2 for all $t \geq t_0$.*

PROOF OF LEMMA 1. Suppose that Lemma 1 is false. Let $t^* > t_0$ be the first time at which either x or y is zero. Assume that x is zero first. Then evaluating the first equation of (1) at $t = t^*$ gives $\dot{x}(t^*) = b_1 c_1 y(t^*)$. This quantity is positive. (Note that $y(t^*)$ cannot equal zero since $x = 0$, $y = 0$ is an equilibrium solution of (1).) Hence $x(t)$ is less than zero for t close to and less than t^*, but this contradicts our assumption that t^* is the first time at which $x(t)$ equals zero. We run into the same contradiction if $y(t^*) = 0$. Thus both $x(t)$ and $y(t)$ are positive for $t \geq t_0$. □

PROOF OF LEMMA 2. Suppose that Lemma 2 is false. Let $t^* > t_0$ be the first time at which either $x = c_1$ or $y = c_2$. Suppose that $x(t^*) = c_1$. Evaluating the first equation of (1) at $t = t^*$ gives $\dot{x}(t^*) = -a_1 c_1$. This quantity is negative. Hence, $x(t)$ is greater than c_1 for t close to and less than t^*, but this contradicts our assumption that t^* is the first time at which $x(t)$ equals c_1. We run into the same contradiction if $y(t^*) = c_2$. Thus $x(t)$ is less than c_1 and $y(t)$ is less than c_2 for $t \geq t_0$. □

Having shown that the system of equations (1) is a plausible model of gonorrhea, we now see what predictions it makes concerning the future course of this disease. Will gonorrhea continue to spread rapidly and uncontrollably as the data in Figure 7.1 seem to suggest, or will it level off eventually? The following extremely important theorem of epidemiology provides the answer to this question.

Theorem. (a) *Suppose that $a_1 a_2$ is less than $b_1 b_2 c_1 c_2$. Then every solution $x(t)$, $y(t)$ of (1) with $0 < x(t_0) < c_1$ and $0 < y(t_0) < c_2$, approaches the equilibrium solution*

$$x = \frac{b_1 b_2 c_1 c_2 - a_1 a_2}{a_1 b_2 + b_1 b_2 c_2}, \qquad y = \frac{b_1 b_2 c_1 c_2 - a_1 a_2}{a_2 b_1 + b_1 b_2 c_1}$$

as t approaches infinity. In other words, the total numbers of infective males and infective females will ultimately level off.

(b) *Suppose that $a_1 a_2$ is greater than $b_1 b_2 c_1 c_2$. Then every solution $x(t)$, $y(t)$ of (1) with $0 < x(t_0) < c_1$ and $0 < y(t_0) < c_2$, approaches zero as t approaches infinity. In other words, gonorrhea will ultimately die out.*

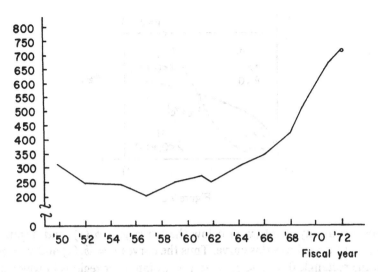

Figure 7.1. Reported Cases of Gonorrhea, in Thousands, for 1950–1973.

The first step in our proof is to split the rectangle $0 < x < c_1, 0 < y < c_2$ into regions in which both dx/dt and dy/dt have fixed signs. This is accomplished in the following manner. Setting $dx/dt = 0$ in (1) and solving for y as a function of x gives

$$y = \frac{a_1 x}{b_1(c_1 - x)} \equiv \phi_1(x).$$

Similarly, setting $dy/dt = 0$ in (1) gives

$$x = \frac{a_2 y}{b_2(c_2 - y)}, \quad \text{or} \quad y = \frac{b_2 c_2 x}{a_2 + b_2 x} \equiv \phi_2(x).$$

Observe first that $\phi_1(x)$ and $\phi_2(x)$ are monotonic increasing functions of x; $\phi_1(x)$ approaches infinity as x approaches c_1, and $\phi_2(x)$ approaches c_2 as x approaches infinity. Secondly, observe that the curves $y = \phi_1(x)$ and $y = \phi_2(x)$ intersect at $(0, 0)$ and at (x_0, y_0) where

$$x_0 = \frac{b_1 b_2 c_1 c_2 - a_1 a_2}{a_1 b_2 + b_1 b_2 c_2}, \quad y_0 = \frac{b_1 b_2 c_1 c_2 - a_1 a_2}{a_2 b_1 + b_1 b_2 c_1}.$$

Thirdly, observe that $\phi_2(x)$ is increasing faster than $\phi_1(x)$ at $x = 0$, since

$$\phi_2'(0) = \frac{b_2 c_2}{a_2} > \frac{a_1}{b_1 c_1} = \phi_1'(0).$$

Hence $\phi_2(x)$ lies above $\phi_1(x)$ for $0 < x < x_0$, and $\phi_2(x)$ lies below $\phi_1(x)$ for $x_0 < x < c_1$, as shown in Figure 7.2. The point (x_0, y_0) is an equilibrium point of (1) since both dx/dt and dy/dt are zero when $x = x_0$ and $y = y_0$.

Finally, observe that dx/dt is positive at any point (x, y) above the curve $y = \phi_1(x)$, and negative at any point (x, y) below this curve. Similarly, dy/dt

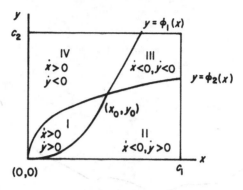

Figure 7.2

is positive at any point (x, y) below the curve $y = \phi_2(x)$, and negative at any point (x, y) above this curve. Thus the curves $y = \phi_1(x)$ and $y = \phi_2(x)$ split the rectangle $0 < x < c_1, 0 < y < c_2$ into four regions in which dx/dt and dy/dt have fixed signs (see Figure 7.2).

Next, we require the following four simple lemmas.

Lemma 3. *Any solution $x(t), y(t)$ of (1) which starts in region I at time $t = t_0$ will remain in this region for all future time $t \geq t_0$ and approach the equilibrium solution $x = x_0, y = y_0$ as t approaches infinity.*

PROOF. Suppose that a solution $x(t), y(t)$ of (1) leaves region I at time $t = t^*$. Then either $\dot{x}(t^*)$ or $\dot{y}(t^*)$ is zero, since the only way a solution of (1) can leave region I is by crossing the curve $y = \phi_1(x)$ or $y = \phi_2(x)$. Assume that $\dot{x}(t^*) = 0$. Differentiating both sides of the first equation of (1) with respect to t and setting $t = t^*$ gives

$$\frac{d^2 x(t^*)}{dt^2} = b_1(c_1 - x(t^*))\frac{dy(t^*)}{dt}.$$

This quantity is positive, since $x(t^*)$ is less than c_1 and dy/dt is positive on the curve $y = \phi_1(x), 0 < x < x_0$. Hence $x(t)$ has a minimum at $t = t^*$. This is impossible, since $x(t)$ is increasing whenever the solution $x(t), y(t)$ is in region I. Similarly, if $\dot{y}(t^*) = 0$, then

$$\frac{d^2 y(t^*)}{dt^2} = b_2(c_2 - y(t^*))\frac{dx(t^*)}{dt}.$$

This quantity is positive, since $y(t^*)$ is less than c_2, and dx/dt is positive on the curve $y = \phi_2(x), 0 < x < x_0$. Hence $y(t)$ has a minimum at $t = t^*$. This is impossible, since $y(t)$ is increasing whenever the solution $x(t), y(t)$ is in region I.

The previous argument shows that any solution $x(t), y(t)$ of (1) which starts in region I at time $t = t_0$ will remain in region I for all future time $t \geq t_0$. This implies that $x(t)$ and $y(t)$ are monotonic increasing functions of time for $t \geq t_0$, with $x(t) < x_0$ and $y(t) < y_0$. Consequently, both $x(t)$ and $y(t)$ have limits ξ, η, respectively, as t approaches infinity. This, in turn, implies that (ξ, η) is an equilibrium point of (1). Now, as is easily seen from Figure 7.2, the only equilibrium points of (1) are $(0, 0)$ and (x_0, y_0), but (ξ, η) cannot equal $(0, 0)$ since both $x(t)$ and $y(t)$ are increasing functions of time. Hence $(\xi, \eta) = (x_0, y_0)$, and this proves Lemma 3.   □

Lemma 4. *Any solution $x(t), y(t)$ of (1) which starts in region III at time $t = t_0$ will remain in this region for all future time and ultimately approach the equilibrium solution $x = x_0, y = y_0$.*

PROOF. Exactly the same as Lemma 3 (see Exercise 1).   □

Lemma 5. *Any solution $x(t), y(t)$ of (1) which starts in region II at time $t = t_0$, and remains in region II for all future time must approach the equilibrium solution $x = x_0, y = y_0$ as t approaches infinity.*

PROOF. If a solution $x(t), y(t)$ of (1) remains in region II for $t \geq t_0$, then $x(t)$ is monotonic decreasing and $y(t)$ is monotonic increasing for $t \geq t_0$. Moreover, $x(t)$ is positive and $y(t)$ is less than c_2, for $t \geq t_0$. Consequently, both $x(t)$ and $y(t)$ have limits ξ, η, respectively, as t approaches infinity. This, in turn, implies that (ξ, η) is an equilibrium point of (1). Now, (ξ, η) cannot equal $(0, 0)$ since $y(t)$ is increasing for $t \geq t_0$. Therefore, $(\xi, \eta) = (x_0, y_0)$, and this proves Lemma 5.   □

Lemma 6. *Any solution $x(t), y(t)$ of (1) which starts in region IV at time $t = t_0$ and remains in region IV for all future time must approach the equilibrium solution $x = x_0, y = y_0$ as t approaches infinity.*

PROOF. Exactly the same as Lemma 5 (see Exercise 2).

We are now in a position to prove our Theorem.

PROOF OF THEOREM. (a) Lemmas 3 and 4 state that every solution $x(t), y(t)$ of (1) which starts in region I or III at time $t = t_0$ must approach the equilibrium solution $x = x_0, y = y_0$ as t approaches infinity. Similarly, Lemmas 5 and 6 state that every solution $x(t), y(t)$ of (1) which starts in region II or IV and which remains in these regions for all future time must also approach the equilibrium solution $x = x_0, y = y_0$. Now, observe that if a solution $x(t), y(t)$ of (1) leaves region II or IV, then it must cross the curve $y = \phi_1(x)$ or $y = \phi_2(x)$, and immediately afterwards enter region I or region III. Consequently, all solutions $x(t), y(t)$ of (1) which start in regions II and IV or on the curves $y = \phi_1(x)$ and $y = \phi_2(x)$, must also approach the equilibrium solution $x(t) = x_0, y(t) = y_0$.   □

(b) PROOF 1. If $a_1 a_2$ is greater than $b_1 b_2 c_1 c_2$, then the curves $y = \phi_1(x)$

and $y = \phi_2(x)$ have the form described in Figure 7.3. In region I, dx/dt is positive and dy/dt is negative; in region II, both dx/dt and dy/dt are negative; and in region III, dx/dt is negative and dy/dt is positive. It is a simple matter to show (see Exercise 3) that every solution $x(t)$, $y(t)$ of (1) which starts in region II at time $t = t_0$ must remain in this region for all future time, and approach the equilibrium solution $x = 0$, $y = 0$ as t approaches infinity. It is also trivial to show that every solution $x(t)$, $y(t)$ of (1) which starts in region I or region III at time $t = t_0$ must cross the curve $y = \phi_1(x)$ or $y = \phi_2(x)$, and immediately afterwards enter region II (see Exercise 4). Consequently, every solution $x(t)$, $y(t)$ of (1), with $0 < x(t_0) < c_1$ and $0 < y(t_0) < c_2$, approaches the equilibrium solution $x = 0$, $y = 0$ as t approaches infinity.   □

(b) PROOF 2. We would now like to show how we can use the Poincaré–Bendixson[1] theorem to give an elegant proof of part (b). Observe that the system of differential equations (1) can be written in the form

$$\frac{d}{dt}\begin{bmatrix} x \\ y \end{bmatrix} = \begin{bmatrix} -a_1 & b_1 c_1 \\ b_2 c_2 & -a_2 \end{bmatrix}\begin{bmatrix} x \\ y \end{bmatrix} - \begin{bmatrix} b_1 xy \\ b_2 xy \end{bmatrix}. \tag{2}$$

Thus the stability of the equilibrium solution $x = 0$, $y = 0$ of (2) is determined by the stability of the equilibrium solution $x = 0$, $y = 0$ of the linearized system

$$\frac{d}{dt}\begin{bmatrix} x \\ y \end{bmatrix} = A\begin{bmatrix} x \\ y \end{bmatrix} = \begin{bmatrix} -a_1 & b_1 c_1 \\ b_2 c_2 & -a_2 \end{bmatrix}\begin{bmatrix} x \\ y \end{bmatrix}.$$

The characteristic polynomial of the matrix A is

$$\lambda^2 - (a_1 + a_2)\lambda + a_1 a_2 - b_1 b_2 c_1 c_2$$

whose roots are

$$\lambda = \frac{-(a_1 + a_2) \pm [(a_1 + a_2)^2 - 4(a_1 a_2 - b_1 b_2 c_1 c_2)]^{1/2}}{2}.$$

It is easily verified that both these roots are real and negative. Hence the equilibrium solution $x = 0$, $y = 0$ of (2) is asymptotically stable. This implies that any solution $x(t)$, $y(t)$ of (1) which starts sufficiently close to the origin $x = y = 0$ will approach the origin as t approaches infinity. Now, suppose that a solution $x(t)$, $y(t)$ of (1), with $0 < x(t_0) < c_1$ and $0 < y(t_0) < c_2$, does not approach the origin as t approaches infinity. By the previous remark, this solution must always remain a minimum distance from the origin. Consequently, its orbit for $t \geq t_0$ lies in a bounded region in the $x - y$ plane which contains no equilibrium points of (1). By the Poincaré–Bendixson theorem, therefore, its orbit must spiral into the orbit of a periodic solution of (1). However, the system of differential equations

[1] Martin Braun, *Differential Equations and Their Applications*. New York: Springer-Verlag, 1975, Section 4.8.

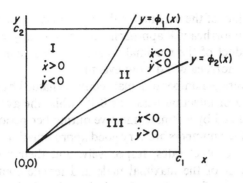

Figure 7.3

(1) has no periodic solution in the first quadrant $x \geq 0$, $y \geq 0$. This follows from the fact that

$$\frac{\partial}{\partial x}[-a_1 x + b_1(c_1 - x)y] + \frac{\partial}{\partial y}[-a_2 y + b_2(c_2 - y)x]$$

$$= -(a_1 + a_2 + b_1 y + b_2 x)$$

is strictly negative if both x and y are nonnegative.[2] Consequently, every solution $x(t), y(t)$ of (1), with $0 < x(t_0) < c_1$ and $0 < y(t_0) < c_2$ approaches the equilibrium solution $x = 0$, $y = 0$ as t approaches infinity.   □

Now, it is quite difficult to evaluate the coefficients a_1, a_2, b_1, b_2, c_1, and c_2. Indeed, it is impossible to obtain even a crude estimate of a_2, which should be interpreted as the average amount of time that a female remains infective. (Similarly, a_1 should be interpreted as the average amount of time that a male remains infective.) This is because most females do not exhibit symptoms. Thus a female can be infective for an amount of time varying from just one day to well over a year. Nevertheless, it is still possible to ascertain from public health data that $a_1 a_2$ is less than $b_1 b_2 c_1 c_2$, as we now show. Observe that the condition $a_1 a_2 < b_1 b_2 c_1 c_2$ is equivalent to

$$1 < \left[\frac{b_1 c_1}{a_2} \times \frac{b_2 c_2}{a_1} \right].$$

The quantity $b_1 c_1 / a_2$ can be interpreted as the average number of males that one female infective contacts during her infectious period, if every male is susceptible. Similarly, the quantity $b_2 c_2 / a_1$ can be interpreted as the average number of females that one male infective contacts during his infectious period, if every female is susceptible. The quantities $b_1 c_1 / a_2$ and $b_2 c_2 / a_1$ are called the maximal female and male contact rates, respectively, and the theorem can now be interpreted in the following manner.

[2] See Problem 11 of Section 4.8 in the author's text *Differential Equations and Their Applications*, Springer-Verlag, 1975.

(a) If the product of the maximal male and female contact rates is greater than one, then gonorrhea will approach a nonzero steady state.

(b) If the product of the maximal male and female contact rates is less than one, then gonorrhea will die out eventually.

In 1973, the average number of female contacts named by a male infective during his period of infectiousness was 0.98, while the average number of male contacts named by a female infective during her period of infectiousness was 1.15. These numbers are very good approximations of the maximal male and female contact rates, respectively, and their product does not exceed the product of the maximal male and female contact rates. (The number of contacts of a male or female infective during their period of infectiousness is slightly less than the maximal male or female contact rates. However, the *actual* number of contacts is often greater than the number of contacts named by an infective.) The product of 1.15 with 0.98 is 1.0682. Thus gonorrhea will ultimately approach a nonzero steady state.

Remark. Our model of gonorrhea is rather crude since it lumps all promiscuous males and all promiscuous females together, regardless of age. A more accurate model can be obtained by separating the male and female populations into different age groups and then computing the rate of change of infectives in each age group. This has been done recently, but the analysis is too difficult to present here. We just mention that a result completely analogous to our theorem is obtained: either gonorrhea dies out in each age group, or it approaches a constant, positive level in each age group.

Exercises

In Exercises 1 and 2, we assume that $a_1 a_2 < b_1 b_2 c_1 c_2$.

1. (a) Suppose that a solution $x(t)$, $y(t)$ of (1) leaves region III of Figure 7.2 at time $t = t^*$ by crossing the curve $y = \phi_1(x)$ or $y = \phi_2(x)$. Conclude that either $x(t)$ or $y(t)$ has a maximum at $t = t^*$. Then, show that this is impossible. Conclude, therefore, that any solution $x(t)$, $y(t)$ of (1) which starts in region III at time $t = t_0$ must remain in region III for all future time $t \geq t_0$.

   (b) Conclude from (a) that any solution $x(t)$, $y(t)$ of (1) which starts in region III has a limit ξ, η as t approaches infinity. Then, show that (ξ, η) must equal (x_0, y_0).

2. Suppose that a solution $x(t)$, $y(t)$ of (1) remains in region IV of Figure 7.2 for all time $t \geq t_0$. Prove that $x(t)$ and $y(t)$ have limits ξ, η, respectively, as t approaches infinity. Then conclude that (ξ, η) must equal (x_0, y_0).

In Exercises 3 and 4, we assume that $a_1 a_2 > b_1 b_2 c_1 c_2$.

3. Suppose that a solution $x(t)$, $y(t)$ of (1) leaves region II of Figure 7.3 at time $t = t^*$ by crossing the curve $y = \phi_1(x)$ or $y = \phi_2(x)$. Show that either $x(t)$ or $y(t)$ has a

maximum at $t = t^*$. Then show that this is impossible. Conclude, therefore, that every solution $x(t)$, $y(t)$ of (1) which starts in region II at time $t = t_0$ must remain in region II for all future time $t \geq t_0$.

4. (a) Suppose that a solution $x(t)$, $y(t)$ of (1) remains in either region I or II of Figure 7.3 for all time $t \geq t_0$. Show that $x(t)$ and $y(t)$ have limits ξ, η, respectively, as t approaches infinity.
   (b) Conclude that $(\xi, \eta) = (0, 0)$.
   (c) Show that (ξ, η) cannot equal $(0, 0)$ if $x(t)$, $y(t)$ remains in region I or region III for all time $t \geq t_0$.
   (d) Show that any solution $x(t)$, $y(t)$ of (1) which starts on either $y = \phi_1(x)$ or $y = \phi_2(x)$ will immediately afterwards enter region II.

5. Assume that $a_1 a_2 < b_1 b_2 c_1 c_2$. Prove directly that the equilibrium solution $x = x_0$, $y = y_0$ of (1) is asymptotically stable. Warning: The calculations are extremely tedious.

6. Assume that the number of homosexuals remains constant in time. Call this constant c. Let $x(t)$ denote the number of homosexuals who have gonorrhea at time t. Assume that homosexuals are cured of gonorrhea at a rate α_1, and that new infectives are added at a rate $\beta_1(c_1 - x)x$.
   (a) Show that $\dot{x} = -\alpha_1 x + \beta_1 x(c - x)$.
   (b) What happens to $x(t)$ as t approaches infinity?

7. Suppose that the number of homosexuals $c(t)$ grows according to the logistic law $\dot{c} = c(a - bc)$, for some positive constants a and b. Let $x(t)$ denote the number of homosexuals who have gonorrhea at time t, and assume (see Exercise 6) that $\dot{x} = -\alpha_1 x + \beta_1 x(c - x)$. What happens to $x(t)$ as t approaches infinity?

Notes for the Instructor

Objectives. To show that ultimately the incidence of gonorrhea will level off to constant values.

Prerequisites. Concept of differential equations and equilibrium points. Calculus.

Time. One to two lectures.

CHAPTER 8

DNA, RNA, and Random Mating: Simple Applications of the Multiplication Rule

Helen Marcus–Roberts*

1. Introduction

Sometimes simple applications of mathematics can give us insight into some very interesting biological phenomena. As an example we shall consider the multiplication rule. Understanding potential possibilities by being able to count them in a simple way will give us greater understanding about the vast diversity in nature and about the great differences among people.

The kinds of questions we will want to answer are: How many cell divisions (mitoses) must take place to attain the full complement of cells in an adult? Why does the basic code of RNA consist of three bases? Why is there so much diversity among sexually reproducing organisms? How does a cell store all the information required for organisms to develop into functioning organisms? How can random mating account for the fact that members of the same family can have such different characteristics? We will find that we can answer these questions if we can account for the possibilities that can occur. These possibilities can be counted by applying a simple counting rule known as the multiplication rule.

2. Multiplication Rule

2.1 The Rule

Counting rules and, in our particular case, the multiplication rule permit us to count without the need to enumerate and list all possible outcomes. We

* Department of Mathematics and Computer Science, Montclair State College, Upper Montclair, NJ 07043.

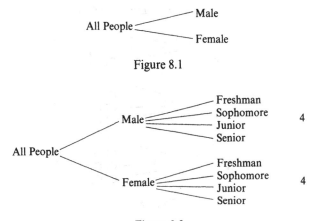

Figure 8.1

Figure 8.2

motivate the multiplication rule by considering the following example. Assume that you are taking a survey to determine the number of students in various categories. The categories of interest are sex (male or female) and class standing (freshman, sophomore, junior, and senior). How many different categories are possible? We start first by enumerating the possibilities and then we will develop a general rule. We note first that we can subdivide all the people by sex into two categories, which we represent by using the tree diagram given in Figure 8.1.

Using the same approach we find that we can subdivide the males by class and do the same for the females. We therefore get the tree diagram given in Figure 8.2. If we add up all the possibilities, we find that the males can be classified in four categories and so can the females. The total number of classifications is given by $4 + 4 = 4(1 + 1) = 4 \times 2 = 2 \times 4 = 8$. If we look at the numbers we are multiplying, we can attach some meaning to them. In the multiplications 2×4, we notice that 2 corresponds to the number of possibilities for the sex of individuals and 4 corresponds to the number of classifications for the students. Therefore, it appears that we can count the number of classifications by considering the number of possibilities for the first choice and the number of possibilities for the second choice and then multiplying the two together. In general, we can represent this rule in the following way:

(# of choices for 1st thing) $\times$ (# of choices for 2nd thing).

We consider one more example before we state our rule formally. In a primary election there are three candidates for Governor and four candidates for Lieutenant Governor on the ballot of one of the parties. The winning combination will be one of how many possible winning teams? We start by enumerating all the possibilities by using a tree diagram. (See Figure 8.3.) If we count the possible slates we find that there are 12 possibilities. We note that we can arrive at this number by considering $4 + 4 + 4 = 4(1 + 1 + 1) = 4 \times 3 = 3 \times 4$. Again we find that we are in the same pattern of deter-

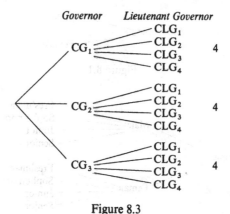

Figure 8.3

mining the number of possibilities for each choice and then multiplying the two together. Now we can formally define the multiplication rule.

Multiplication Rule. *Suppose something can happen in n_1 ways, and suppose that no matter in which way it does happen, something else can happen in n_2 ways. Then the number of ways in which both can happen together is $n_1 \times n_2$:*

$$(\# \text{ of ways } 1) \times (\# \text{ of ways } 2).$$

Multiplication Rule Extension. *If one thing can be done in exactly n_1 different ways, for each of these a second thing can be done in exactly n_2 different ways, and for each of the first two a third can be done in exactly n_3 different ways, then the sequence of things can be done in the product of the number of ways in which the individual things can be done, that is $n_1 \times n_2 \times n_3$ ways. The extension to more than three things follows in a similar manner, i.e., we have $n_1 \times n_2 \times n_3 \times n_4 \times n_5 \times \cdots$ ways.*

We now see that if we want to extend the first example and include a classification by major we will be able to apply the multiplication rule extension. Assume, in your survey that you want to classify students by sex (male or female), class standing (freshman, sophomore, junior, or senior) and major (social science, business administration, mathematical sciences, biology, chemistry, or physics). We note that if we were to try to use a tree diagram to enumerate all possibilities, it would become rather cumbersome and messy, but if we apply the extension of the multiplication rule it becomes rather trivial to count the number of possible classifications. Using the multiplication rule we find that there are two choices for the first category, four for the second category, and six for the third category; therefore, the total number of classifications is given by $2 \times 4 \times 6 = 48$. (These types of questions are important in making up a questionnaire and knowing the number of possible answers that could be received.)

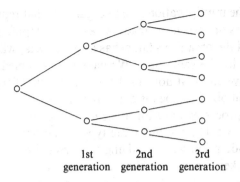

1st   2nd   3rd
generation   generation   generation

Figure 8.4. Binary Fission.

2.2 Application to Binary Fission

Consider a process like binary fission, for example, in amoebas or paramecia.[1] If these organisms continue to reproduce without any interruption or disturbances, how many paramecia or amoebas will there be at the end of five generations or 10 generations or 20 generations if we start with a single amoeba or paramecium? As in many applications of mathematics to the real world, it is important that one understands the process about which we are asking questions. Once we can understand a particular phenomenon it may become easier to ask a mathematical question. In this particular case, we have to understand what happens when an amoeba or paramecium undergoes binary fission. The end result of binary fission is that a single amoeba or paramecium becomes 2 amoebas or 2 paramecia, as shown in Figure 8.4. To ascertain how many amoebas (paramecia) there will be at the end of five generations, we simply apply the multiplication rule. In the first generation there are two possible offspring. For each of these, there are two possible offspring in the second generation. For each of the offspring in the second generation there are two possible offspring in the third generation, and so on. Therefore, the number of amoebas (paramecia) at the end of five generations can be determined by applying the multiplication rule in the following way:

$$\begin{pmatrix} \text{\# for} \\ \text{1st gen.} \end{pmatrix} \times \begin{pmatrix} \text{\# for} \\ \text{2nd gen.} \end{pmatrix} \times \begin{pmatrix} \text{\# for} \\ \text{3rd gen.} \end{pmatrix} \times \begin{pmatrix} \text{\# for} \\ \text{4th gen.} \end{pmatrix} \times \begin{pmatrix} \text{\# for} \\ \text{5th gen.} \end{pmatrix}$$

Substituting the correct numbers we find that at the end of five generations we can expect $2 \times 2 \times 2 \times 2 \times 2 = 2^5 = 32$ amoebas (paramecia) if we start out with a single amoeba (or paramecium). Using the same type of analysis, it follows that at the end of 10 generations, we can expect $2 \times 2 \times 2 \times 2 \times 2 \times 2 \times 2 \times 2 \times 2 \times 2 = 2^{10} = 1024$ amoebas (paramecia).

It is very important when one applies mathematics to real world phenomena to be aware of the oversimplifications that are being made. In our

---

[1] Amoebas and paramecia are single-celled organisms.

application of the multiplication rule to organisms that reproduce by under-
going binary fission, we have made a few oversimplifications. We have
assumed that all the organisms (amoebas or paramecia) will undergo binary
fission at basically the same time. We have also assumed that all the new
organisms survive and that none of them die. In spite of the oversimplifications, we can still obtain some insight into a process that keeps on doubling
its size. (Such processes have an amazing potential growth. What other
processes in our world have this same type of mechanism?) An extremely
important consideration when studying processes that double periodically
is the time it takes for the doubling to occur. If an organism undergoes
binary fission once every 100 years, then it produces 1024 new organisms
in 1000 years. But if binary fission occurs once every week, then in about 10
weeks there will be 1024 organisms, and in just one year there would be
4, 503, 599, 627, 370, 496 new organisms! Amoebas and paramecia are
members of the phylum protozoa and the number of divisions for members
of this phylum ranges from 0.03 per day to 10.9 per day, with quite a few
members of this phylum dividing 2, 3, 4, or 6 times a day. (See Spector [2].)

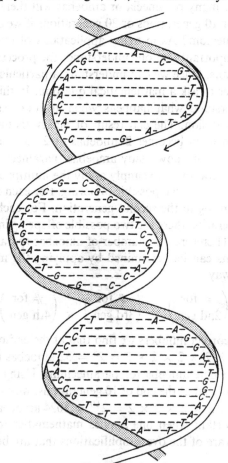

Figure 8.5. DNA Chain (Double Helix).

3. DNA and RNA

In this section we address the questions posed in Section 1. Once again we will see that if we understand something about the process we are interested in we will be able to use mathematics to gain some insight into the phenomenon.

We start by taking a brief look at a molecule called DNA (deoxyribonucleic acid), which is the basic unit of inheritance. The power of this molecule is that it contains the blueprint for the functions and development of life (including human life). The DNA molecule is often referred to as the double helix. (See Figure 8.5.) A DNA molecule consists of two chains that are chemically bonded together. The bonding occurs in such a way that the two chains are complementary. If the chemical composition of one of the chains is determined, then the chemical composition of the second chain is fully determined. Chains of DNA molecules consist of phosphate, sugar, and a

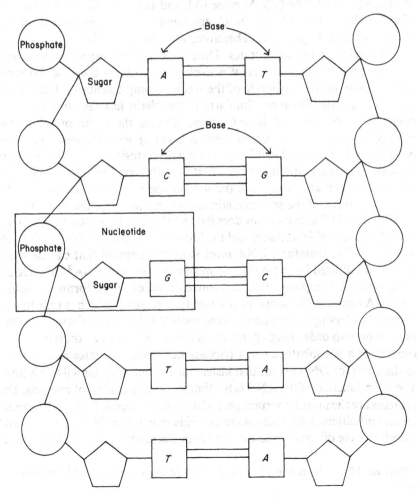

Figure 8.6. Schematic of DNA Molecule.

Table 1. The 20 Commonly
Occurring Amino Acids
Which Make Up Proteins

Phenylalanine	Histidine
Leucine	Glutamine
Isolucine	Asparagine
Methionine	Lysine
Valine	Aspartic Acid
Serine	Glutamic Acid
Proline	Cysteine
Threonine	Tryptophan
Alanine	Arginine
Tryosine	Glycine

base. The only variable part of the chain is the base. There are four bases: Thymine (T), Cytosine (C), Adenine (A), and Guanine (G). The basic unit of a phosphate, sugar (deoxyribose), and one of the four bases is known as a *nucleotide*. (See Figure 8.6.) Therefore, a chain of the DNA molecule is simply a collection of nucleotides. The complementary aspect of the chains is determined by the fact that if a nucleotide contains the base Adenine, then the base in the nucleotide of the second (complementary) strand must contain the base Thymine. Similarly if the chain has Guanine then the complementary chain will have Cytosine. That is, the chains of the double helix pair up in such a way that Adenine pairs up with Thymine, Thymine pairs up with Adenine, Guanine pairs up with Cytosine, and Cytosine pairs up with Guanine. It should be clear that we only have to study one chain of the double helix at a time since the second one is totally determined. (We can almost think of the second chain as a mirror image of the first chain.)

What does DNA do and how does it do it? Previously, we stated that DNA is the basic unit of inheritance and the blueprint for the functions and development of life; therefore, DNA must store information that can be interpreted and utilized by our bodies. A molecule known as RNA[2] (ribonucleic acid), which is complementary to a single strand of DNA, forms. Basically, the DNA contains the actual instruction (information) which is transmitted to the RNA (acting as a messenger) and the RNA then transmits the information on how to order long chains of amino acids known as proteins. RNA consists of a phosphate, a sugar (ribose) and bases; the bases are the same as the bases for DNA except that instead of Thymine (T), Uracil (U) is used. The main function of the RNA is to stimulate the formation of proteins. The proteins are the most important part of the whole process. Different arrangements and different numbers of amino acids represent different proteins and therefore have different functions and uses. Proteins have two primary func-

[2] There are different types of RNA. To keep things simple, we shall speak of them all as the same.

tions: 1) differently structured proteins represent the array of building materials to construct living matter (building blocks) and 2) they produce enzymes that speed up chemical reactions in the body. Certain chemical reactions can take seconds or minutes in the presence of enzymes when otherwise they might take years or centuries. Proteins are composed of 20 commonly occurring amino acids, listed in Table 1. RNA has two functions in forming proteins: 1) selecting the appropriate number of each amino acid, and 2) arranging the amino acids in a specific order (in order to perform a specific function). RNA must somehow have a code unique for a particular amino acid in order to accomplish its functions. Specifically, we want to address the following question: How does RNA create a code which distinguishes among the different amino acids?

3.1 Number of Bases Necessary for the Genetic Code

If we refer to Figures 8.5 and 8.6 we see that the only part of the DNA molecule that can be changed is the sequence of bases (Thymine, Guanine, Cytosine, and Adenine). In RNA the variable units are the bases Uracil, Guanine, Cytosine, and Adenine. How can an RNA chain (a single strand) such as the one given in Figure 8.7, transmit information about how to put the amino acids together? Is it possible for a single nucleotide to select one of the 20 amino acids? Effectively, we are asking if a single nucleotide can contain 20 different codes. This really boils down to determining how many different nucleotides are possible. The answer is obvious. Since there are four bases, and the only variable part of the nucleotide is the base, it follows that there can only be four distinct nucleotides. Therefore, a single nucleotide cannot possibly code for all 20 commonly occurring amino acids: it can code for, at most, four of them. The next question to consider is, Can two nucleotides together code for the 20 amino acids? We can answer this by trying to consider whether two nucleotides together can yield 20 codes. We can count the number of possible codes for two nucleotides by using the multi-

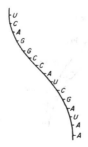

Figure 8.7. RNA Chain.

plication rule. In this case we count the number of possibilities for each nucleotide and then multiply them together. We know that there are four possibilities for each nucleotide so that the total number of possibilities for the two nucleotides together is given by (4 for 1st nucleotide) × (4 for 2nd nucleotide) = 16. Since there are more than 16 amino acids it is clear that more than two nucleotides must be used in order to code for all the amino acids. We can confirm this result by using a tree diagram. Figure 8.8 yields all possibilities. We can count the number of codes, and we find 16 distinct possible codes. Thus two nucleotides are not adequate for coding for all 20 amino acids. We again note that applying the multiplication rule involved much less effort than using a tree diagram to enumerate all the possibilities.

If we consider three nucleotides, and apply the multiplication rule, we see that we can get (4 for 1st nucleotide) × (4 for 2nd nucleotide) × (4 for 3rd nucleotide) = 64 different arrangements and more than enough codes. In fact, three nucleotides together form what is known as a *codon*, and the

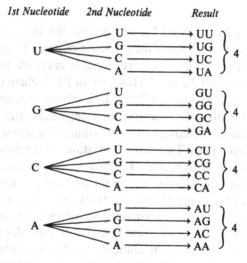

Figure 8.8

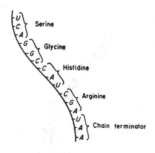

Figure 8.9

Table 2. Codons for Amino Acids (Genetic Code)

Phenylalanine	UUU, UUC
Leucine	UUA, UUG, CUU, CUC, CUA, CUG
Isolucine	AUU, AUC, AUA
Methionine	AUG
Valine	GUU, GUC, GUA, GUG
Serine	UCU, UCC, UCA, UCG, AGU, AGC
Proline	CCU, CCC, CCA, CCG
Threonine	ACU, ACC, ACA, ACG
Alanine	GCU, GCC, GCA, GCG
Tyrosine	UAU, UAC
Histidine	CAU, CAC
Glutamine	CAA, CAG
Asparagine	AAU, AAC
Cysteine	UGU, UGC
Trytophan	UGG
Arginine	CGU, CGC, CGA, CGG, AGA, AGG
Glycine	GGU, GGC, GGA, GGG
Lysine	AAA, AAG
Aspartic Acid	GAU, GAC
Glutamic Acid	GAA, GAG
Chain terminator	UAA, UAG, UGA

codon is a code specific for a particular amino acid. The string of codons next to each other form the order that the amino acids are arranged in and hence the specific protein. The codons for the amino acids are given in Table 2. (Note that almost all the amino acids have more than one codon. It is also very interesting to note that these codons are probably universal for all species, they are not unique for human beings.) Using Table 2, we see that the RNA chain of Figure 8.7 yields the chain of amino acids given in Figure 8.9.

3.2 Number of Possible Chains and the Complexity of Life

Applying the multiplication rule has given us the insight to understand why codons consist of three bases rather than a sequence of less than three bases. We can gain further insights into the power of DNA and RNA chains by once again applying the multiplication rule. The power of these molecules in terms of the number of potential chains is due to the possibility of placing one of four different bases in each nucleotide. Specifically we want to ask how many different chains are possible in a DNA chain of specified length or an RNA chain of specified length. We have already discovered that for an RNA chain of length three, that is three nucleotides, there are 64 possible chains. How many different chains are possible in an RNA chain that would code for two amino acids, that is, have six nucleotides? Applying the multiplication rule we find that there are $4 \times 4 \times 4 \times 4 \times 4 \times 4 = 4^6 = 4096$ different possible chains and the number of possible arrangements of amino acids would be $20 \times 20 = 400$. If an RNA chain is nine nucleotides long (codes for three amino acids), there are by a similar calculation $4^9 = 262,144$ possible different chains. The number of possible arrangements of amino acids that could result from an RNA chain of length nine, that is, three codons, would be $20 \times 20 \times 20 = 8000$.

The really interesting question is: How long is a typical RNA chain? A typical RNA chain is between 300 and 3000 nucleotides long.[3] A chain which is 300 nucleotides long can be any one of 4^{300} different chains, and the chain that is 3000 nucleotides long can be any one of 4^{3000} different chains. How large are the numbers 4^{300} and 4^{3000}? We think in base 10, that is $100 = 10^2$ and $1000 = 10^3$ and $1,000,000 = 10^6$. Can we get some feeling for the magnitude of numbers that are given in base 4? If we play around with the powers of base 4 we find that $4^2 = 16$, $4^3 = 64$, $4^4 = 256$, $4^5 = 1024$, and $4^6 = 4096$. Since $4^5 = 1024 > 1000 = 10^3$, it makes sense to use 10^3 as a lower approximation for 4^5 and translate the numbers to base 10. If we use this approximation, we find that

$$4^{300} = (4^5)^{60} > (10^3)^{60} = 10^{180},$$

that is $4^{300} > 10^{180}$, which is 10 followed by 180 zeros, a very large number! Even when expressed as a number in base 10, it is still hard to comprehend the magnitude of a number like 10^{180}. As a basis for comparison let us consider the following situation. It is known that the number of molecules in a teaspoon of water is about 10^{23}. If we take 10 teaspoons there would be $10 \times 10^{23} = 10^{24}$ molecules. In fact in a gallon there are 768 teaspoons and therefore $768 \times 10^{23} = 7.68 \times 10^{25}$ molecules in a gallon. How many gallons would be needed to attain 10^{180} molecules? It follows that 10^{180} molecules is approximately $10^{180}/(7.68 \times 10^{25}) = 1.302 \times 10^{154}$ gallons. To see how large this number is, note that the average person in the U.S. uses about 50 gallons of water a day (for baths, showers, toilet flushing, eating, drinking, etc.). At this rate, 1.302×10^{154} gallons would last the United States population (200,000,000) 3.57×10^{141} years. This is still too huge a number to be comprehensible. We pose the same questions about the potential number of distinct chains if the number of nucleotides is 3000. There are 4^{3000} possible molecules. Using the same lower approximation $4^5 > 10^3$, we find that $4^{3000} > 10^{1800}$. (Using the same analogy to the number of molecules in a teaspoon of water, we find that it would take 1.302×10^{1774} gallons of water contain 10^{1800} molecules, and it would last the U.S. population 3.57×10^{1761} years.) We see the potential for diversity

---

[3] There are some RNA chains of 75 nucleotides, whereas others have as many as 5000 nucleotides.

and different information that the mechanisms for RNA permit. The diversity really staggers the mind. It all boils down to the flexibility that is attained by having four different bases to place in the appropriate position of the nucleotide.

Similar calculations are done for typical DNA chains and are given in Table 3.

We now ask how many different sequences of amino acids can an RNA chain actually code? Once again, we can obtain answers by applying the multiplication rule. An RNA chain of 900 bases can code for 300 amino acids, since a codon consists of three bases. Since each position of the chain of 300 amino acids can be filled by any of the 20 commonly occurring amino acids, the total number of possible chains of amino acids is given by 20^{300}. Since $20 = 2 \times 10$, and since $2^{10} > 10^3$ we find that $20^{300} > 10^{390}$. (Why?) Therefore, an RNA chain of 900 bases (nucleotides) has the potential to code for more than 10^{390} (10 followed by 390 zeros) different sequences of amino acids. Similarly, an RNA chain of 1500 bases (nucleotides) can code for 20^{500} different amino acid sequences (why?), which is greater than 10^{650} different chains. The power of such a simple setup is really quite staggering and very difficult to fully comprehend.

Hemoglobin is a pigment in red blood cells which causes the cells to appear red, and it is the substance that allows the red blood cells to affect the vital exchange of oxygen and carbon dioxide in the lungs and tissues. Hemoglobin is a complex protein that consists of 574 amino acids (it therefore requires an RNA chain of 1722 bases (nucleotides) to code for it). Hemoglobin appears in two forms: normal hemoglobin, known as hemoglobin A, and hemoglobin S which is found in persons with the disease sickle cell anemia (which can often be fatal). The only difference between these two types of hemoglobin is the difference of one amino acid in the chain of 574. In hemoglobin S, valine has been substituted for glutamic acid found in hemoglobin A. (This occurs in a specific location of the amino acid chain.) The codons for glutamtic acid are GAA and GAG, while those for valine are GUA or GUG. Therefore, the change of a single base, that is, a U substituted for an A, apparently can create a tremendous and drastic effect on human beings. (To be precise, this substitution of valine for glutamic acid occurs twice in the chain, since the same sequence of amino acids appears twice in the hemoglobin molecule.)

4. Random Mating

The next questions we want to answer are, How is the information contained in RNA transmitted? and Why does so much diversity exist even among members of the same family? We do not plan to go into a whole biology course here, but we will briefly discuss some highlights and also give some more insight into the phenomenon by applying the multiplication rule.

Table 3. Lengths of DNA Chains

Entity	x = No. of Nucleotides per Cell	y = No. of Possible Chains with x Nucleotides	No. of Gallons of Water to Contain y molecules
1. E. coli	4.2×10^6	$4^{4.2 \times 10^6} > 10^{2.52 \times 10^6} =$ $10^{2,520,000}$	$1.302 \times 10^{2,519,974}$
2. Chicken Embryo Cells	5×10^9	$4^{5 \times 10^9} > 10^{3 \times 10^9} =$ $10^{3,000,000,000}$	$1.302 \times 10^{2,999,999,974}$
3. Mouse (Bone marrow)	1.3×10^{10}	$4^{1.3 \times 10^{10}} > 10^{7.8 \times 10^9} =$ $10^{7,800,000,000}$	$1.302 \times 10^{7,799,999,974}$
4. Guinea Pig	1.7×10^{10}	$4^{1.7 \times 10^{10}} > 10^{1.02 \times 10^{10}} =$ $10^{10,200,000,000}$	$1.302 \times 10^{10,199,999,974}$
5. Drosophila	8×10^7	$4^{8 \times 10^7} > 10^{4.8 \times 10^7} =$ $10^{48,000,000}$	$1.302 \times 10^{47,999,974}$
6. Human (Fibroblasts—connective tissue cells—part of tendon)	2.1×10^{10}	$4^{2.1 \times 10^{10}} > 10^{1.26 \times 10^{10}} =$ $10^{12,600,000,000}$	$1.302 \times 10^{12,599,999,974}$

Table 4. Chromosome Numbers

Opossum	11 pairs
Drosophila (fruit fly)	4 pairs
Rat	21 pairs
Mouse	20 pairs
Dog	39 pairs
Cat	19 pairs
Cow	30 pairs
Horse	33 pairs
Chimpanzee	24 pairs
Man	23 pairs
Crayfish	200 pairs

4.1 Mitosis

Human life (as well as life in muticellular or higher organisms) starts from a single cell. The single cell contains genes in the chromosomes. Organisms have a characteristic number of pairs of chromosomes. These chromosomes contain the genetic information that is contained or stored in the DNA and RNA. Some characteristic numbers of chromosomes for different organisms are given in Table 4. We have to understand how the genetic information (DNA and RNA) is transmitted from parents to their offspring. Two basic types of cell division take place in organisms. These are mitosis and meiosis. The two types of cell division are necessary to maintain this characteristic number of chromosomes that are unique to a particular organism. For simplicity, we will illustrate the concepts by using fruit flies, since they only have four pairs of chromosomes. Let us start by considering a fertilized cell, that is, an egg cell that has been fertilized by a sperm cell. This fertilized cell undergoes many divisions until it ultimately becomes in some sense a "copy" of its parents. Since it must be a copy of its parents, it must also have the same number of chromosomes that its parents have. Therefore, we must have a cell division that maintains the characteristic number of chromosomes of that particular species. This type of cell division is known as *mitosis*. That is, from a fertilized fruit fly cell (egg) with four pairs of chromosomes, mitosis results in cells that will also have four pairs of chromosomes. This idea is illustrated in Figure 8.10. Mitosis is simply a process of cell division which results in two cells with the identical genetic information of the original and the same number of chromosomes.

Full-grown adults contain about 10^{14} cells. How many times does the original fertilized cell have to undergo mitosis to reach the full complement of cells? Once again, we have an application of the multiplication rule. If we assume that there are no interruptions and that no cells die off, we have the same situation we discussed in the example on binary fission. The question reduces to, How many generations must there be in order to get 10^{14}

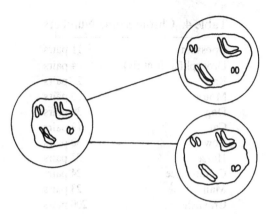

Figure 8.10. Figurative Results of Mitosis in Fruit Flies.

cells? We have each cell dividing into two so we get $2 \times 2 \times 2 \times \cdots \times 2 =$
$\underbrace{\qquad\qquad\qquad}_{n \text{ times}}$
$2^n = 10^{14}$, and we want to find n. What power n is such that 2^n will be equal
to 10^{14}? To answer this, note that 2^{10} is approximately 10^3, so $2^{40} = (2^{10})^4$
is approximately $(10^3)^4 = 10^{12}$. Since $10^{14} = 10^{12} \times 10^2$, we shall determine the value of x so that $2^x \sim 10^2$. We find that $2^6 = 64$ and $2^7 = 128$,
so we see that 2^7 is approximately 10^2. Therefore we find that $2^{47} = 2^{40} \times$
2^7 is approximately $10^{12} \times 10^2 = 10^{14}$. Thus we can conclude that 47
mitotic divisions must occur to achieve 10^{14} cells. We can also calculate this
another way. We have $2^n = 10^{14}$, so $n \log_{10} 2 = 14 \log_{10} 10 = 14$, so $n =$
$14/\log_{10} 2$. Since $\log_{10} 2 \approx 0.30103$, $n \approx 47$. By applying the multiplication
rule, we see very simply that about 47 mitotic cell divisions are required in
order to achieve the full complement of cells in an adult human being.

4.2 Meiosis

We still have not answered the question posed in the introduction about
how the hereditary material from both parents is transmitted and why
members of the same family can look so different. What would happen if
we were to get a sperm cell and an egg cell from the two parents, and each
cell contained the full complement of chromosomes? If the sperm cell from
a man contained 23 pairs of chromosomes and an egg cell from a woman
contained 23 pairs of chromosomes, the resulting fertilized egg would contain 46 pairs of chromosomes (twice the number of normal chromosomes),
and if this could continue then with each generation the number of chromosomes would double. Clearly, something must happen in the sperm and
egg cells so that the full set of chromosomes is reduced by half. Then when
the egg cell is fertilized by the sperm cell, the resulting fertilized cell will
contain the correct number of chromosomes. This reduction of the number
of chromosomes by a factor of half is accomplished by the cell division

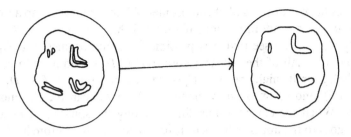

Figure 8.11. Schematic of End Results of Meiosis for Fruit Flies.

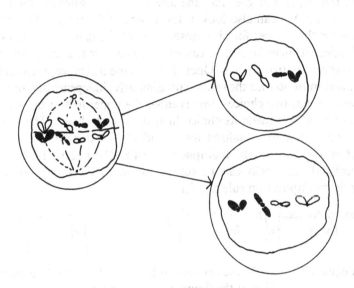

Figure 8.12. Chromosomes Lining Up across the Spindle and Then Separating.

known as *meiosis*. Schematically, this is represented for fruit flies in Figure 8.11. The cells that result from meiosis are said to have the haploid number of chromosomes (1/2 the number). The full complement of chromosomes is known as the diploid number. As a result of meiosis, we get the variation that exists among members of the same family. Each fertilized egg gets half its complement of chromosomes from each parent (1/2 from the sperm and 1/2 from the egg) and in repeated matings when the egg is fertilized the chromosomes involved may not be the same ones.

How many different gametes (sperm or egg) could be formed during meiosis? Once more we can apply the basic multiplication rule and get an understanding of the extreme variation that can exist. Consider once again the fruit fly. During meiosis the chromosomes line up in a random fashion across an imaginary line known as a spindle (see Figure 8.12). Then the cell divides in two in such a way that one member of each pair of the chromosomes goes in each half of the cell, forming the sperm or egg cell. Thus we can study the number of choices one of the chromosomes in each pair can make. (The second chromosome of the pair must go to the other half.)

Fruit flies have four pairs of chromosomes. All four pairs line up across the spindle in some random fashion. If we label the pairs $A_1 A_2$, $B_1 B_2$, $C_1 C_2$, and $D_1 D_2$, then we see that it is possible for chromosomes $A_2 B_1 C_1 D_1$ to line up in one half of the cell (therefore $A_1 B_2 C_2 D_2$ would have to be in the other half), or it might be $A_1 B_1 C_1 D_2$ in one half (and $A_2 B_2 C_2 D_1$ in the other half), and so on. In how many possible ways can the chromosomes line up? When the chromosomes line up along the spindle, let us assume that A_1 goes to the upper half (then A_2 has to go into the bottom half). Then either B_1 or B_2 can go into the upper half with A_1 and the one that does not go into the upper half goes into the lower half, and similarly for C and D chromosomes. We can also look at this from a different point of view. Let us consider the choices for chromosome A_1 of the pair of A's. How many possibilities are there for A_1? A_1 can either go into the top half or the bottom half, so there are two choices. Once A_1 has made its choice, then A_2 has no choice and must go into the other half. Similarly, independently of what A_1 has done, B_1 has two choices, that is either the upper half or the lower half. Again once B_1 has made its choice then B_2 has no choice. The same type of procedure can be visualized for C and D. We therefore have again a perfect application for the multiplication rule. The question is how many genetically distinct cells can be formed when a cell undergoes meiosis? Using the multiplication rule, we find

$$\begin{pmatrix} \text{no. of choices} \\ \text{for } A_1 \\ 2 \end{pmatrix} \times \begin{pmatrix} \text{no. of choices} \\ \text{for } B_1 \\ 2 \end{pmatrix} \times \begin{pmatrix} \text{no. of choices} \\ \text{for } C_1 \\ 2 \end{pmatrix} \times \begin{pmatrix} \text{no. of choices} \\ \text{for } D_1 \\ 2 \end{pmatrix}$$

which equals $2^4 = 16$. These results can be verified using a tree diagram as in Figure 8.13. Looking at the figure, we can verify that it is possible for 16

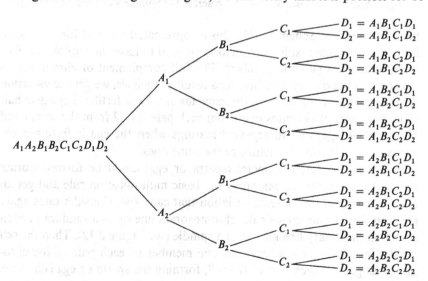

Figure 8.13. Possible Cells Formed during Meiosis.

distinct sperm or egg cells to be formed during meiosis. During meiosis all 16 types are not formed at any one time during a single meiotic division.

How many distinct sperm (or egg) cells can be formed during meiosis in human beings? Human beings have 23 pairs of chromosomes. Therefore, noting that one chromosome from each of 23 pairs will have a choice to make (that is, upper or lower) and applying the multiplication rule, we find that the total number of distinct sperm (or egg) cells that can potentially form during meiosis is given by $2 \times 2 \times \cdots \times 2 = 2^{23} = 8,388,608$. We still have not completely answered the question of why people, even members of the same family, tend to look (and act) different. The question we really want to answer is not how many sperm or egg cells can be formed, but how many fertilized eggs can be formed? If we assume that one of the $8,388,608 = 2^{23}$ sperm cells will fertilize one of the $8,388,608 = 2^{23}$ egg cells that can be potentially formed, then we have again an application of the multiplication rule. The total number of fertilized eggs that could potentially be formed is given by

$$\begin{pmatrix} \text{no. of sperm cells} \\ \text{to choose from} \\ 2^{23} \end{pmatrix} \times \begin{pmatrix} \text{no. of egg cells} \\ \text{to choose from} \\ 2^{23} \end{pmatrix} = 2^{46} = 70,368,744,177,664$$

That is an incredibly large number of possibilities.[4]

We can generalize this discussion to the case of n pairs of chromosomes. If an organism has n pairs of chromosomes, then by applying the multiplication rule we find that 2^n possibly distinct sperm (or egg) cells can be formed during meiosis, and that it is possible for $2^n \times 2^n = 2^{2n}$ possible fertilized eggs to be formed. These simple calculations can help give us a feeling for why there exists so much variation among organisms.

Exercises

1. An octapeptide is a chain of eight amino acids (each can be one of 20 naturally occurring amino acids). How many octapeptides are theoretically possible?

2. Cows have 30 pairs of chromosomes, spider monkeys have 17 pairs, and opossums have 11 pairs.
   (a) How many distinct germ cells (sperm or egg cells) are possible for cows, spider monkeys, and opossums?
   (b) If the male and female of each can be assumed to have completely different chromosomes, what is the maximum number of distinct zygotes (fertilized eggs)? Answer for cows, spider monkeys, and opossums.

---

[4] One comment should be made, and that is that these huge numbers may not be completely accurate estimates. If all the genetic content in the male and female is not different, then the number of distinct zygotes (fertilized cells) will be decreased. For a simple introduction to this subject see Mosimann [1].

3. A restaurant menu lists three soups, ten meat dishes, five desserts, and three bever-
   ages. In how many ways can a meal (consisting of soup, meat dish, a dessert and
   beverage) be ordered?

4. A typical selective service number is 4-4-47-648, where the first two digits cannot
   be zero. How many selective service numbers are possible?

5. Suppose you take a 10-question true/false test. In how many ways can you turn in
   your answer sheet if you are guessing?

6. Consider a DNA molecule of fixed length. How many nucleotides would there
   have to be in a DNA chain if it has been determined that there are 1024 possible
   different arrangements?

7. (a) RNA codes for the production of amino acids. There are 20 commonly occur-
       ring amino acids. Why is it necessary to use a sequence of three nucleotides
       (or bases) rather than two or one?
   (b) If an RNA molecule is 240 nucleotides long, for how many possible sequences
       of amino acids can it code?

8. In a mating of two hybrid tall plants, $Tt \times Tt$ (where T is dominant tall, and t is
   recessive short) the possible results are TT (tall), Tt (tall), and tt (short). These are
   known as the genotypic results (actual genetic composition—not the visible trait).
   (a) If plants hybrid for two traits (e.g., height and color of seed) are mated, with
       the two traits inherited totally independently, how many distinct genotypes are
       possible?
   (b) If plants hybrid for three traits are mated, how many distinct genotypes are
       possible?
   (c) If plants hybrid for five traits are mated, how many distinct genotypes are
       possible?
   (d) If plants hybrid for n traits are mated, how many distinct genotypes are possible?

9. In *complete dominance*, the hybrid appears to have the dominant trait. For example,
   if T is dominant tall and t is recessive short, the observable outcomes (phenotypes)
   are tall (TT and Tt) and short (tt).
   (a) If plants hybrid for two traits both of which exhibit complete dominance are
       mated, how many distinct phenotypes are possible?
   (b) If plants hybrid for three traits all of which exhibit complete dominance are
       mated, how many distinct phenotypes are possible?
   (c) If plants hybrid for five traits all of which exhibit complete dominance are
       mated, how many distinct phenotypes are possible?
   (d) If plants hybrid for n traits all of which exhibit complete dominance are mated,
       how many distinct phenotypes are possible?

10. If we start with a single amoeba, how many will we have at the end of five genera-
    tions? Eight generations?

References

[1] J. E. Mosimann, *Elementary Probability for the Biological Sciences*. New York:
     Appleton-Century-Crofts, 1968.
[2] W. S. Spector, Ed., *Handbook of Biological Data*. Philadelphia, PA: Saunders,
     1956.

Notes for the Instructor

Objectives. This chapter is appropriate for courses in precalculus, mathematics, for liberal arts (topics type course), finite mathematics, probability for biology majors, probability for mathematics majors.

Time. An hour or two, depending on the level of the students.

Prerequisite. High school algebra.

CHAPTER 9
Cigarette Filtration

Donald A. Drew*

In spite of the warnings of the Surgeon-General and various cancer research organizations, people are smoking more cigarettes than ever. Considering the strength of the tobacco lobby and the economic reliance of many areas of the country on tobacco, it is unlikely that cigarette smoking will ever be banned. Thus it seems essential from a public health point of view that we study such mitigating processes as the use of filters in cigarettes.

Let us consider what happens to some component T in the tobacco smoke. T may represent tar, or nicotine, or some other component of tobacco smoke which is released by burning the tobacco. In the process which we wish to model, T is released by burning and travels down the cigarette, where it is absorbed (at least partially) by both the unburned tobacco and the filter. Any T which is absorbed by the tobacco is rereleased at a later time when that section of tobacco is burned. Thus all the T which is initially in the tobacco is released by burning.

We shall now make some modeling assumptions about the cigarette and the smoking procedure. Exactly how much smoke goes through the filter and how much goes directly into the air from the burning end depends on the smoker. If the smoker just holds the cigarette, none of the smoke passes through the filter. On the other hand, a chain smoker draws smoke through the filter with every inhalation. The average smoker is somewhere between these two extremes.

We wish to bypass this complex process with our model. We do this by assuming that a machine is smoking the cigarette. We assume that the smoke is traveling at a constant speed through the cigarette. We shall also assume that of the smoke released by burning the cigarette, only a fraction a passes

* Department of Mathematical Sciences, Rensselaer Polytechnic Institute, Troy, NY 12181.

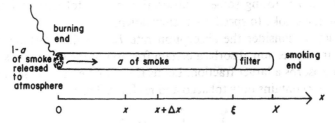

Figure 9.1. The Cigarette. For the Analysis of the Rate of Deposition of T, We Assume that the Burning End Remains at $x = 0$.

into the cigarette; the remaining $1 - a$ of the smoke is released to the atmosphere. In our discussion we will assume $a \neq 1$.

We shall also assume that the smoke moves through the cigarette and out the filter with a much larger velocity than the velocity at which the burning part of the cigarette progresses down the cigarette. This is equivalent to the assumption that whatever deposition of T in the tobacco and filter occurs, it occurs at the instant of its release by burning.

The last assumption essentially breaks the problem up into two parts. First we consider the rate of deposition of T in the cigarette, *assuming that the burning end does not move*. Second, we compute the total flow of T through the end of the cigarette during the burning of the cigarette.

The cigarette, and the coordinate system used for the computation of the rate of deposition of T are shown in Figure 9.1.

Now let us write a balance law for the mass of smoke in a section of the cigarette lying between some arbitrary points x and $x + \Delta x$. (A balance law is a statement that accounts for all changes in some quantity. In this case the quantity is the mass of T in the section of cigarette lying between x and $x + \Delta x$.) In words, the balance law is

the rate of flow of T through $x + \Delta x$ is equal to
the rate of flow of T through x minus
the rate of loss of T due to absorption.

We note that this statement of balance assumes that no amount of T accumulates in the section between x and $x + \Delta x$ *in the smoke itself*. Of course, T is accumulating in its bound form in the tobacco or filter, or whatever occupies the section between x and $x + \Delta x$.

Let us now consider the flow rate q of the component T. Suppose V is the velocity of the smoke and $\rho(x)$ is the mass density of T per unit length of *smoke* (in the cigarette). Then the flow rate through the point x is

$$q(x) = \rho(x)V. \tag{1}$$

See the Appendix for a detailed discussion of density and flow rate.

We have assumed that the velocity of the smoke V is constant. Essentially, we assume that as much *smoke* passes through the filter as starts down the cigarette at the burning end. The component T is only a small fraction of the total smoke; losing some to absorption by the tobacco or filter does not cause the smoke to speed up or slow down.

Now let us consider the absorption rate L. We shall assume that the tobacco in any section absorbs a certain fraction of the smoke present, and the filter absorbs a larger fraction. Let us first assume that the section from x to $x + \Delta x$ contains only tobacco and no filter. Then

$$L = b \int_x^{x+\Delta x} \rho(\tilde{x}) \, d\tilde{x}, \tag{2}$$

where b is the rate of mass absorption by the tobacco, and $\int_x^{x+\Delta x} \rho(\hat{x}) \, d\hat{x}$ is the mass of T in the section from x to $x + \Delta x$.

On the other hand, if the section lies completely in the filter,

$$L = \beta \int_x^{x+\Delta x} \rho(\hat{x}) \, d\hat{x}, \tag{3}$$

where β is the rate of mass absorption by the filter. To consider sections containing both tobacco and filter is not necessary. (See Exercise 1.)

In terms of the symbols, the balance law becomes

$$q(x + \Delta x) = q(x) - L. \tag{4}$$

Let us consider the case when the section from x to $x + \Delta x$ lies entirely in the tobacco. Using (1) and (2) in (4) gives

$$\rho(x) - \rho(x + \Delta x) = \frac{b}{V} \int_x^{x+\Delta x} \rho(\hat{x}) \, d\hat{x}. \tag{5}$$

Now, Δx is arbitrary. Let us divide by Δx and let $\Delta x \to 0$. Then

$$\frac{\rho(x) - \rho(x + \Delta x)}{\Delta x} = \frac{b}{V} \frac{1}{\Delta x} \int_x^{x+\Delta x} \rho(\hat{x}) \, d\hat{x}. \tag{6}$$

As $\Delta x \to 0$, the right-hand side approaches $(b/V) \rho(x)$. Consider the left-hand side. We write

$$\frac{\rho(x) - \rho(x + \Delta x)}{\Delta x} = -\frac{\rho(x + \Delta x) - \rho(x)}{\Delta x} \tag{7}$$

and let $\Delta x \to 0$. The second difference quotient above approaches $d\rho/dx$.

Thus the equation for the mass density is

$$\frac{d\rho(x)}{dx} = -\frac{b}{V} \rho(x). \tag{8}$$

This differential equation is valid for $0 < x < \xi$, where ξ is the location of the beginning of the filter.

For the filter, we have

$$\frac{d\rho(x)}{dx} = -\frac{\beta}{V} \rho(x) \tag{9}$$

for $\xi < x < X$. See Exercise 2.

If we solve the equations in the different regions, we get

$$\rho(x) = \begin{cases} \rho_0 e^{-(b/V)x}, & 0 < x < \xi \\ Re^{-(\beta/V)x}, & \xi < x < X. \end{cases} \tag{10}$$

See Exercise 3.

To determine ρ_0, we assume that the rate of burning to release T gives H units of mass per unit time, of which aH enters the end $x = 0$ per unit time. (The remaining $(1 - a)H$ is released to the air.) Thus the flux (mass per unit time) at $x = 0$ is aH, but the flux is also given by $V\rho_0 e^{-(b/V)\cdot 0} = V\rho_0$. Thus

$$\rho_0 = \frac{aH}{V}. \tag{11}$$

To determine R, we impose the condition that the flux through the cross section dividing the tobacco from the filter is continuous. Thus

$$\rho_0 e^{-(b/V)\xi} = Re^{-(\beta/V)\xi}, \tag{12}$$

so that

$$R = \rho_0 e^{(\beta-b)\xi/V}. \tag{13}$$

The flux of component T through the end $x = X$ is given by

$$q(X) = \rho(X)V, \tag{14}$$

which is

$$\begin{aligned} q(X) &= aHe^{[(\beta-b)/V]\xi - \beta X/V} \\ &= aHe^{-[\beta/V](X-\xi)}e^{-[b/V]\xi}. \end{aligned} \tag{15}$$

This concludes the analysis of the deposition of T. Before we move on to the analysis of the burning of the whole cigarette, let us interpret our result (15).

First, we note that the flux of T through the end depends on a and H not independently, but in the combination aH. Thus for this analysis, at least, we do not need to know a and H independently. We also note that we can make the filter more effective by increasing its absorption rate β or by increasing its length $X - \xi$. In either case, because the quantity appears in the exponent, the increase in effectiveness will be dramatic.

We now wish to model the situation when the whole cigarette is smoked. Thus we must account for the release, deposition, and rerelease of T as the cigarette is smoked. We note that of the T that is released on burning a given section of the cigarette, $1 - a$ is released to the atmosphere and the remaining a passes into the cigarette. Of the amount that enters the cigarette, some is absorbed by the tobacco, some by the filter, and the rest passes through the smoking end. That which is absorbed by the tobacco will be released again later when that section is burned.

In order to account for the amount of T which is absorbed by the tobacco, we must write a balance law for $W(x, t)$, the density of T in the tobacco (mass per unit length). Notice now that we include time t as a variable of interest.

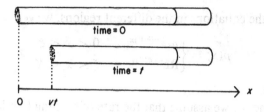

Figure 9.2. New Coordinate System.

For this problem, we shall measure distance x from the initial position of the burning end (see Figure 9.2).

We denote the burning velocity (that is, the velocity of the burning end) by v. Thus in time interval t, the burning end has moved from $x = 0$ to $x = vt$. Our assumption about *slow* burning is that $v \ll V$, that is, the velocity of the burning end is much smaller than the inhalation or smoke velocity V.

Let us now compute the rate of release of T by burning. If we burn for Δt time units, that is, we burn the section from $x = vt$ to $x = v(t + \Delta t)$, the *amount* of T released is approximately

$$\int_{vt}^{v(t+\Delta t)} W(x, t) \, dx. \tag{16}$$

The *rate* of release of T by burning, then, is

$$\lim_{\Delta t \to 0} \frac{1}{\Delta t} \int_{vt}^{vt+v\Delta t} W(x, t) \, dx = vW(vt, t), \tag{17}$$

but this is precisely what was meant by H in the previous analysis:

$$H = vW(vt, t). \tag{18}$$

Let us now consider the balance law for $W(x, t)$. Consider a section of the cigarette lying between x and $x + \Delta x$. The rate of change of the mass of T in the tobacco is

$$\frac{d}{dt} \int_{x}^{x+\Delta x} W(\tilde{x}, t) \, d\tilde{x}. \tag{19}$$

Since the tobacco does not move, T does not flow in or out while it is in the tobacco; it flows into the section in the *smoke* and is deposited in the tobacco. Thus the flux terms are zero. The rate of gain of mass of T in the tobacco is precisely equal to the rate of loss of mass of T from the smoke.

We have calculated the rate of deposition of T in the tobacco (equation 2); it is

$$b \int_{x}^{x+\Delta x} \rho(\tilde{x}, t) \, d\tilde{x} = \frac{abH}{V} \int_{x}^{x+\Delta x} e^{-b(\tilde{x}-vt)/V} \, d\tilde{x}$$

$$= \frac{abv}{V} W(vt, t) e^{(bv/V)t} \int_{x}^{x+\Delta x} e^{-b\tilde{x}/V} \, d\tilde{x}. \tag{20}$$

We have assumed that the burning occurs so slowly that the deposition can be treated through the previous analysis. Thus the balance law becomes

$$\frac{d}{dt} \int_x^{x+\Delta x} W(\tilde{x}, t)\, d\tilde{x} = \frac{abv}{V} W(vt, t) e^{(bv/V)t} \int_x^{x+\Delta x} e^{-b\tilde{x}/V}\, d\tilde{x}. \qquad (21)$$

If we integrate with respect to t, divide by Δx, and let $\Delta x \to 0$, we obtain

$$W(x, t) = W(x, 0) + \frac{abv}{V} e^{(-bx/V} \int_0^t e^{(bv/V)\tau} W(v\tau, \tau)\, d\tau. \qquad (22)$$

See Exercise 4.

Solving the integral equation (22) is not as difficult as one might first think. If we assume that $W(x, 0)$, the initial density of T in the tobacco, is constant, substitute $x = vt$, and multiply (22) by $e^{(bv/V)t}$, we have

$$W(vt, t) e^{(bv/V)t} = W_0 e^{(bv/V)t} + \frac{abv}{V} \int_0^t e^{(bv/V)\tau} W(v\tau, \tau)\, d\tau. \qquad (23)$$

If we denote $W(vt, t) e^{(bv/V)t} = f(t)$, we have

$$f(t) = W_0 e^{(bv/V)t} + \frac{abv}{V} \int_0^t f(\tau)\, d\tau. \qquad (24)$$

Differentiating with respect to t gives

$$f'(t) - \frac{abv}{V} f(t) = \frac{bv}{V} W_0 e^{(bv/V)t}. \qquad (25)$$

If we substitute $t = 0$ in (24) we obtain

$$f(0) = W_0. \qquad (26)$$

The solution of the ordinary differential equation (25) subject to (26) gives

$$f(t) = \frac{W_0}{1 - a} e^{bvt/V} (1 - ae^{(a-1)bvt/V}) \qquad (27)$$

and hence

$$W(vt, t) = \frac{W_0}{1 - a} (1 - ae^{(a-1)bvt/V}). \qquad (28)$$

See Exercise 5.

Substitution of $W(vt, t)$ in (22) gives

$$W(x, t) = W_0 \left[1 + \frac{a}{1 - a} e^{-bx/V} (e^{+bvt/V} - e^{abvt/V}) \right]. \qquad (29)$$

See Exercise 6.

From the results so far, let us calculate the total flow of T through the smoking end. The flux (mass per unit time) is

$$q(X) = V\rho(X). \qquad (30)$$

In the old coordinates (no time change), the smoking end remained in the same place. Now $X = X_0 - vt$, and $\xi = \xi_0 - vt$, where X_0 is the initial length of the cigarette and ξ_0 is the initial position of the filter. Using the expression for $\rho(x)$, we have the result that the flux is

$$q(X) = \frac{V \cdot a \cdot v \cdot W(vt, t)}{V} \exp\left[-\frac{b}{V}\xi_0 - \frac{\beta}{V}(X_0 - \xi_0) + \frac{b}{V}vt\right], \quad (31)$$

but

$$W(vt, t) = \frac{W_0}{1 - a}[1 - ae^{-(b/V)(1-a)vt}]. \quad (32)$$

Thus the total mass Q_β of the T which passes through the smoking end in smoking the cigarette *down to the filter* (so that $t = \xi_0/v$) is

$$Q_\beta = \int_{t=0}^{t=\xi_0/v} avW(vt, t)\exp\left[-\left(\frac{b}{V}\right)\xi_0 - \left(\frac{\beta}{V}\right)(X_0 - \xi_0) + \frac{bvt}{V}\right]dt$$

$$= \frac{avW_0}{1 - a}\exp\left[-\left(\frac{b}{V}\right)\xi_0 - \left(\frac{\beta}{V}\right)(X_0 - \xi_0)\right]\int_{t=0}^{\xi_0/v} e^{bvt/V} - ae^{abvt/V}\, dt$$

$$= \frac{aW_0 V}{b(1 - a)}e^{-(\beta/V)(X_0-\xi_0)}(1 - e^{-(1-a)(b/V)\xi_0}) \quad (33)$$

See Exercise 7.

We would like to use the above result to evaluate the effectiveness of having a filter. If there is no filter, then the cigarette is filled with tobacco from $x = 0$ to $x = X_0$. We can then use (33) to compute the total flow Q_b of T through the cigarette by setting $\beta = b$, since the absorption rate β of the "filter" is the same as the absorption rate of the tobacco.

Thus the ratio of total flow with the filter to the total flow without the filter is

$$\frac{Q_\beta}{Q_b} = e^{-[(\beta-b)/V](X_0-\xi_0)} \quad (34)$$

We can draw several conclusions from (34). First, since $V > 0$ and $X_0 > \xi_0$, we note that if $\beta > b$, $Q_\beta/Q_b < 1$, but if $\beta < b$, $Q_\beta/Q_b > 1$. Thus to be more effective than no filter at all, the filter must be more effective at absorption of T than the tobacco is. Most filter materials used do satisfy this requirement. Some foreign cigarettes, however, have a hollow paper tube instead of a filter. For those cigarettes, $\beta = 0$, and $Q_0/Q_b = e^{(b/V)(X_0-\xi_0)}$ is greater than one. Thus as far as the health of the smoker is concerned, it is better to have a tobacco filled "filter" than none at all, provided the "filter" is not smoked.

We also see that for constant filter length $X_0 - \xi_0$, the ratio Q_β/Q_b decreases exponentially fast with increasing absorption rate $\beta - b$. We further see that for constant absorption rate $\beta - b$, the ratio Q_β/Q_b decreases exponentially with increasing filter length $X_0 - \xi_0$. Since increasing the absorption rate of the filter material usually requires research into the effectiveness and practicality of new materials, and such research is expensive, we might suggest that an easier way to obtain the same effect is to increase the length of the filter. Cigarette manufacturers, however, have other constraints, such as having to use existing machinery for manufacturing, and the more nebulous problem of having to sell the longer filter to the smoking public. (What could you use as advertising?)

Let us now consider another analysis which is within our grasp using (31) and (32). It has been said that one reason for having a filter at all is to keep the smoker from smoking all of the cigarette, and thereby getting all the T which is inhaled. In doing this analysis, let us assume that the filter is only as effective in absorption of T as the tobacco itself; so that $\beta = b$.

If we smoke only to the filter, the total flow of T through the smoking end is

$$Q_b = \frac{aW_0 V}{b(1-a)} e^{-(b/V)(X_0 - \xi_0)} (1 - e^{-(1-a)(b/V)\xi_0}). \tag{35}$$

If we smoke the cigarette to the end $x = X_0$, we must integrate (31) from $t = 0$ to $t = X_0/v$. The result is that Q_T the total flux of T through the cigarette is

$$\begin{aligned} Q_T &= \frac{avW_0}{1-a} e^{-(b/V)X_0} \int_{t=0}^{t=X_0/v} e^{bvt/V} - ae^{abvt/V}\, dt \\ &= \frac{aW_0 V}{b(1-a)} (1 - e^{-(1-a)(b/V)X_0}). \end{aligned} \tag{36}$$

The ratio of the flux of T through the smoking end for smoking the "filter" cigarette to that for smoking the total length is

$$\frac{Q_b}{Q_T} = e^{-(b/V)(X_0 - \xi_0)} \left(\frac{1 - e^{-(1-a)(b/V)\xi_0}}{1 - e^{-(1-a)(b/V)X_0}} \right). \tag{37}$$

See Exercise 8.

To see the important trends in this equation, let us expand Q_b/Q_T as a function of ξ_0 in a Taylor series about $\xi_0 = X_0$. Then

$$Q_b/Q_T = 1 + (\xi_0 - X_0) \frac{b}{V} \left(\frac{1 - ae^{-(1-a)(b/V)X_0}}{1 - e^{-(1-a)(b/V)X_0}} \right) + K(\xi_0 - X_0)^2. \tag{38}$$

where K is a constant. See Exercise 9.

For ξ_0 near X_0, we can ignore the term $K(\xi_0 - X_0)^2$. Since $a < 1$, we see that $Q_b/Q_T < 1$.

We might also use the model to attempt to indicate effective ways for people to cut down on their consumption of T without stopping smoking altogether. One suggested way is to smoke only some fraction, such as one-half, of the cigarette. Exercise 10 outlines the analysis of this technique of cutting down consumption of T.

Exercises

1. (a) Write an appropriate expression for L in the case when the section from x to
   $x + \Delta x$ contains some tobacco (from x to ξ) and some filter (from ξ to $x + \Delta x$).
   (b) In the analysis leading to equation (8), we let $\Delta x \to 0$. Explain what happens
   to the expression in part (a) for L as $\Delta x \to 0$.

2. Derive equation (9).

3. Solve the differential equations (8) and (9) to get the expressions in equation (10).

4. Derive equation (22).

5. Solve the differential equation (25) subject to the initial condition (26) to get (27).
   Also, derive equation (28).

6. Derive equation (29).

7. Derive (33).

8. Derive (37).

9. Expand Q_b/Q_T in a Taylor series in $\xi_0 - X_0$ to get (38).

10. By integrating the expression (31) for $q(X)$ from $t = 0$ to $t = \xi_0/2v_0$, compute the
    total flux $Q_{1/2}$ of T which passes through the cigarette by smoking one-half of it.
    Find the ratio $Q_{1/2}/Q_b$. (Use $\beta = b$ for the above analysis.)

11. Butts and Ashes, a hypothetical cigarette company, manufactures a cigarette which
    contains 800 milligrams (mg) of tar. The length of the tobacco section is 8 cm, and
    the length of the filter is 2 cm. The absorption rate of tar by the tobacco is $b = 0.02$
    per second, while the absorption rate of the filter is $\beta = 0.08$ per second. Compute
    the total flux of tar through the cigarette when smoked by a machine which draws
    smoke through the cigarette at a speed of 5 cm/sec. The fraction of smoke lost to
    the air at any instant during the smoking is 0.7.

12. Butts and Ashes wish to take the $1,000,000 that they usually give to the American
    Cancer Society annually and invest it wisely in research on making a better ciga-
    rette. They find that the present research community estimates that they are able
    to improve both the tobacco by lowering the total tar content W_0 and the filter by
    increasing the absorption rate β. The research community estimates that it would
    cost $1000 per milligram to reduce the tar in the tobacco, while it would cost
    $10,000 per 0.01 units of β to increase β. How should they spend their money?
    That is, how should they divide the $1,000,000 between tobacco research and filter
    research?

Appendix: Discussion of Density and Flow Rate

Let us discuss the mass density of T per unit length. Consider a "snapshot"
of the smoke in the cigarette at any instant. Let x be any point in the cigarette,
not an end point. Consider the section of the cigarette from $x - (\varepsilon/2)$ to

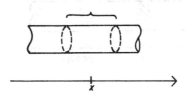

Figure 9.3

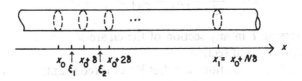

Figure 9.4

$x + (\varepsilon/2)$. For different values of ε, the mass of T in the smoke in this section is different, since more mass will be included in the section if ε is larger (Figure 9.3).

If we let $m(x, \varepsilon)$ denote the mass of T in the section, we define the *density* at x (mass per unit length) by

$$\rho(x) = \lim_{\varepsilon \to 0} \frac{m(x, \varepsilon)}{\varepsilon} \qquad (A1)$$

Let us now consider the relationship between total mass and mass density. Note that if x_0 and x_1 are arbitrary points in the cigarette, the mass of T between x_0 and x_1 is $m((x_0 + x_1)/2, x_1 - x_0)$. However, this mass is also equal to the sum of the masses of T of the sections from x_0 to $x_0 + \delta$, from $x_0 + \delta$ to $x_0 + 2\delta$, $\cdots$, where $\delta = (x_1 - x_0)/N$, where N is an integer (see Figure 9.4). Thus

$$m\left(\frac{x_0 + x_1}{2}, x_1 - x_0\right) = m(\xi_1, \delta) + m(\xi_2, \delta) + \cdots + m(\xi_N, \delta),$$

$$(A2)$$

where ξ_1 is the midpoint of the segment between x_0 and $x_0 + \delta$, and ξ_2 is the midpoint between $x_0 + \delta$ and $x_0 + 2\delta$, $\cdots$.

Now write

$$m(\xi_j, \delta) = \frac{m(\xi_j, \sigma)}{\delta} \cdot \delta. \qquad (A3)$$

The mass becomes

$$m\left(\frac{x_0 + x_1}{2}, x_1 - x_0\right) = \sum_j \frac{m(\xi_j, \delta)}{\delta} \cdot \delta. \qquad (A4)$$

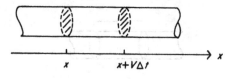

Figure 9.5

If we now let $N \to \infty$, so that $\delta \to 0$, the summation becomes

$$m\left(\frac{x_0 + x_1}{2}, x_1 - x_0\right) = \int_{x_0}^{x_1} \rho(x)\,dx. \tag{A5}$$

Thus the mass of T in any section of the cigarette is equal to the integral of the density over that section.

Now let us discuss the flow rate. Let V be the (constant) velocity of smoke measured to the right. That is, if a certain "slice" of smoke is identified by coloring or some kind of tracer at x at time t, then that slice is found at $x + V\Delta t$ at time $t + \Delta t$ (Figure 9.5).

We see that in time Δt, $V \cdot \Delta t$ is the length of the section of smoke which has moved through the location x. That is, at time t, the first "slice" of smoke to move through x is at x; and that slice has moved to $x + V\Delta t$ after Δt time units. The last slice to make it through x is still at x, having just made it there. All slices originally in between moved across x at some intermediate time.

The mass of smoke which moved through the section x during this time interval is the sum of the masses of each slice, which becomes

$$\int_{x}^{x+V\Delta t} \rho(\hat{x})\,d\hat{x}. \tag{A6}$$

The rate of flux of mass $q(x)$ through x is

$$q(x) = \lim_{\Delta t \to 0} \left[\frac{1}{\Delta t} \int_{x}^{x+V\Delta t} \rho(\hat{x})\,d\hat{x}\right]. \tag{A7}$$

If we denote $I(\xi) = \int_{x}^{x+\xi} \rho(\hat{x})\,d\hat{x}$, then by the fundamental theorem of calculus

$$\left.\frac{dI}{d\xi}\right|_{\xi=0} = \rho(x) = \lim_{\xi \to 0} \frac{I(\xi) - I(0)}{\xi} = \lim_{\xi \to 0} \frac{I(\xi)}{\xi}. \tag{A8}$$

The rate of mass flux $q(x)$ through x can be written as

$$q(x) = V \cdot \lim_{\Delta t \to 0} \frac{1}{V\Delta t} \int_{x}^{x+V\Delta t} \rho(\hat{x})\,d\hat{x} = V\rho(x). \tag{A9}$$

Reference

[1] B. Noble, *Applications of Undergraduate Mathematics in Engineering*. MAA and Macmillan, 1967.

Notes for the Instructor

Objectives. The problem of calculating the release of a component of tobacco smoke by burning is studied. This chapter discusses the concepts of density and flux.

Prerequisites. Multivariable calculus, differential equations.

Time. Two lectures.

Remarks. This chapter makes liberal use of calculus concepts like the fundamental theorem, Riemann integral and derivatives. A simple first-order ordinary differential equation must be solved to obtain the answer. This problem appeared in a shorter form in Ben Noble's book, *Applications of Undergraduate Mathematics in Engineering.*

PART III

ECOLOGY

CHAPTER 10

Efficiency of Energy Use in Obtaining Food, I: Humans

Fred S. Roberts*

1. Introduction

1.1 The Problem

The world population has reached four billion people and continues to grow rapidly; it is expected to reach seven billion by the year 2000 [26]. There is increasing concern about the ability of mankind to feed itself. A large percentage of mankind is already malnourished ([32], [1]), and famine in sub-Saharan Africa and parts of Asia has been in the headlines in recent years. Undoubtedly, more serious starvation has been avoided so far by the incredible productivity of agricultural systems, such as that of the United States, and by the application of modern technology to world-wide food production. (We have all heard about the "green revolution.") As a measure of how successful we have been in increasing productivity, it is estimated that under modern cropping systems, the yield of an acre planted in corn in the U.S. has increased from 26 bushels in 1909 to 87 bushels in 1971. The major part of this increase has been since about 1950 (Pimentel *et al.* [29, pp. 444–445]).

Unfortunately, this increased productivity of modern agriculture has been obtained at a price: the use of vast amounts of energy. In the early days of agriculture, the only energy used in food production was human labor. Gradually, man found that he could substitute animals for some of his own work. Later on, he added machines. Today, fossil fuel has become a major input in agricultural production [12]. Energy is used not only in driving tractors around a farm, it is also used in irrigation, in producing

* Department of Mathematics, Rutgers University, New Brunswick, NJ 08903.

and applying chemical fertilizers, in pesticides, and so on. (This does not even take into account the amount of energy used to process food, to transport it to the supermarket, to store it and prepare it at home, etc.) All of this use of energy was fine while energy was inexpensive and abundant (or appeared to be abundant). Now, however, man has begun to see the end of cheap, easily obtained energy. There are sober implications for our future ability to feed the increasing human population.

It is clearly becoming necessary for man to be more efficient in the use of energy. By way of contrast, a body of ecological literature suggests that animals are very efficient in their use of energy. Hainsworth and Wolf [10] suggest that animals evolve so as to be efficient in their use of energy in foraging for food. Schoener [38] argues that for a class of predators identical except in size, that predator will be optimal in size (and will evolve) which obtains energy to support its food requirements in an optimal way. Emlen [8] assumes that natural selection favors the development of feeding preferences which will maximize caloric intake per unit time.

In this first of two chapters, we will consider ways to measure efficiency of energy use in obtaining food energy. We will then consider strategies for optimizing energy efficiency. In the final section, we will apply the earlier discussion to human food production. In the follow-up chapter (Roberts and Marcus-Roberts [36]), we will apply strategies for optimizing the efficiency of energy use to construct a series of mathematical models of the behavior of animals in searching for food. We will try to model the predator which is energy efficient and make some predictions about his feeding habits, his body size, and so on. These biological models will be *descriptive* in nature, describing the behavior of a predator trying to be energy efficient. The discussion of human energy use, in contrast, will be *prescriptive* or *normative* in nature, discussing how decisions about energy use in food production *should* be made.

It should be mentioned that, while we emphasize energy content of food, there are more goals in eating than simply obtaining energy. Animals and humans need a "balanced diet," which has not only enough calories of food energy, but also a combination of proteins, vitamins, and so on. We shall briefly mention the need for a balanced diet in our considerations at one point. However, we will concentrate on calories.

1.2 Organization of the Chapter

This chapter is divided into four sections, the first of which is this Introduction. Section 2 gives a very brief background to some of the biology and physics which we use in the following. We hope that much of what follows will be understandable with just this brief background. However, it should be emphasized that if one is to seriously consider expanding on what is presented here, or doing one's own modeling, a more serious grounding in biology and physics will be needed. Section 3 introduces the notion of efficiency and discusses alternative ways to define it. This section formulates the "global optimum efficiency problem" and discusses ways to solve it. The final section of this chapter, Section 4, discusses the energy efficiency of human food production and then investigates whether the procedures described for solving the global optimum efficiency problem are appropriate for human food production. Finally, Section 4 also considers a variety of strategies for increasing energy efficiency in food production and analyzes some of these strategies mathematically.

2. Energy and Food: Some Biological and Physical Background

All work performed by humans or animals is made possible by the release of energy through *metabolism*: the combustion or oxidation of food by respiratory processes. The term work includes the flexing or relaxing of muscles and it also includes the synthesizing of proteins to build new body cells. The energy used in metabolism has its original source in the sun. Solar energy is captured by plants and, through the process of *photosynthesis*, is converted into chemical energy. In turn, this chemical energy is passed on from plants to small animals, from these to larger animals, and so on through *food chains*. Some of this energy eventually reaches man.

Ecology is that science which deals with food chains and, more generally, with the relationships between living things and their interrelations with their physical environment [28]. The organisms and the physical environment in which they exist form what is called an *ecosystem*. We shall be concerned with the flow of energy through an ecosystem. The branch of science which deals with this subject is called *energetics* and involves a mixture of physics, chemistry, and biology.

Energy, as the physicists define it, is the capacity to do work. Energy comes in various forms, including mechanical, chemical, radiant, and heat energy. The critical fact about energy is that it can neither be created nor destroyed, only changed from one form to another. This is the *first law of thermodynamics*.

Energy, since it takes various forms, is measured in various units. For example, work done in raising an object is usually measured by multiplying weight lifted by height raised. The work done in raising a one gram weight a distance of one centimeter up against the force of gravity is called one *erg*. The erg is a measure of the mechanical energy used in work. Similarly, heat energy can be measured. The heat required to raise the temperature of one gram of water one degree centigrade is called a *calorie* and is abbreviated *cal*. One thousand calories are called a *kilogram calorie*, or *kilocalorie*, abbreviated *kcal* or *Cal*. By studying transformations between mechanical energy and heat energy (in particular, how much work it took to heat up water), Joule determined the relationship between heat energy and energy performed in working: 4.2×10^7 ergs are equivalent to 1 calorie. In studying the energy inputs into agriculture, it will be very important for us to convert the different forms of energy used into the same units. In accordance with the literature of energetics, we shall always use the kcal as a measure of energy.

References. Much of this section is based on Phillipson [28]. Most basic ecology texts have sections on energy flow. Some good references are Colinvaux [4], Ricklefs [35], Odum [27], and Reid [34]. Books more specifically on energetics include Kleiber [16], Lehninger [19], Miller [24], and Wesley [43].

3. Efficiency and Optimally Efficient Behavior

3.1 Definition of Efficiency

Consider a process or an activity a which uses a certain amount of input $I(a)$ to produce a certain amount of output $O(a)$. The *efficiency* of the activity can be measured as

$$e(a) = \frac{O(a)}{I(a)}. \tag{1}$$

For example, an oil burner used to heat a room burns a certain amount of oil. The input energy can be measured as the heat produced by burning, the output energy as the heat which actually reaches the room. The efficiency of the oil burner is the ratio. Normally, this is about 0.60 to 0.65, so we say the oil burner is 60–65% efficient [6, p. 39]. Similarly, an investment which yields $200 for an initial input of $100 has an efficiency of $200/100 = 2$, or 200%. In general, we want our investments to have efficiencies of more than one. Finally, an agricultural procedure which yields 6000 kilocalories of food energy if 500 kilocalories of energy are used to grow the food has an efficiency of 6000/500 or 12.

This notion of efficiency is very common in thermodynamics and is a natural way of measuring the relative values of output and input. Of course, efficiency can be defined in other ways. Commoner [6, p. 39] thinks that the efficiency of the oil burner, for example, should be measured by considering all possible procedures for heating the room to the desired temperature and computing the least amount of work which would have accomplished the desired task (heating the room to, say, 70°). The least amount of work is calculated using the most efficient conceivable procedure, and then the efficiency of the oil burner is the ratio of the least amount of work conceivable to the actual amount of work involved if the oil burner is used to perform the task. This efficiency Commoner calls, following a team from the American Physical Society, the "efficiency according to the second law of thermodynamics." In this sense, the oil burner turns out to be only 8.2% efficient.[1] Another way of measuring efficiency would be to consider *net output*, i.e., output less input, and divide by input:

$$\frac{O(a) - I(a)}{I(a)}.$$

Still other measures bring in time, or another factor, and measure the net output per unit of time, or per unit of this other factor. Consider for instance

$$\frac{O(a) - I(a)}{T(a)},$$

where $T(a)$ might represent the time taken by the activity a.

We shall return to this latter notion in the exercises and in Chapter 11 of this volume (Roberts and Marcus-Roberts [36]). But here, we shall investigate the efficiency $e(a)$ defined by Eq. (1). We shall seek ways to choose from a collection of activities those which maximize the total efficiency and achieve certain goals.

3.2 The Global Optimum Efficiency Problem

Suppose we are faced with a choice among possible activities or processes or items. Each activity i has an input I_i and an output O_i, and its efficiency is defined, in accordance with equation (1), as

$$e_i = O_i/I_i.$$

Suppose we are required to perform enough of these activities (choose enough of the processes or items) so that during the course of the day (or year), the total output is equal to some number M. In Section 4, we shall encounter this problem where O_i is the food energy produced by a given process on a given piece of land, and I_i is the energy used in that process on the piece of land. (We will need to add the restriction that no piece of land may be used with more than one process. This is easily incorporated.) We shall encounter a similar problem in [36, Section 4.7] from the point of view of a predator. O_i will be the food energy attainable from the ith item in a set of potential food items, and I_i the energy required to capture and eat the ith food item. The predator wants to choose food items to eat so

[1] The most efficient way to heat a room is to use a heat pump, a device which does the reverse of what a refrigerator does: it cools the out-of-doors to warm the room.

that he eats enough food to meet his daily requirements M. A third interpretation is to think of I_i as the number of dollars invested in the ith potential investment, and O_i as the expected return on this investment. We want to choose investments over the course of a year so that we get a return of M dollars.

The major problem we shall consider is not only how to choose processes, items, or investments to meet a desired total output, but how to do so most efficiently. Suppose S is a set of processes, items, or investments which yield the desired output. According to our general principle (1), the efficiency of the set of activities S can be calculated as the output divided by the input, or as

$$e(S) = \frac{\sum_{i \in S} O_i}{\sum_{i \in S} I_i}. \tag{2}$$

We shall seek that set of processes, items, or investments which has maximum efficiency. Our problem can be stated formally as follows:

$$\left. \begin{array}{c} \text{maximize } e(S) = \dfrac{\sum_{i \in S} O_i}{\sum_{i \in S} I_i} \\[2em] \text{subject to } \sum_{i \in S} O_i = M \end{array} \right\}. \tag{3}$$

Of course, (3) reduces to the problem of minimizing $\sum_{i \in S} I_i$ subject to the requirement that $\sum_{i \in S} O_i = M$. However, it will be convenient to state the problem in the form (3) as we shall encounter it in this form later.

Modifying (3) to read

$$\left. \begin{array}{c} \text{maximize } e(S) = \dfrac{\sum_{i \in S} O_i}{\sum_{i \in S} I_i} \\[2em] \text{subject to } \sum_{i \in S} O_i \geq M \end{array} \right\} \tag{4}$$

might be more reasonable. Problem (4) says we obtain at least the desired output, while (3) says we obtain it exactly. We shall discuss (4) later. We concentrate on (3) because in the predation interpretation, we think (3) (or the modification (6) to follow) is the more reasonable problem: solutions to (4) could require the predator to spend too much time eating or eat too much for his own good. Either (3) or (4) is reasonable for our other interpretations.

Problem (3) can easily be stated as a linear programming problem, in fact a problem in integer linear programming. Let x_i count the number of times that i is included. Of course, x_i will be either 0 or 1. Then (3) becomes

$$\left.\begin{array}{c} \text{maximize } \dfrac{\sum_i x_i O_i}{\sum_i x_i I_i} \\[2em] \text{subject to } \sum_i x_i O_i = M \\[1.5em] 0 \le x_i \le 1, \text{ all } i \\[1em] x_i \text{ an integer, all } i \end{array}\right\}. \qquad (5)$$

This is equivalent to the linear programming problem

$$\left.\begin{array}{c} \text{minimize } \sum_i x_i I_i \\[1.5em] \text{subject to } \sum_i x_i O_i = M \\[1.5em] 0 \le x_i \le 1, \text{ all } i \\[1em] x_i \text{ an integer, all } i \end{array}\right\}.$$

Thus the usual techniques of (integer) linear programming may be brought to bear on this problem. There is, however, a special method which sometimes solves it, as we shall see.

We shall call (3) the *global optimum efficiency problem*, or the *GOE problem*, for short. Of course, analogous problems can be stated using other definitions of efficiency, such as those mentioned in Section 3.1. If the definition net output per unit of input is used, then the problem is equivalent to the present one. For

$$\frac{O - I}{I}$$

is maximized whenever O/I is maximized. The GOE problem when the net output per unit of time is being maximized will be discussed in the exercises.

One way to go about solving the GOE problem is to be "greedy." First choose that process or item i for which O_i/I_i is as large as possible (choose arbitrarily in case of ties). Next, choose that process i for which O_i/I_i is next highest. Continue until the desired output is attained. This procedure corresponds to what we often do. We try to optimize the efficiency of our choices one step at a time. In trying to optimize our investments, we choose first the best potential investment. Then, if we have more money to invest, we choose our next best investment, and so on.

Unfortunately, if we are required to attain the desired sum of outputs M *exactly*, the *greedy procedure* or *greedy algorithm* we have described may force us to overshoot. Let us give an example. Table 1 gives a collection of processes and their inputs and outputs. Suppose the required M is 1000. The greedy algorithm would work as follows. First choose process 2, since $e_2 = 8.6$ is the largest efficiency. Then choose process 3, since $e_3 = 8.3$ is the next highest efficiency. Unfortunately, $O_2 + O_3$ is already larger than $M = 1000$.

Table 1. $M = 1000$

Process i	1	2	3	4	5	6
Output O_i	100	600	500	200	400	300
Input I_i	100	70	60	80	50	70
Efficiency $e_i = O_i/I_i$	1.0	8.6	8.3	2.5	8.0	4.3

Table 2. Feasible Solutions to the GOE Problem with the Data of Table 1.

Subset S of Processes	$e(S) = \sum_{i \in S} O_i / \sum_{i \in S} I_i$
1, 2, 6	1000/240
1, 3, 5	1000/210
1, 4, 5, 6	1000/300
2, 5	1000/120
3, 4, 6	1000/210

Thus the greedy algorithm does not give a *feasible solution* to the GOE problem (3), a solution satisfying the constraints

$$\sum_{i \in S} O_i = M.$$

A variant of the greedy algorithm, which we might call the *slightly less greedy algorithm*, is the following. Pick at each step the process with the highest available efficiency which does not cause an overshoot of M by $\sum O_i$ (as usual, choosing arbitrarily in case of ties). This procedure leads to the solution of picking process 2 first and then process 5. Exercise 7 asks the reader to construct an example where the slightly less greedy algorithm does not lead to a *feasible solution*, although there are feasible solutions to the problem. Exercise 8 further investigates this algorithm.

Table 2 lists all feasible solutions for the problem of Table 1, namely all sets S of processes for which

$$\sum_{i \in S} O_i = 1000.$$

(The reader should check that he agrees with this table.)

Clearly, the subset consisting of processes 2 and 5 gives the optimal solution, since 1000/120 is maximal among the $e(S)$. This happens to be the solution provided by the slightly less greedy algorithm. This algorithm does not always lead to an optimal solution to the GOE problem, even if it leads to a feasible solution. The reader is asked to show this in Exercise 8.

If the data of Table 1 is used but the required M is changed from 1000 to 1100, then the greedy algorithm does lead to a feasible solution. This solution is to choose processes 2 and 3. Table 3 lists all feasible solutions in this case. (Once again, the reader should check that he agrees with this table.) We

Table 3. Feasible Solutions to the GOE
Problem with the Data of Table 1 if M
is Changed to 1100.

Subset S of Processes	$e(S) = \sum_{i \in S} O_i / \sum_{i \in S} I_i$
1, 2, 5	1100/220
1, 3, 4, 6	1100/310
2, 3	1100/130
2, 4, 6	1100/220
3, 4, 5	1100/190

can easily see that the greedy solution leads to the maximum $e(S)$ and hence
provides an optimal solution to the GOE problem in this case. This is no
accident.

Theorem. *If the greedy algorithm leads to a feasible solution of the GOE problem, then it leads to an optimal solution.*[2]

We shall prove this theorem in Section 3.3. What it says is that by attempting to optimize locally (i.e., at every step), we can sometimes optimize glob-
ally. The result is really quite surprising, because in general the expression

$$\frac{\sum O_i}{\sum I_i}$$

is quite different from the expression

$$\sum \frac{O_i}{I_i}.$$

As we have seen, the greedy algorithm does not always give a feasible
solution to the GOE problem (3). In Section 4, we shall ask whether it gives
a feasible solution in the case of human use of energy to produce food. On
the other hand, many of us, in trying to be efficient, are using the greedy
algorithm in making choices, for example in choosing investments. Perhaps
this can be explained by arguing that we do not care if we go a little bit over
the required amount of output (energy or return on investment) M. Perhaps
we are trying to solve the following variant of the GOE problem:

$$\left. \begin{array}{l} \text{maximize } e(S) = \dfrac{\sum\limits_{i \in S} O_i}{\sum\limits_{i \in S} I_i} \\[2em] \text{subject to } \sum\limits_{i \in S} O_i \geq M \\[1.5em] \sum\limits_{i \in T} O_i < M \quad \text{for all proper subsets } T \text{ of } S \end{array} \right\} \quad (6)$$

[2] If there are ties, then each solution obtained using the greedy algorithm is optimal.

Table 4. $M = 760$

i	1	2	3
O_i	750	250	10
I_i	100	50	5
$e_i = O_i/I_i$	7.5	5	2

In this problem we pick S so as to maximize global efficiency $e(S)$ and meet the requirements, but just barely in the sense that leaving out any process in S will not meet the requirements. The greedy algorithm always leads to feasible solutions of this problem, if such solutions exist. However, surprisingly, these solutions may not be optimal! To give an example, consider the data of Table 4 with $M = 760$. The greedy algorithm leads to a selection of processes 1 and 2. The corresponding global efficiency is $1000/150 = 6.7$. However, the feasible solution of choosing processes 1 and 3 has a higher global efficiency of $760/105 = 7.2$. Thus, if we are trying to solve (6), using the greedy algorithm may not give us optimal solutions.

Some of the mathematical models we shall present in Chapter 11 of this volume (Roberts and Marcus-Roberts [36]) will assume that animals perform the greedy algorithm in trying to optimize their energy efficiency. Philosophers of science try to distinguish between descriptive models of behavior and prescriptive or normative models of behavior. *Descriptive* models try to describe how an organism behaves, *prescriptive* models how it *should* behave. Since we have seen that the greedy algorithm may not in fact optimize, these models which assume the greedy algorithm should most probably be considered descriptive rather than prescriptive. They are based on the assumption that organisms *try* to optimize and adopt a natural procedure for doing so (perhaps the only one their minds can cope with on a step by step basis). However, they may not be optimizing with their procedure.

Earlier we observed that the proper problem to consider may not be the GOE problem (3), but problem (4):

$$\left. \begin{array}{l} \text{maximize } \dfrac{\sum\limits_{i \in S} O_i}{\sum\limits_{i \in S} I_i} \\[2em] \text{subject to } \sum\limits_{i \in S} O_i \geq M \end{array} \right\} . \tag{4}$$

Note that if we change the objective in (3) to read minimize $\sum_{i \in S} I_i$, we get a problem equivalent to (3). Making the same change in (4) leads to the problem

$$\left. \begin{array}{l} \text{minimize } \sum\limits_{i \in S} I_i \\[1.5em] \text{subject to } \sum\limits_{i \in S} O_i \geq M \end{array} \right\} . \tag{4a}$$

We shall call (4a) the *input minimization problem*. The reader should note that (4) and (4a) are not equivalent (Exercise 15).

One can ask if the greedy algorithm solution to problem (6) necessarily leads to an optimal solution to (4). The answer is no, as the reader is asked to show in Exercise 14a. One can also talk about a different kind of greedy algorithm, a *greedy minimization algorithm*, for (4): pick first that activity of minimum I_i, next that activity of minimum I_i among those left, until just reaching or exceeding M in outputs. Exercise 14b will ask the reader to show that the greedy minimization algorithm may not lead to an optimal solution of this problem.

EXERCISES

1. Consider the data of Table 5. Solve the GOE problem and compare the solution to a solution found by the greedy algorithm, if there is one.

Table 5. $M = 800$

i	1	2	3	4	5	6
O_i	200	400	350	200	400	450
I_i	150	250	175	40	100	150

2. Find a slightly less greedy solution to the GOE problem defined by Table 5, and compare to the optimal solution.

3. Solve (6) using the data of Table 5, and compare the optimal solution to a greedy solution.

4. Repeat Exercise 1 for the data of Table 6.

Table 6. $M = 1000$

i	1	2	3	4	5	6
O_i	800	400	600	800	200	200
I_i	400	200	400	500	50	40

5. Repeat Exercise 2 for the data of Table 6.

6. Repeat Exercise 3 for the data of Table 6.

7. Show that the slightly less greedy algorithm may not lead to a feasible solution of the GOE problem, even though feasible solutions do exist.

8. Show that the slightly less greedy algorithm may lead to a feasible solution of the GOE problem which is not optimal.

9. Show that if there is ambiguity because of ties, one choice in the greedy algorithm can lead to a feasible solution of the GOE problem while another choice can lead to an infeasible solution.

10. The GOE problem and its variant, problem (6), are related to an important class of problems in applied operations research known as knapsack problems. To be concrete, suppose that p different pieces of equipment are being considered for inclusion on a space ship traveling to Mars. The ith item has a certain scientific value s_i and a certain weight w_i. We would like to choose which items of equipment to take so that the scientific value of the total is as large as possible, but the total weight of the equipment taken is no greater than a certain maximum amount M. The problem can be formulated mathematically by letting x_i be the number of units of the ith item taken; then $x_i = 0$ or 1. We wish to

$$\text{maximize} \sum_{i=1}^{p} x_i s_i$$

subject to the constraints:

$$
\left.
\begin{aligned}
& \sum_{i=1}^{p} x_i w_i \leq M \\
& 0 \leq x_i \leq 1, \qquad i = 1, 2, \cdots, p \\
& x_i \text{ an integer}, \qquad i = 1, 2, \cdots, p
\end{aligned}
\right\}
\tag{7}
$$

Problem (7) is a typical problem in integer linear programming and is called the *knapsack problem* (think of a knapsack rather than a space ship). The problem can easily be converted into a problem where we minimize rather than maximize, into a problem where the x_i are allowed to be any nonnegative integers, not just 0 or 1, or into a problem where we want $\Sigma x_i w_i \geq M$ or $\Sigma x_i w_i = M$. An extensive discussion of knapsack problems is given in Garfinkel and Nemhauser [9].

(a) Formulate a greedy algorithm for solving the knapsack problem (7).

(b) Consider the concrete problem where four items are under consideration for the space ship, and the values and weights of these items are given in Table 7. Let M be 5. Find all feasible solutions to this problem, and an optimal solution. Find a greedy solution and determine if it is optimal.

Table 7. $M = 5$

i	1	2	3	4
s_i	8	6	10	11
w_i	5	1	3	2

(c) Change the data of Table 7 so that s_1 becomes 15 instead of 8. Find all feasible solutions, an optimal solution, and a greedy solution, and determine if the greedy solution is optimal. (Note: Magazine *et al.* [22] discuss conditions under which the greedy algorithm does solve the knapsack problem.)

11. Use of the greedy algorithm to solve the GOE problem suggests consideration of the following problem:

$$
\left.
\begin{aligned}
& \text{maximize} \sum_{i \in S} \frac{O_i}{I_i} \\
& \text{subject to} \sum_{i \in S} O_i = M
\end{aligned}
\right\}
\tag{8}
$$

This problem might be called the *local optimum efficiency problem*, or *LOE problem*. Solve this problem for

(a) the data of Table 1;
(b) the data of Table 1 with M changed to 1100;
(c) the data of Table 4;
(d) the data of Table 5;
(e) the data of Table 6.

12. Translate the LOE problem of Exercise 11 into a knapsack problem (Exercise 10).

13. Although the GOE problem and the LOE problem of Exercise 11 are closely related, solutions to them can be quite different. Show that the greedy algorithm can lead to a feasible solution of both of these problems, and hence an optimal solution of the first problem, without leading to an optimal solution of the second! This shows that our intuition about optimizing efficiency is not very good. (Hint: Consider your answers to Exercise 11b.)

14. (a) Show that the greedy algorithm solution to (6) does not necessarily lead to an optimal solution to the corresponding problem (4).
    (b) Show that the greedy minimization algorithm does not necessarily lead to an optimal solution to problem (4).

15. Show that problems (4) and (4a) are not equivalent.

16. Discuss the relation between the greedy minimization solution to (4) and the optimal solutions to problems (3) and (6).

17. Modify the knapsack problem of Exercise 10 as follows. The trip to Mars will not be worthwhile unless the total scientific value of all items carried along is at least a certain minimum amount M. The idea is to choose equipment to take along whose total scientific value is at least M, while minimizing the weight.
    (a) Formulate this as a linear programming problem. (This problem is also called the *knapsack problem*.)
    (b) Discuss the relation between this problem and (4a).
    (c) Find an optimal solution to this problem if the weights, scientific values, and M are as in Exercise 10. Compare a greedy solution.

18. Consider the problem of optimizing net output per unit time. Each process has an input I_i, an output O_i, and a time T_i. The efficiency of the process would be defined as

$$\frac{O_i - I_i}{T_i},$$

while the efficiency of a set S of processes would be defined as

$$\frac{\sum_{i \in S}(O_i - I_i)}{\sum_{i \in S} T_i}.$$

(a) Formulate the analogue of the GOE problem.
(b) Describe what you would mean by the greedy algorithm and the slightly less greedy algorithm.
(c) Discuss the relation between the greedy solutions (if they exist), the slightly less greedy solutions, and the optimal solutions.

(d) Do the same for the analogue of (6).

(e) Do the same for the analogue of the LOE problem (8) of Exercise 11.

3.3 Proof of the Optimality of Greedy Solutions of the GOE Problem[3]

We shall prove that if a greedy solution to the GOE problem (3) is feasible, it is also optimal. The proof will be by induction on the number of processes in S. We require the following two lemmas.

Lemma 1. *Suppose* $a_i > 0$, $b_i > 0$, *and* $a_i/b_i \geq x$ *for* $i = 1, 2, \cdots, p$. *Then*

$$\frac{\sum_{i=1}^{p} a_i}{\sum_{i=1}^{p} b_i} \geq x.$$

PROOF. We have $a_i \geq b_i x$ for all i. Thus

$$\frac{\sum a_i}{\sum b_i} = \frac{a_1 + a_2 + \cdots + a_p}{b_1 + b_2 + \cdots + b_p}$$

$$\geq \frac{b_1 x + b_2 x + \cdots + b_p x}{b_1 + b_2 + \cdots + b_p}$$

$$= x. \qquad \square$$

Lemma 2. *Suppose* $c_i > 0$, $d_i > 0$, *and* $c_i/d_i \leq x$ *for* $i = 1, 2, \cdots, r$. *Then*

$$\frac{\sum_{i=1}^{r} c_i}{\sum_{i=1}^{r} d_i} \leq x.$$

PROOF. Similar. $\qquad \square$

Suppose S is a feasible greedy solution to the GOE problem. We are assuming that S is feasible. Suppose T is any other feasible solution. Let (a_1, b_1) be (O, I) for the first element of S (i.e., for which O/I is maximal), let (a_2, b_2) be (O, I) for the second element of S, and so on up until (a_p, b_p) is (O, I) for the last element of S. Thus

$$\frac{a_1}{b_1} \geq \frac{a_2}{b_2} \geq \cdots \geq \frac{a_p}{b_p}. \tag{9}$$

---

[3] This section may be omitted without loss of continuity.

Let the (O, I) pairs from processes in T be denoted as $(c_1, d_1), (c_2, d_2), \cdots,$ (c_r, d_r), with

$$\frac{c_1}{d_1} \geq \frac{c_2}{d_2} \geq \cdots \geq \frac{c_r}{d_r}. \tag{10}$$

(Note that r may or may not be equal to p.) We wish to prove that

$$\frac{\sum\limits_{i=1}^{p} a_i}{\sum\limits_{i=1}^{p} b_i} \geq \frac{\sum\limits_{j=1}^{r} c_j}{\sum\limits_{j=1}^{r} d_j}. \tag{11}$$

Suppose S has just one process, i.e., $p = 1$. Then

$$\frac{a_1}{b_1} \geq \frac{c_j}{d_j}, \quad \text{all } j,$$

for otherwise S would not be a greedy solution. By Lemma 2 with $x = a_1/b_1$, (11) follows. This proves the theorem for solutions S with one process.

Let us now assume the theorem is true if S has less than p processes and show it for S of p processes. We consider two cases:

Case 1 $\dfrac{a_p}{b_p} \geq \dfrac{c_1}{d_1}$

Case 2 $\dfrac{c_1}{d_1} > \dfrac{a_p}{b_p}.$

Case 1. In this case, by (9), $a_i/b_i \geq c_1/d_1$ for all i, and so by Lemma 1,

$$\frac{\sum\limits_{i=1}^{p} a_i}{\sum\limits_{i=1}^{p} b_i} \geq \frac{c_1}{d_1}.$$

Therefore, by (10),

$$\frac{\sum\limits_{i=1}^{p} a_i}{\sum\limits_{i=1}^{p} b_i} \geq \frac{c_j}{d_j}, \text{ all } j.$$

If we let $x = \Sigma a_i/\Sigma b_i$, Lemma 2 implies that

$$\frac{\sum\limits_{i=1}^{p} a_i}{\sum\limits_{i=1}^{p} b_i} \geq \frac{\sum\limits_{j=1}^{r} c_j}{\sum\limits_{j=1}^{r} d_j},$$

as desired.

Case 2. We know that $c_1/d_1 > a_p/b_p$. If u is the process with output–input pair (c_1, d_1), then u is in S. Otherwise we could have chosen u over the process with pair (a_p, b_p). Thus set S would not be a greedy solution. Hence for some k, u has output–input pair (a_k, b_k) and $a_k = c_1$ and $b_k = d_1$. Let S' consist of all processes in S except u and T' of all processes in T except u. Then it is easy to show that S' is a feasible greedy solution to the new GOE problem obtained by removing the process u from the list of possible processes, and reducing M by the appropriate amount a_k. Similarly, T' is a feasible solution to this GOE problem. By inductive assumption applied to S' and T', we have

$$\frac{\sum_{i \neq k} a_i}{\sum_{i \neq k} b_i} \geq \frac{\sum_{j \neq 1} c_j}{\sum_{j \neq 1} d_j}. \tag{12}$$

Now since S' and T' are both feasible solutions to the same GOE problem,

$$\sum_{i \neq k} a_i = \sum_{j \neq 1} c_j.$$

Hence (12) implies that

$$\sum_{i \neq k} b_i \leq \sum_{j \neq 1} d_j.$$

Finally, since $a_k = c_1$ and $b_k - d_1$, we have

$$\sum_i a_i = \sum_j c_j \tag{13}$$

and

$$\sum_i b_i \leq \sum_j d_j. \tag{14}$$

Equations (13) and (14) together give us (11), which completes the proof.

EXERCISES

19. Prove Lemma 2.

20. Show that, in general, it is possible to have

$$\frac{\sum_{i=2}^{p} a_i}{\sum_{i=2}^{p} b_i} \geq \frac{\sum_{j=2}^{r} c_j}{\sum_{j=2}^{r} d_j},$$

$$a_1 = c_1,$$

$$b_1 = d_1,$$

and

$$\frac{\sum_{i=1}^{p} a_i}{\sum_{i=1}^{p} b_i} < \frac{\sum_{j=1}^{r} c_j}{\sum_{j=1}^{r} d_j}.$$

(Thus the obvious method of proof fails.)

4. Human Energy Use for Food

4.1 Total Energy Accounting[4]

As we pointed out in the Introduction, while animals might be very efficient users of energy in the process of obtaining food, human beings, at least modern human beings, tend not to be. In this section, we shall try to determine just how efficient modern agriculture is and discuss strategies for providing enough food for the world's billions, given limitations on energy available for the production of food.

Heichel [12] defines the business of agriculture as collecting and storing solar energy as food energy in plant and animal products. Very primitive agriculture used only human energy as an input in producing food. Humans derived all of their energy from food. Hence it was incumbent upon them to be as efficient as possible in an energetic sense. Their *energetic efficiency*, defined as

$$e = \frac{\text{energy obtained from food}}{\text{human energy used in obtaining or raising food}}, \qquad (15)$$

had to be at least one, and indeed had to be quite a bit larger than one for there to be enough energy left over to grow, build shelter, fight off enemies, etc. Gradually, man found that he could use foraging animals to replace some of his work in raising food. At this point, his energetic efficiency e of (15) increased: he raised the same or a greater amount of food with less of his own energy. Much later on, when man began to use fossil-fuel-powered machines to help him with his agriculture, his energetic efficiency e increased even further. The same thing happened when man began using chemical fertilizers and extensive irrigation to increase food yields and decrease time spent raising food. The additional fuel invested through animals, chemicals, machines to plow or irrigate, etc., is called by Heichel [12] *auxiliary* or *cultural energy*. With an increasing awareness that many forms of cultural energy are scarce has come the realization that calculating the efficiency of agriculture by means of the formula (15) does not tell the whole story. If we want to know how efficiently we use energy in obtaining food, we probably should use the formula

$$e = \frac{\text{energy obtained from food}}{\text{total energy used in obtaining or raising food}}. \qquad (16)$$

The attempt to measure e of Equation (16) is called *total energy accounting*. Let us briefly investigate how one might obtain a total energy accounting for agriculture.[5]

---

[4] This subsection borrows heavily from the papers by Hayes [11], Heichel [12], Hirst [13], Pimentel *et al.* [29], Pimentel *et al.* [30], Pimentel *et al.* [31], and Rapoport [33].

[5] Total energy accounting is sometimes called *net energy analysis*, and there is a rather extensive recent literature on this subject. Some comprehensive references are Bullard *et al.* [3], Connolly and Spraul [7], Leach [18], and Roberts [37].

Table 8. Inputs into U.S. Corn Production for Selected Years on an Average Hectare Corn Field[†]

Inputs (units)	1945	1950	1954	1959	1964	1970
Labor (hours)	57	44	42	35	27	22
Machinery (kcal)	444,600	617,500	741,000	864,500	1,037,400	1,037,400
Fuel (liters)	140	159	178	187	197	206
Nitrogen (kg)	8	17	30	46	65	125
Phosphorus (kg)	8	11	13	18	20	35
Potassium (kg)	6	11	20	34	46	67
Seeds for planting (kg)	11	13	16	19	21	21
Irrigation (kcal)	103,740	128,440	148,200	170,430	187,720	187,720
Insecticides (kg)	0	0.11	0.34	0.78	1.12	1.12
Herbicides (kg)	0	0.06	0.11	0.28	0.43	1.12
Drying (kcal)	9,880	34,580	74,100	163,020	247,000	296,400
Electricity (kcal)	79,040	133,380	247,000	345,800	501,410	765,700
Transportation (kcal)	49,400	74,100	111,150	148,200	172,900	172,900
Corn yield (kg/ha)	2,132	2,383	2,572	3,387	4,265	5,080

[†] Source: Pimentel et al. [30], data revised from Pimentel et al. [29]. Reprinted with permission of Center for Environmental Quality Management, Cornell University.

Pimentel et al. [29] do a total energy accounting for corn production in the United States during various years from 1945 through 1970. They begin by considering the various inputs into corn production. Their data on these inputs were revised and published in Pimentel et al. [30] and are shown in Table 8. (Obtaining such a total energy accounting is rather difficult. For example, it is necessary to estimate how much energy is used in transporting machinery and supplies to corn fields, how much energy is used in irrigation, etc.)[6]

The data in Table 8 is rather revealing. For example, it shows that the labor input per hectare (1 hectare = about 2.5 acres, 1 acre = about 0.4 hectares) decreased more than 60% between 1945 and 1970. At the same time, yields of corn increased from 2132 kg per hectare to about 5080. In terms of bushels, this is an increase from about 85 bushels per hectare in 1945 to about 203 in 1970. Combining the yield and labor figures, one determines that the average farmer spent 40 minutes to produce one bushel of corn in 1945, and 6 1/2 minutes to produce one bushel in 1970, a dramatic reduction.

Still looking at Table 8, we see that fuel consumption for all machinery rose from 140 liters (37 gallons) per hectare in 1945 to about 206 liters (53 gallons) in 1970. The use of nitrogen fertilizer has gone up much more

[6] The study by Pimentel et al. has been criticized by a number of authors for various reasons, for instance for neglecting technological improvements in fertilizer and machinery production and in cultivation, counting some nonagricultural energy uses such as fuels for farm families' automobiles, and double counting electricity (including it separately and in its primary use in irrigation). Smil et al. [39] have recently attempted to rectify the shortcomings in the Pimentel et al. study and also to demonstrate the difficulties and fuzziness inherent in such energy analyses.

dramatically, from 8 kg (about 18 pounds) of nitrogen per hectare in 1945 to about 125 kg (about 280 pounds) in 1970.

For us to be able to make much use of the data in Table 8 each of the entries has to be translated into a common unit. The natural unit to choose is the kcal. Translating all of the figures in Table 8 into kcals involves some difficult decisions. For example, one pound of nitrogen is estimated to be equivalent to 8400 kcal if production and processing of nitrogen fertilizer is included. Similar considerations enter into the translation of man-hours into kcals, use of herbicides into kcals, etc. Some of the decisions are very difficult. For example, if animals are used, does one use as an energy equivalent the food they eat while on the cropland, the food they eat during the whole growing season, or the food they eat all year? In any case, Pimentel *et al.* [29] have tried to translate the data of Table 8 into kcal units. The result, updated and reprinted in Pimentel *et al.* [30], is shown as Table 9. We see from Table 9 that in 1945, one hectare used for corn produced 7,504,640 kcal, with an input of 2,314,442 kcal, for an energetic efficiency (16) of 3.24. By 1970, the yield had increased dramatically to 17,881,600 kcal per hectare. However, the energy input had also increased dramatically to 7,104,612 kcal, for an energetic efficiency of 2.52, less than the 1945 efficiency.

By way of contrast, Table 10 shows the energy inputs in corn production in Mexico using only manpower. The energetic efficiency is 10.13.

Table 11 shows the yields and energetic efficiencies for a variety of crops under different agricultural processes. In corn produced in Mexico with oxen, for example, the energetic efficiency goes down to 3.38, compared to

Table 9. Energy Inputs into U.S. Corn Production per Hectare in Selected Years in kcal[†]

Inputs	1945	1950	1954	1959	1964	1970
Labor	31,022	23,947	22,859	19,049	14,695	11,974
Machinery	444,600	617,500	741,000	864,500	1,037,400	1,037,400
Fuel	1,339,800	1,521,630	1,703,460	1,789,590	1,885,290	1,971,420
Nitrogen	140,800	299,200	528,000	809,600	1,144,000	2,200,000
Phosphorus	25,520	35,090	41,470	57,420	63,800	111,650
Potassium	13,200	24,200	44,000	74,800	101,200	147,400
Seeds for planting	77,440	91,520	112,640	133,760	147,840	147,840
Irrigation	103,740	128,440	148,200	170,430	187,720	187,720
Insecticides	0	2,662	8,228	18,876	27,104	27,104
Herbicides	0	1,452	2,662	6,776	10,406	27,104
Drying	9,880	34,580	74,100	163,020	247,000	296,400
Electricity	79,040	133,380	247,000	345,800	501,410	765,700
Transportation	49,400	74,100	111,150	148,200	172,900	172,900
Total inputs	2,314,442	2,987,701	3,784,769	4,601,821	5,540,765	7,104,612
Corn yield	7,504,640	8,388,160	9,053,440	11,922,240	15,012,800	17,881,600
kcal return/kcal input	3.24	2.81	2.39	2.59	2.71	2.52

[†] Source: Pimentel *et al.* [30], data revised from Pimentel *et al.* [29]. Reprinted with permission of Center for Environmental Quality Management, Cornell University.

Table 10. Energy Inputs in Corn Production
in Mexico per Hectare per Year Using Only
Manpower[†]

Input	Quantity	Kilocalories
labor	1,144 hrs	622,622
Axe and hoe	16,500 kcal	16,500
Seeds	10.4 kg	36,608
Total		675,730
Corn yield	1,944 kg	6,842,880
kcal return/kcal input		10.13

[†] Source: Pimentel et al. [30]. Data from Lewis [20].
Reprinted with permission of Center for Environmental
Quality Management, Cornell University.

Table 11. Yields and Energetic Efficiencies of Different Crops under
Different Systems of Production

Food	How Produced	Yield (kcal/ha/year)	Energy Input (kcal/ha/year)	Energetic Efficiency (Yield/Input)
Corn[a]	U.S., 1945	7,504,640	2,314,442	3.24
Corn[a]	U.S., 1970	17,881,600	7,104,612	2.52
Corn[a]	Mexico, with manpower	6,842,880	675,730	10.13
Corn[b]	Mexico, with oxen	3,312,320	979,456	3.38
Rice[a]	U.S., present day	21,039,480	15,352,015	1.37
Rice[a]	Phillipines, present day	6,004,020	1,831,298	3.28
Rice[b]	Phillipines, with water buffalo	1,500,000	93,750	16.00
Sugar beets[b]	U.S., present day	250,000	?	less than 1
Yams[c]	Tsembaga Indians, New Guinea, using manpower	1,440,260	87,288	16.5

[a] Pimental et al. [30].
[b] Heichel [12], translated into hectares using 1 ha = 2.5 acres.
[c] Rapoport [33], translated into hectares using 1 ha = 2.5 acres.

an efficiency of 10.13 with manpower alone, and 2.52 in modern U.S.
agriculture. Even more revealing from this data is how the energetic efficiencies of different crops can differ. For example, in modern U.S. agriculture, the energetic efficiency of rice production is a little more than 1,
considerably less than that of corn production. Sugar beets have an energetic
efficiency of less than 1: more calories of energy are spent in producing
sugar beets than are gained from eating them! By way of comparison, rice

Table 12. Summary of Basic Statistics

	Optimistic	Pessimistic
Yearly caloric requirement per person	10^6 kcal	
(Usable) arable land in the world	3.6×10^9 ha	1.6×10^9 ha
Solar energy hitting a typical field per hectare per year	11×10^9 kcal	5×10^9 kcal

production in the Phillipines using just water buffalo is estimated to have an energetic efficiency of about 16. Rapoport [33] estimated the energetic efficiency of yam production by primitive methods by the Tsembaga Indians in New Guinea to be about 16.5.[7] In general, the most primitive forms of agriculture have been the most energetically efficient, by far.

4.2 Applying the Greedy Algorithm

Suppose man were trying to be energetically efficient in his production of food. How would he do it? Let us try to use the methods of Section 3 and formulate man's problem as a global optimum efficiency problem. We will first have to calculate the energy requirements M for mankind. The daily caloric requirement for a moderately active 170 pound man is about 3000 kcal (Kleiber [16], Brown [2]). We will show how this number is arrived at in Section 2.3 of the next chapter of this volume. Less active or lighter people can get away with fewer calories, while more active or larger ones need more.[8] A daily requirement of 3000 kcal translates into a yearly requirement of about 1.1×10^6 kcal. Let us, for the sake of discussion, use the number 10^6 or one million as the yearly caloric requirement (in kcal) per human being. We shall begin to tabulate such information in Table 12 for later reference. For a population of p persons, the yearly caloric requirements are $p \times 10^6$ kcal. These are the energy requirements M for the GOE problem.

To attain M kcal of food energy, we need to choose a crop and method of production for each acre or hectare of available land. Suppose we use the greedy algorithm, and choose for each hectare the most efficient crop and method of production suitable to it. For the sake of discussion, suppose we limit ourselves to the crops and processes of Table 11, and assume that their yields and efficiencies are independent of the nature of the land— a big oversimplification. Then the greedy algorithm would say to grow yams in the Tsembaga fashion or perhaps rice in the primitive Phillipines fashion,

[7] Some foods can be grown with even higher efficiencies in especially appropriate areas. For example, cassavas can be grown, with nonmachine and nonanimal methods, at an efficiency as high as 37.5 in the Congo Leopoldville region (Pimentel et al. [30, p. 29]).

[8] At present, at least 50% of the world's population eats under 2250 kcal per day, barely enough to sustain life (Brown [2], U.N. Food and Agriculture Organization [40]).

with just water buffalo, on each hectare. Either method would, according to Table 11, yield about 1.5×10^6 kcal per hectare per year. Would this algorithm lead to a "solution" of the GOE problem, if it is required that we feed p people and hence attain $M = p \times 10^6$ kcal of food energy? To see, we shall have to calculate how many hectares of arable land are available for planting crops. There are about 36×10^9 acres of land on the planet Earth. Of this, only about one quarter, or 9×10^9 acres, or 3.6×10^9 hectares, are good or fair for agricultural production (Brown [2, pp. 130–131]). The President's Science Advisory Panel on the World Food Supply [32] estimates 3.2×10^9 hectares. Approximately half that land, the richest and most accessible part, is cultivated today (Meadows et al. [23]). This is nearly all of the reasonable arable land (Pimentel et al. [30, p. 1]). Prime agricultural land is being converted into urban use very rapidly. Thus a more pessimistic estimate of the usable arable land is 1.6×10^9 hectares. At 1.5×10^6 kcal per hectare per year, we could expect a total production of $(3.6 \times 10^9) \times (1.5 \times 10^6) = 5.4 \times 10^{15}$ kcal per year, if all arable land is used for agriculture, including marginal land. Since 10^6 kcal per year are required per person (Table 12), this yield would feed a total of

$$\frac{5.4 \times 10^{15}}{10^6} = 5.4 \times 10^9 \text{ people,}$$

or about 5.4 billion people, assuming the world's food is divided up equally. This is more than the current world population, but less than the world population of seven billion projected for the year 2000 (National Academy of Sciences [26]). In short, for the current requirement M, the greedy solution would provide more than enough yield or productivity, but for the year 2000 requirement M, it would not. We have made strong assumptions: 1) that the yields of the greedy solution processes (yams or rice using water buffalo) would be as high everywhere as they are on the most favorable land; 2) that the most optimistic estimate for the amount of arable land is used and that all arable land is cultivated; 3) that food is divided up equally. Thus we might even wonder if this sort of agriculture could really feed all of today's population. In short, using the greedy algorithm may not lead to a solution of the global optimum efficiency problem, because it may not lead to enough food production.

To obtain a solution to the GOE problem under these conditions, we will need to use methods of linear programming. To illustrate how this might work, let us suppose, for simplicity, that we wish to meet the caloric requirements of feeding 10 billion people with just rice, and suppose we limit our selection to two of the methods of rice production described in Table 11: (1) modern Phillipines and (2) Phillipines using water buffalo. Let h_i be the number of hectares where rice is grown using method (i). Assuming that all arable land is available, we have

$$h_1 + h_2 \le 3.6 \times 10^9, \tag{17}$$

the number of arable hectares in the world (Table 12). The total food yield would be approximately, using Table 11,

$$O = (6 \times 10^6)h_1 + (1.5 \times 10^6)h_2 \text{ kcal} \tag{18}$$

and the total energy input would be approximately

$$I = (1.8 \times 10^6)h_1 + (9 \times 10^4)h_2 \text{ kcal.} \tag{19}$$

We require that O feed a population of 10 billion people, which has a caloric requirement (using Table 12) of

$$10^{10} \times 10^6 = 10^{16} \text{ kcal.}$$

Thus we require that

$$(6 \times 10^6)h_1 + (1.5 \times 10^6)h_2 = 10^{16}, \tag{20}$$

again assuming that the world's food can be split up equally. Our problem boils down to minimizing I of (19) subject to the restrictions (17) and (20) and, of course, the restrictions that

$$h_1 \geq 0, \qquad h_2 \geq 0, \qquad h_1, h_2 \text{ integers.}$$

The solution to the problem is easily obtained using graphical techniques. The solution is

$$h_1 \approx 1 \times 10^9 \text{ ha.}$$

$$h_2 \approx 2.6 \times 10^9 \text{ ha.}$$

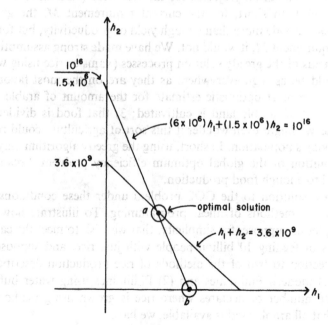

Figure 10.1. The Feasible Region Consists of the Line Segment from a to b.

(The reader should check this solution; Figure 10.1 might help here.) According to this solution, much of the land would be cultivated using water buffalo agriculture, and the rest by modern Phillipine agriculture.

It is interesting to note that the solution will be the same if we formulate our problem as an input minimization problem (Problem (4a) of Section 3). Here, we require (17) holds but modify (20) to read

$$(6 \times 10^6)h_1 + (1.5 \times 10^6)h_2 \geq 10^{16}. \tag{21}$$

We still wish to minimize I of (19). The reader can easily check graphically why the solution to this problem is the same as before.

The reader should see by now, at least in principle, how he might solve similar problems of a more realistic nature. With each hectare of land, for each possible crop and each possible agricultural method, would be information about corresponding energy inputs and yields. One of the possibilities could be not to use that hectare at all. However, for simplicity, one would assume that it could be used with no more than one crop and no more than one method of production, i.e., that it could not be split up further. The problem of meeting food production requirements with a minimum of energy use could be reduced to a large linear programming problem. The practical problem would be harder than the mathematical one: how would the world ever get together to agree on implementing the solution to this linear programming problem?

4.3 Alternative Strategies

The GOE problem has so far been attacked with the assumption that a fixed set of alternative processes are given from which to choose. We can think of modifying the process set to make it lead to a more energy-efficient solution. Hayes [11], Heichel [12], Hirst [13], Pimentel et al. [29], Pimentel et al. [30], and Pimentel et al. [31] all talk about possible strategies for replacing existing agricultural processes with less energy-intensive ones, i.e., ones using less energy but producing comparable yields. Some of the possible strategies are the following:

(1) Increase the use of human labor.
(2) Use more horses and mules.
(3) Use livestock manure as fertilizer.
(4) Plant legumes like sweet clover ("green manure") in rotation with crops like corn, in order to replace some fertilizers.
(5) Change dietary habits to favor more energy-efficient foods.
(6) Use crop residues or animal wastes as fuel.
(7) Introduce additional fertilizer and other high-energy inputs into production where they have the highest possible impact in yield.

Table 13. Energy Use in the U.S. Food System[†]

Activity	Percent of Total Use
Food processing	33
Household storage and preparation	30
Agriculture	18
Wholesale and retail trade	16
Transportation	3

[†] Source: Hirst [13].

We shall discuss alternatives (5) and (7) in the following subsections. Other possible strategies involve looking at energy use in the whole of the food system. For example, Hirst [13] estimates that agriculture uses only 18% of the energy used in the U.S. food system. Table 13 gives percentages for the other uses of energy in the U.S. food system. Wholesaling and retailing food uses almost as much energy as agriculture, while food processing uses much more and storage and preparation of food in households uses almost as much as food processing. Thus, for example, there are significant energy savings possible by making retail stores more energy-conscious, by decreasing our dependence on processed foods such as TV dinners, and by using refrigerators with better insulation.

4.3.1 *Changing Diets.* An individual animal or plant must be energetically efficient in the sense that the ratio of energy obtained to energy expended must be at least one. If, for a period of time, this is not the case, then the animal will not be able to survive. In contrast, one can look at animals or plants or even whole ecosystems as "producers" of energy. They take in a certain amount of energy (radiant energy from the sun in the case of plants, chemical energy in the case of animals), and they pass on a certain amount of energy to the animals which eat them. One can think of an animal's or plant's or ecosystem's efficiency as a producer as a ratio:

$$L = \frac{\text{energy yielded when eaten}}{\text{energy obtained when eating (or from the sun}^9)}. \tag{22}$$

This efficiency is sometimes called the *Lindeman efficiency* after the pioneering work of Lindeman [21], who tried to measure this efficiency for various ecosystems. The Lindeman efficiencies are of course less than one. Some of the energy obtained when eating is used for activities such as feeding, for respiration, for defending or patrolling territory, and so on. Some of it is wasted. Only a percentage of the energy obtained by a lower animal or plant in eating is passed along to higher animals who happen to eat it. Experiments have shown that on the average only about 10% of that energy is passed along. Thus the Lindeman efficiencies L are about 0.1.

[9] In the case of plants.

(They vary from about 0.05 to about 0.2 or more.) For example, let us use a typical food chain as described by Lamont Cole (Hayes [11]), with the 10% rule of thumb for L. Of 1000 calories (kcal) in algae in a lake, small aquatic animals can obtain about 100 calories. Smelt, eating these animals, obtain about 10 calories. If a man eats the smelt, he gets about one calorie. If he waits for a trout to eat the smelt and then eats the trout, he gets about 0.1 calories. This great inefficiency in transferring food energy up a food chain explains why most food chains in nature are no more than five steps long, starting with a plant which receives energy from the sun. (For a more detailed discussion of this point, see Phillipson [28, p. 10], Odum [27, p. 40], or Wilson and Bossert [44, pp. 150–151], who argue that no animals prey on tigers, not because the tigers are so formidable, but because they produce too few calories to make the effort worthwhile!)

Humans stand at the end of food chains. These food chains have been getting longer over the years. Indeed, as Hayes [11] points out, per capita intake of beef in the U.S. has more than doubled in recent decades, and cattle are high on a food chain themselves. Thus the efficiency with which humans obtain food energy has decreased. If people were to change their eating habits and get their calories from lower on food chains, energy would be obtained much more efficiently. For example, Table 14 shows the percentage l of the sun's energy reaching a field which is obtainable through consumption of a given type of food, if the field is used exclusively to produce that kind of food (by perhaps first producing food that food eats, etc.). The number l can be thought of as 100 times the Lindeman efficiency L of the crop relative to the initial solar energy input. The solar energy hitting a typical field in California in one year is about 11×10^9 kcal per hectare (Kleiber [16, p. 341]). This is very high for many parts of the world, but we shall use it to make some simple calculations. The figure 11×10^9 dis-

Table 14. Efficiency of Different Foods in Passing on Solar Energy[†]

Food	Percent of Sun's Energy Obtainable (l)	Number of People Who Could Be Fed on One Hectare in One Year, Using Solar Radiation of 11×10^9 kcal.
1. Potatoes	0.1	11
2. Grain	0.05	5.5
3. Prunes	0.04	4.4
4. Milk	0.04	4.4
5. Pork	0.015	1.65
6. Eggs	0.002	0.22
7. Algae	50.0	5500

† Source: Values of l from Kleiber [16, p. 341]. Values assume pre-1961 style agriculture and do not take into account cultural energy used in producing the food.

regards the fact that a given hectare of land is not used for growing all year long. Pimentel *et al.* [29] estimate that during the growing season for corn, about 2×10^9 kcal reaches one average acre of land, or about 5×10^9 kcal reaches one average hectare. This more pessimistic number is less than half the first estimate.

We have assumed (Table 12) that one person requires 10^6 kcal of food energy per year. Using potatoes, we would obtain, according to Table 14, about 0.10% of the solar energy hitting a given hectare in a year, or about

$$10^{-3} \times 11 \times 10^9 = 11 \times 10^6 \text{ kcal/year.}$$

We would have enough energy with one hectare to feed about 11 people. By Table 12 there are about 3.6×10^9 arable hectares in the world. Thus feeding everyone on potatoes, and assuming the same *l* for all available land, and as usual assuming that food would be split up equally, we could feed a world population of

$$11 \times 3.6 \times 10^9 \approx 40 \text{ billion people.}$$

If we used the more pessimistic estimates of arable land and solar energy available, we would obtain a less optimistic population estimate:

5×10^9 kcal solar energy,
5×10^6 kcal per hectare from potatoes,
1 hectare feeds 5 people,
1.6×10^9 arable hectares,
$5 \times 1.6 \times 10^9 = 8 \times 10^9 = 8$ billion people.

By way of contrast, using eggs, we would obtain in one year 0.002% of the total energy reaching one hectare, or, using the higher solar energy estimate,

$$2 \times 10^{-5} \times 11 \times 10^9 = 22 \times 10^4 \text{ kcal.}$$

Thus we would be able to feed only about

$$\frac{22 \times 10^4}{10^6} = 22 \times 10^{-2} = 0.22 \text{ people per hectare.}$$

We would need almost five hectares just to feed one person. We can feed 50 times the number of people on one hectare using potatoes that we can using eggs. Using only eggs, even under the optimistic assumptions, we could support a world population of only

$$0.22 \times 3.6 \times 10^9 \approx 800 \text{ million people,}$$

considerably less than the present world population. Clearly, given the limitations of available land and energy, and hence yields, diets will have to be modified to become more energy-efficient. (An alternative is to control population growth.) It should also be clear from these considerations why most of the world's population eats mostly grains.

Miller [24, pp. 292 ff] includes a similar discussion in which he points out that, as the world's population increases, the amount of meat which can be eaten must decrease. We may even have to go to the bottom of the food chain, says Miller, and eat "algae-burgers."

Unfortunately, as Miller also points out, simply feeding people algae or indeed just feeding them rice or potatoes will not prevent starvation. Most starvation is caused not by a lack of calories, but by a lack of proteins, resulting in malnutrition and disease. The plant crops that contain the most calories generally contain the least protein. Also, crops of just one species do not contain all of the proteins needed for good health. Thus we want not only to achieve a minimum caloric yield, but also to make sure that each person has a certain minimum amount of such protein-rich foods as milk, eggs, and pork. (Some food scientists feel that a mix of grains will provide sufficient proteins (Pimentel et al. [31, p. 15], Brown [2]).)

Suppose for the sake of discussion that the possible list of foods we can use is limited to those in Table 14 except algae. Suppose we want to have at least a_i kg of food i per person per year in order to have a sufficient protein content in their diets. This would correspond to some number b_i of kcal of food i per year. With b_i as a minimum amount of food i per person, what mix of foods would support the largest number of people, and how many people could be supported in this way?

To answer this question, let us suppose that p people are supported by using h_i hectares for food i ($i = 1, 2, \cdots, 6$). The number of kcal produced per hectare per year using food i is

$$\alpha_i = l_i \times 10^{-2} \times 11 \times 10^9 = 11 l_i \times 10^7 \text{ kcal}, \tag{23}$$

where l_i is the percentage efficiency shown in the second column of Table 14 and 11×10^9 is the solar energy getting through to one hectare of land per year (Table 12). Thus we have (as a variant of the GOE problem) the following requirements:

$$\sum_{i=1}^{6} \alpha_i h_i = p \times 10^6 \tag{24}$$

$$\alpha_i h_i \geq b_i p, \qquad i = 1, 2, \cdots, 6 \tag{25}$$

$$\sum_{i=1}^{6} h_i \leq 3.6 \times 10^9. \tag{26}$$

Constraint (24) says that p people can be supported with a requirement of 10^6 kcal per person per year. Constraint (25) says that enough food of type i is produced so that each person has at least b_i kcal of food i. Constraint (26) says that the total number of hectares used is at most the number of arable hectares in the world. We wish to know how to maximize p subject to the constraints (24)–(26). This is a linear programming problem which involves seven variables, $h_1, h_2, \cdots, h_6$, and p. It is readily reduced to an easier problem as follows. Using as little land as possible for the less efficient foods will only increase the total caloric yield. Thus the optimal solution will involve using only the minimum amount of land for all foods but potatoes. It follows that we may set $\alpha_i h_i = b_i p$ for $i = 2, 3, \cdots, 6$, and hence we have

$$h_i = \frac{b_i}{\alpha_i} p, \qquad i = 2, 3, \cdots, 6. \tag{27}$$

Substituting into (24) and (26), we obtain

$$\alpha_1 h_1 + \sum_{i=2}^{6} b_i p = p \times 10^6 \tag{28}$$

$$h_1 + \sum_{i=2}^{6} \frac{b_i}{\alpha_i} p \leqq 3.6 \times 10^9. \tag{29}$$

Equation (28) gives

$$h_1 = \frac{p \left[10^6 - \sum_{i=2}^{6} b_i \right]}{\alpha_1}. \tag{30}$$

Substituting this value of h_1 into inequality (29) gives the inequality

$$\frac{p \left[10^6 - \sum_{i=2}^{6} b_i \right]}{\alpha_1} + p \sum_{i=2}^{6} \frac{b_i}{\alpha_i} \leqq 3.6 \times 10^9$$

or

$$p \leqq \frac{3.6 \times 10^9}{\left[\dfrac{10^6 - \sum_{i=2}^{6} b_i}{\alpha_1} + \sum_{i=2}^{6} \dfrac{b_i}{\alpha_i} \right]}. \tag{31}$$

The value on the right-hand side of Equation (31) is the maximum value of p, provided there is a feasible solution. The proper values of $h_1, h_2, \cdots, h_6$ can be obtained from this value of p by using Equations (30) and (27).

Let us give an example. Suppose we require that humans obtain at least 10% of their caloric requirements from milk, but otherwise are allowed to be fed totally on potatoes.[10] Then the maximum world population which could be fed is determined as follows. First, $b_4 = 0.1 \times 10^6 = 10^5$, since 10^6 are the total caloric requirements for a given person. The number $b_i = 0$ otherwise. Second, by (23) and Table 14, $\alpha_1 = 1.1 \times 10^7$ and $\alpha_4 = 0.44 \times 10^7 = 4.4 \times 10^6$. Thus, using the number on the right-hand side of (31) as the value of the maximum p, we find

[10] The number 10% is a reasonable number to use, since the daily protein requirement is estimated to be around 70 grams, or the equivalent of 300–400 calories out of the daily 2800 to 3000 calories needed. The requirement is higher if the protein is not at least half of animal origin. (Brown [2, pp. 109, 111], U.N. Food and Agriculture Organization [40]).

$$p = \frac{3.6 \times 10^9}{\left[\dfrac{10^6 - 10^5}{1.1 \times 10^7} + \dfrac{10^5}{4.4 \times 10^6}\right]} \tag{32}$$

$$\approx 34.4 \times 10^9 = 34.4 \text{ billion people.}$$

This is less than the 40 billion people we calculated above could be supported if everyone ate only potatoes, but it is considerably more than the present world population or even that projected for the year 2000. If we used the less optimistic estimates of arable land and solar energy available from Table 12, we would get a maximum population estimate of about one quarter this number. (The reader is asked to check this.) Under the solution (32), the number of hectares which would have to be devoted to milk production would be, by (27),

$$h_4 = \frac{b_4}{\alpha_4} p$$

$$= \frac{10^5}{4.4 \times 10^6} \times 34.4 \times 10^9$$

$$\approx 7.8 \times 10^8.$$

The number of hectares devoted to potato production would be less, namely (by (30)),

$$h_1 = \frac{[34.4 \times 10^9][10^6 - 10^5]}{1.1 \times 10^7}$$

$$= 2.81 \times 10^9.$$

(The numbers h_1 and h_4 do not add up exactly to 3.6×10^9 because of round off error in the computations.)

4.3.2 *Where To Use a Limited Amount of Fertilizer.* Given a limited amount of nitrogen fertilizer, where should it best be used to produce maximal yields of food? To answer this question, one needs to have a model which relates various outputs of production to various inputs. Munson and Doll [25] have studied the yield of corn under various nitrogen inputs in fertilizer. They let other inputs into corn production stay at fixed levels and raised the nitrogen level. The results of their experiment are shown in Figure 10.2, in the dashed lines. Note that yields of corn with all other inputs fixed increased with the addition of more nitrogen, up to a point, 246 kg of nitrogen added per hectare per year. After that, the yields started going down with increased use of nitrogen. (The 1970 average U.S. input of nitrogen (Table 8) is 125 kg.) More interesting is that, as can be observed from the solid lines of Figure 10.2, the ratio of kcal of yield to kcal of nitrogen input starts decreasing with inputs of about 135 kg of nitrogen per hectare per year (or slightly more than the 1970 level). Adding 45 kg of nitrogen per hectare if no nitrogen had previously been used increased yield from 2132 to 3638 kg/ha, but adding

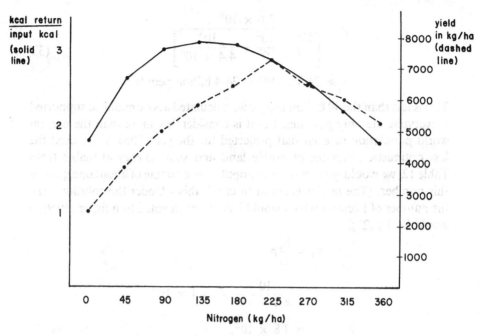

Figure 10.2. Corn Yields with Varying Inputs of Nitrogen. Source: Munson and Doll [25], as Reproduced in Pimentel *et al.* [30]. Reprinted with Permission of Center for Environmental Quality Management, Cornell University.

45 kg of nitrogen per year to a field already receiving 179 kg yielded only a tiny increase, from 6147 to 6335 kg/ha/year. Thus, adding fertilizer to fields receiving little fertilizer would have a significantly greater impact on yield than continuing to add fertilizer to already highly and perhaps over-fertilized fields.[11] It should not be hard to build a mathematical model which would help a "world agricultural agency" decide where to use a fixed supply of nitrogen fertilizer in order to give maximum food yield. We suggest that this would make a good project. Similar analysis could be made for other inputs. However, there are some dangers which are disregarded in these considerations. With inputs such as pesticides, the output per input can be dependent on how much of that input has been used in the past. For example, larger and larger quantities of pesticide often have to be added to maintain yields, once a pesticide program has been started.

4.4 The Problem of Food and Energy in Perspective

Even in the United States, where use of energy in food production is very high, the energy used in producing food is a small percentage of total national energy use. Various authors (Hayes [11], Heichel [12], Hirst [13],

[11] As Commoner [5, Ch. 5, pp. 149–151] points out, the reason more fertilizer does not result in as much more growth is that plants have a certain limited capacity to grow. Not as much of the added fertilizer is taken up by the plants, and this can result in serious pollution of water supplies, rivers, and lakes, from fertilizer runoff.

Pimentel *et al.* [31]) estimate this as 3–5% of the total U.S. energy use—maybe 12% if all aspects of the food system are included, aspects such as transportation, processing, retailing, and household storage and preparation (see Table 13). Thus, if just a small saving were made on other uses of energy in the U.S., there would be a relatively abundant energy supply for food production. In the U.S. then, at current projected levels of energy availability, food production would not suffer much from scarcity of energy, though it would from increasing price of energy, as that could lead to significantly higher prices for food. On the other hand, it is interesting to ask how much energy would be required if all of the world's billions were fed using U.S.-style agriculture. Then, according to Hayes [11], the amount of energy required for agriculture alone in one year would be almost 80% of all the energy used in one year in the world today! A similar point is made in Pimentel *et al.* [31, p. 5]. We consider a related point in Exercise 27 (to follow). In sum, it would clearly be impossible to bring the entire world up to the level of food energy use found in the United States. With cultural energy and arable lands scarce, and population increasing, something has to give.

EXERCISES

To the reader: Most of these exercises will have different answers, depending on the assumptions you make. State your assumptions explicitly before you start. We suggest that you try at least two sets of assumptions for each, the optimistic and the pessimistic of Table 12.

21. Returning to our discussion of how to feed the world's population using a combination of rice production according to modern Phillipine agriculture and water buffalo agriculture,
    (a) determine how you would allocate the two processes in order to feed five billion people and to solve the GOE problem;
    (b) do the same for a population of 30 billion;
    (c) Repeat (a) for the input minimization problem;
    (d) Repeat (b) for the input minimization problem.

22. (a) Solve the GOE problem for a world of 10 billion people which uses either corn production in the Mexican style with just manpower or corn production in the Mexican style with oxen.
    (b) Solve the input minimization problem in this situation.

23. (a) Solve the GOE problem for a world of 10 billion people which is allowed to use any of the methods of corn production in Table 11.
    (b) Solve the input minimization problem in this situation.

24. What population could be fed using just prunes? (Use the data of Table 14.)

25. What is the largest population which could be fed using grain or pork, if at least 15% of the caloric energy had to be obtained from pork? How much land would be used for each?

26. According to Pimentel *et al.* [29], 5×10^9 kcal per hectare of solar radiation reaches a corn field each year. Using the yields in 1945 and 1970 from Tables 8 and 9, calculate the Lindeman efficiencies of the corn field in those two years, compare to the Lindeman efficiency of grain calculated as 1/100 of the value *l* shown in Table 14, and compare the solar energy input to the "cultural" energy input.

27. (Pimentel *et al.* [29]) An estimated 330 million acres were planted in crops in the U.S. in 1970 (U.S. Department of Agriculture [41], [42]). About 20% of the yield was exported.
   (a) Lowering the number of acres planted by 20% because of export and using a U.S. population of about 200 million, calculate the number of hectares planted per capita (1 hectare $\approx$ 2.5 acres).
   (b) Using Table 8, calculate the number of kcal of energy used per person to feed the U.S. population for one year.
   (c) Using a world population of four billion, calculate the number of kcal of energy required to feed this population for one year using U.S.-style agriculture.
   (d) Using the conversion factor of one gallon of gasoline equals 36,225 kcal (*Handbook of Chemistry and Physics*, Chemical Rubber Company, Cleveland, OH, Table D-230), calculate the number of gallons of gasoline required to feed the world population for one year with U.S.-style agriculture.
   (e) For comparison, the world's known reserves of petroleum are estimated (by Jiler [15]) to be 546 billion barrels of gasoline (31.5 gallons per barrel). How many years would the world supply of petroleum last if everyone were fed using U.S.-style agriculture?

28. Using your answer to Exercise 27(a), how many people could be fed if all of the world's arable land were used to plant corn under U.S.-style agriculture?

29. Compare your answer to Exercise 28 to the number of people who could be fed assuming that corn has a Lindeman efficiency (percentage) as shown in Table 14 for grain.

30. What is the largest population which could be fed if we limited our foods to those in Table 14 (excluding algae) but required that at least 10% of the caloric requirements of each person were met by milk and also at least 5% by eggs?

31. At the end of Section 4.2, we considered a problem equivalent to the GOE problem and a related input minimization problem:

$$\text{minimize} \quad ah_1 + bh_2 \qquad\qquad \text{minimize} \quad ah_1 + bh_2$$
$$\text{subject to} \quad h_1 + h_2 \leq \alpha \qquad\qquad \text{subject to} \quad h_1 + h_2 \leq \alpha$$
$$ch_1 + dh_2 = M \qquad\qquad\qquad ch_1 + dh_2 \geq M.$$

If $b < a$, both of these problems are equivalent to maximizing h_2 subject to the constraints. Assume that and assume that both problems have feasible solutions.
   (a) Show by graphical techniques that if $M/d > \alpha$, then these problems have the same optimal solution.
   (b) Do they necessarily have the same optimal solution if $M/d \leq \alpha$?

32. Develop a theory which would allow you to answer questions of the type we have been answering if food were not split equally among all people of the world.

33. How would our computations change for various years in the future if we assumed that arable land was disappearing at some fixed rate each year?

34. Introduce assumptions about rate of population growth, rate of disappearance of arable land, and perhaps rate of increase of "productivity," and determine for what years population will outgrow food supply.

35. Do the same if a limit is placed on available cultural energy each year.

36. The GOE we have been considering can be looked at in general economic terms as the problem of selecting production activities in the presence of one or more scarce inputs. Develop a formulation of the problem if we consider not just land as a scarce resource, but also one other resource, e.g., labor, machinery, transportation, etc. (Note: As more and more scarce inputs are added, the details of the problem become more complex. Economists have developed various theories for dealing with tradeoffs among scarce resources, which generalize the approach discussed here. An interesting discussion of this general problem can be found in Koopmans [17], and an application is made of these ideas in the model developed by Hudson and Jorgenson [14]. The author thanks William F. Hogan for bringing this general formulation and these references to his attention.)

References

[1] G. Borgstrom, *Harvesting the Earth*. New York: Abelard-Schuman, 1973.
[2] H. Brown, *The Challenge of Man's Future*. New York: Viking, 1958.
[3] C. W. Bullard, P. S. Penner, and D. A. Pilati, "Net energy analysis: Handbook for combining process and input–output analysis," *Resources and Energy*, vol. 1, p. 267, 1978.
[4] P. A. Colinvaux, *Introduction to Ecology*. New York: Wiley, 1973.
[5] B. Commoner, *The Closing Circle*. New York: Knopf, 1971.
[6] ——, *The Poverty of Power* (*Energy and the Economic Crisis*). New York: Knopf, 1976.
[7] T. J. Connolly, and J. R. Spraul, Eds., *Report of the NSF-Stanford Workshop on Net Energy Analysis*, conducted by the Institute for Energy Studies of Stanford University and TRW Systems Group for the National Science Foundation. Stanford, CA, 1975.
[8] J. M. Emlen, "The role of time and energy in food preference," *Amer. Natur.*, vol. 100, pp. 611–617, 1966.
[9] R. S. Garfinkel, and G. L. Nemhauser, *Integer Programming*. New York: Wiley, 1972.
[10] F. R. Hainsworth, and L. L. Wolf, "Power for hovering flight in relation to body size in hummingbirds," *Amer. Natur.*, vol. 106, pp. 589–596, 1972.
[11] D. Hayes, "Energy and food," *Sierra Club Bull.*, vol. 61, pp. 29–31, 1976. (Reprinted from "Energy: The case for conservation," by D. Hayes, Worldwatch Paper 4, Worldwatch Institute, Jan. 1976.)
[12] G. H. Heichel, "Energy needs and food yields," *Tech. Rev.*, pp. 19–25, July–Aug. 1974.
[13] E. Hirst, "Energy for food: From farm to home," *Trans. ASAE*, vol. 17, pp. 323–326, 1974.
[14] E. A. Hudson, and D. W. Jorgenson, "U. S. energy policy and economic growth, 1975–2000," *Bell J. of Economics and Management Science*, vol. 5, pp. 461–514, 1974.
[15] H. Jiler, *Commodity Yearbook*. New York: Commodity Research Bureau, Inc., 1972, pp. 252–253.

[16] M. Kleiber, *The Fire of Life (An Introduction to Animal Energetics)*. New York: Wiley, 1961.

[17] T. C. Koopmans, Ed., *Statistical Inference in Dynamic Economic Models*. New York: Wiley, Cowles Commission, Monograph 10, 1960.

[18] G. Leach, "Net energy analysis—Is it any use?" *Energy Policy*, vol. 3, p. 332, 1975 (special issue of the journal devoted to energy analysis).

[19] A. L. Lehninger, *Bioenergetics*. Menlo Park, CA: W. A. Benjamin, 1973.

[20] O. Lewis, *Life in a Mexican Village: Tepoxtlán Revisited*. Urbana, IL: Univ. of Illinois Press, 1951.

[21] R. L. Lindeman, "The trophic dynamic aspects of ecology," *Ecology*, vol. 23, pp. 399–418, 1942.

[22] M. J. Magazine, G. L. Nemhauser, and L. E. Trotter, "When the greedy solution solves a class of knapsack problems," *Operations Research*, vol. 23, pp. 207–217, 1975.

[23] D. H. Meadows, D. L. Meadows, J. Randers, and W. W. Behrens, III, *The Limits to Growth*. New York: Universe, 1972.

[24] G. T. Miller, *Energetics, Kinetics, and Life: An Ecological Approach*. Belmont, CA: Wadsworth, 1971.

[25] R. D. Munson, and J. P. Doll, "The economics of fertilizer use in crop production," in A. G. Norman, Ed., *Adv. in Agr. XI*, 1959, pp. 133–169.

[26] National Academy of Sciences, *Rapid Population Growth*, vols. I, II. Baltimore, MD: Johns Hopkins Press, 1971.

[27] E. P. Odum, *Ecology*, New York: Holt, Rinehart, and Winston, 1966.

[28] J. Phillipson, *Ecological Energetics*. New York: St. Martin's, 1966.

[29] D. Pimentel, L. E. Hurd, A. C. Bellotti, M. J. Forster, I. N. Oka, O. D. Sholes, and R. J. Whitman, "Food production and the energy crisis." *Science*, vol. 182, pp. 443–449, 1973.

[30] D. Pimentel, W. R. Lynn, W. K. MacReynolds, M. T. Hewes, and S. Rush, "Workshop on research methodologies for studies of energy, food, man and environment, Phase I," Tech. Rep., Cornell Univ. Center for Environmental Quality Management, Ithaca, NY, June 1974.

[31] D. Pimentel, W. R. Lynn, W. K. MacReynolds, and M. Dattner, "Workshop on research methodologies for studies of energy, food, man and environment, Phase II," Tech. Rep., Cornell Univ. Center for Environmental Quality Management, Ithaca, NY, Nov. 1974.

[32] President's Science Advisory Panel on the World Food Supply, *The World Food Problem*, vol. II. U. S. Government Printing Office, 1967.

[33] R. A. Rapoport, "The flow of energy in an agricultural society," *Scientific American*, pp. 117–132, Sept. 1971.

[34] K. Reid, *Nature's Network*. London: Aldus, 1969.

[35] R. E. Ricklefs, *Ecology*. Newton, MA: Chiron, 1973.

[36] F. S. Roberts and H. Marcus-Roberts, "Efficiency of energy use in obtaining food, II: Animals," this volume, chapter 11.

[37] F. S. Roberts, Ed., *Energy Modeling and Net Energy Analysis*. Chicago: Institute of Gas Technology, 1979.

[38] T. W. Schoener, "Models of optimal size for solitary predators," *Amer. Natur.*, vol. 103, pp. 277–313, 1969.

[39] V. Smil, P. Nachman, and T. V. Long, *Energy Analysis and Agriculture*. Boulder, CO: Westview, 1982.

[40] U. N. Food and Agriculture Organization, *Provisional Indicative World Plan for Agricultural Development*. Rome: U. N. Food and Agriculture Organization, 1970.

[41] U. S. Department of Agriculture. *Agr. Econ. Rep. 147*, 1968.

[42] U. S. Department of Agriculture. *Stat. Bull. 233*, 1972.

[43]   J. P. Wesley, *Ecophysics: The Application of Physics to Ecology.* Springfield, IL: Charles C. Thomas, 1974.

[44]   E. O. Wilson and W. H. Bossert, *A Primer of Population Biology.* Stamford, CT: Sinauer Associates, 1971.

Notes for the Instructor

Prerequisites. Background in linear programming at the level of a finite mathematics course will suffice for the understanding of this chapter.

Time. Several class periods.

Remarks. This is the first of two chapters on efficiency of energy use in obtaining food. The second chapter (Chapter 11 in this volume) deals with animal behavior. The two chapters are essentially independent, except that the second chapter depends in places on a few parts of Sections 2 and 3 of this chapter.

This chapter could be used in a finite mathematics course, a linear programming course, or an introductory operations research course. Parts of the second chapter (Chapter 11) might be appropriate in a calculus course, in particular the model of the pure pursuer and the treatment of the allometric law. The two together, or either chapter alone, would be suitable for a modeling course with the appropriate prerequisites. An attempt is made, especially in Chapter 11, to show the development of a mathematical model through several iterations, with predictions from earlier versions tested against information about behavior. Each of the chapters is prepared with possible "open-ended" use in mind. That is, students could be involved in extending the models presented, investigating alternative approaches, and the like.

If these chapters are used in modeling courses, attention should be drawn to the following:

(1) the difference between the normative or prescriptive approach to human energy use and the descriptive approach to animal energy use;

(2) the difference between the deterministic models of the pure pursuer and the stochastic models of the pure searcher;

(3) the large number of different mathematical techniques which are brought to bear on one problem;

(4) the constant attempt, at least in the descriptive models, to test predictions of models, and to modify them if the predictions do not measure up.

CHAPTER 11

Efficiency of Energy Use in Obtaining Food, II: Animals

Fred S. Roberts* and Helen Marcus-Roberts**

1. Introduction: The Problem

Human beings, at least modern human beings, often use their energy in obtaining food in very inefficient ways. Animals, on the other hand, at least according to a body of ecological literature, are very efficient users of energy in obtaining food.

In their efforts to obtain food, primitive human beings were dependent only on their muscle power. The only energy they could use to obtain food had its source in food previously eaten. Then, in general, men had to be relatively efficient users of energy in obtaining food. Modern man has replaced much of the muscle power used in food production with machines, chemical fertilizers, irrigation, and so on. He has dramatically increased his ability to obtain food, but only through using a great deal of energy: energy to run his farm machines, to produce and spread fertilizers, to irrigate, and so on. In the previous chapter (Roberts [33]), ways to measure energy efficiency are discussed, and the efficiency of human energy use in food production is described.

A number of ecologists have suggested that animals are very efficient in their energy use. They evolve so as to be efficient in their use of energy in foraging (Hainsworth and Wolf [12]); their size develops in such a way as to optimize the efficiency of obtaining energy (Schoener [36]); or they develop feeding preferences which maximize their caloric intake per unit

* Department of Mathematics, Rutgers University, New Brunswick, NJ 08903.

** Department of Mathematics and Computer Science, Montclair State College, Upper Montclair, NJ 07043.

time (Emlen [10]).[1] In this module, we develop a series of mathematical models of the energy efficient animal. The models are *descriptive* rather than *prescriptive*—they seek to describe how such an animal behaves or looks, rather than how it *should* behave or look in order to be energy efficient. We will also see that some types of predatory animals are naturally described using *deterministic models*, models where we predict their exact behavior given a certain distribution of food, while other types of predatory animals are more naturally described using *stochastic models*, models which introduce an element of uncertainty or probability into their behavior. The models presented here are used to derive predictions. These predictions are then subjected to some form of verification, for example through comparison to real data or through "thought experiment." Many of these models will be rejected right away. The ones that are not should be regarded as tentative and subject to further test. Many of the assumptions used in building these models can easily be modified by the reader, who is encouraged to do so and to construct alternative models of the energy-efficient animal.

Before reading further, the reader should consult Section 2 of Roberts [33] for a brief statement of the biological and physical background needed to understand what follows. Of course, anyone who seriously applies mathematics to other disciplines must become more well-grounded in these disciplines than he can by reading a few pages of background material. However, this background should suffice to get the reader started.

The reader might also wish to consult the discussion of efficiency in Section 3.1 of Roberts [33], for much of what we say is based on methods of defining energy efficiency. However, this material does not have to be read early on, and most of it is repeated here. No other part of Roberts [33] is needed for the following.

In the next section, we derive a basic law of biology, the allometric law, which will be used in several places in our model-building. In Section 3, we discuss how to define energy-efficient behavior. Then, we will model two types of energy-efficient predatory animals, the pure pursuer in Section 4 and the pure searcher in Section 5.

2. The Allometric Law

2.1 Relative Growth Rates[2]

Suppose x is some biological variable, such as body mass, body length, metabolic rate, etc. The *growth rate* or *absolute growth rate* of x is the derivative dx/dt of x with respect to time t. Sometimes it is convenient to speak of

---

[1] These models disregard other requirements from food such as proteins, vitamins, etc. See Roberts [33, section 4.3.1].
[2] This section borrows from Batschelet [3, pp. 285, 305–307].

the *relative* or the *specific growth rate*, the ratio of dx/dt to x, or

$$\frac{1}{x}\frac{dx}{dt}.$$

For example, suppose an animal is growing at a constant rate of 48 gm in each 24-hour period, or at the rate of 2 gm an hour. Is this a large or a small rate of growth? The answer is relative to the animal's current weight. If the animal currently weighs 24 gm this is a very rapid growth rate. If it currently weighs 100 kg (10,000 gm), it is a very slow growth rate. Hence the relative growth rate can give more information than the absolute growth rate. In the first case, it is

$$\frac{2 \text{ gm/hr}}{24 \text{ gm}} = \frac{1}{12}\text{ hr}^{-1},$$

while in the second case it is

$$\frac{2 \text{ gm/hr}}{10,000 \text{ gm}} = \frac{1}{5000}\text{ hr}^{-1}.$$

With a relative growth rate of $1/12 \text{ hr}^{-1}$, the 100-kg animal would gain more than 8 kg an hour!

Allometry is the study of comparative growth rates of different biological quantities, for example the growth rates of the head and of the hands of a person. Suppose $x(t)$ is the size of one biological quantity at time t, and $y(t)$ the size of a second. It is usually convenient to compare relative growth rates of x and y rather than absolute growth rates. Much biological data suggests that relative growth rates are proportional, i.e., that

$$\frac{1}{y}\frac{dy}{dt} = c\frac{1}{x}\frac{dx}{dt}, \tag{1}$$

where c is a constant of proportionality. The differential equation (1) is called the *allometric law*.

To solve this differential equation, we note that by the chain rule,

$$\frac{dy}{dt}\bigg/\frac{dx}{dt} = \frac{dy}{dx}.$$

Thus we obtain

$$\frac{dy}{dx} = c\frac{y}{x}.$$

This equation can be solved by separation of variables. We obtain

$$\ln y = c \ln x + k, \tag{2}$$

where k is a constant. Equation (2) translates into

$$y = e^{c \ln x + k} = e^k x^c,$$

or

$$y = Kx^c,\tag{3}$$

where $K = e^k$. That is, y is a power function of x. Equations (2) and (3) are also sometimes called the *allometric law*.

Note that the allometric law does not say that every biological quantity grows as a power function of time. Rather, it says that one biological quantity grows as a power function of a second.

The allometric law has been studied by many authors. Some references are Grande and Taylor [11], Huxley [18], Rosen [34, ch. 5], Simpson, *et al.* [38, p. 396 ff], Teissier [40], von Bertalanffy [44, p. 311–332], and Wilbur and Owen [47]. For a very interesting mathematical discussion of some allometric laws, see Smith [39, ch. 1].

In our models of predatory animals, we shall apply the allometric law to the relation between metabolic rate and body weight, and use this relation to estimate energy requirements. We turn to this relation in the next subsection.

2.2 Metabolic Rate and Body Weight[3]

The *metabolic rate* (MR) is defined to be the rate of heat produced by the body per unit of time, and of course it varies with the type of activity the organism is performing. Unless otherwise mentioned, metabolic rate will be thought of as the rate when the organism is resting and fasting. This is called the *basal metabolic rate*. According to the allometric law, MR should be related to body weight by a power function

$$MR = KW^c,\tag{4}$$

for appropriate constants K and c.

Starting in the 1830's (Kleiber [22, p. 180]), it was believed that MR was proportional to surface area S of the body. That is,

$$MR = \alpha S,\tag{5}$$

where α is a constant. (This is again an example of the allometric law.) If the law (5) is right, then we can determine the exponent c in (4) by considering the relation between surface area and body weight. Body weight is often assumed to be roughly proportional to body volume V. (However, see the discussion in Section 4.1.1 below.) What is the relation between S and V? The answer is easy for animals with shapes like cubes or spheres! For a sphere,

$$S = 4\pi r^2\tag{6}$$

$$V = \tfrac{4}{3}\pi r^3,\tag{7}$$

---

[3] This subsection is based in large part on Kleiber [22, ch. 10].

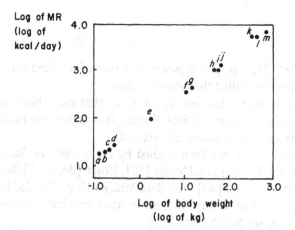

Figure 11.1. Log-log Plot of Metabolic Rate against Body Weight. From Kleiber [22, p. 201]. Reprinted with Permission of John Wiley & Sons, Inc. *Key*: a = Dove; b = Female Rat; c = Male Rat; d = Pigeon; e = Hen; f = Female Dog; g = Male Dog; h = Sheep; i = Woman; j = Man; k = Steer; l = Cow; m = Steer.

where r is the radius. It follows that

$$S = \beta V^{2/3}, \tag{8}$$

where β is a constant. Since V is proportional to W,

$$S = \gamma W^{2/3}, \tag{9}$$

for still another constant γ. It follows from (5) and (9) that

$$MR = \delta W^{2/3}, \tag{10}$$

where δ is a constant. A similar result holds for a cube. (The details are left to the reader as Exercise 6.) For animals without perfectly regular geometric shapes, the calculation of volume and surface area is more complicated. However, one can argue that (8) and hence (9) and (10) hold in general, at least as an approximation. (One might approximate a body by small cubes or spheres in the argument. See Batschelet [3, pp. 78–80] for an indication of how this argument might go.)

The "law" (10) was accepted for many years until Kleiber [20] began to attack the surface law (5) because surface area is not very well-defined. For example, in rabbits, do we count the ears as contributing to surface area? The answer to this question can change surface area by as much as 20%. Kleiber suggested relating MR directly to body weight, and began measuring MR and W to test the law (10) directly. Although early data (for example that of Voit [43]) seemed to confirm the law (10), later data suggested strongly that the exponent 2/3 was quite far off. What does such data look like and how can one estimate the proper exponent?

Let us return to the power law (3), and take logs of both sides. We obtain

$$\log_{10} y = c \log_{10} x + K_1.$$

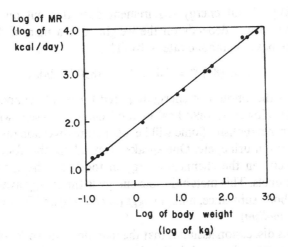

Figure 11.2. Straight Line Fitted to Log-log Plot of Figure 11.1. From Kleiber [22, pp. 201]. Reprinted with Permission of John Wiley & Sons, Inc.

This says that if $\log_{10} y$ is plotted against $\log_{10} x$ the plot should be a straight line with slope c. Figure 11.1 shows a plot of logarithm of MR against logarithm of body weight for various species. Figure 11.2 shows a straight line fitted to these data points. This "best" straight line was obtained using the method of least squares.[4,5] The slope of this line was more nearly 3/4 than 2/3. (Can you see why?) In any case, this data rejects the 2/3 law (Equation (10)) and hence the surface law (Equation (5)) or the law (8) or the assumption that weight is proportional to volume. Similar data have given rise to exponents anywhere between 0.63 and 1.0 (Lasiewski and Dawson [23], Zeuther [48]). Hemmingsen [13], [14] and Kleiber [22] argue that because of the strength of the evidence, an exponent of 3/4 should be generally adopted. Kleiber also argues that if W is measured in kg and MR in kcal per day, then the second constant K in the power law (4) should be about 70. (Why does this follow from Fig. 11.2?) Hence the basal metabolic rate is given by

$$MR = 70W^{3/4}. \tag{11}$$

2.3 Relation to Food Requirements

Since MR is the rate of heat production per unit time, the requirement of food energy (for resting) during given length of time T corresponds to MR times the time T, i.e., to

$$MR \times T$$

---

[4] For a reference on this method, see for example Alder and Roessler [1].

[5] It would perhaps be more appropriate to plot the log of MR against the log of W for different individuals within a species. Good results are harder to get with this, since weights and metabolic rates do not differ greatly for individuals. However, the results are similar to the ones to be discussed for the interspecies comparison. See Kleiber [22, pp. 207ff].

(Kleiber [21]). What energy requirement does this put on a person or animal? The answer depends on the weight. For a man of 81 kg (about 178 lbs.), the basal metabolic rate is, by (11),

$$70 \times (81)^{3/4} = 70 \times 27 = 1890 \text{ kcal/day}.$$

Hence this is the amount of energy required for basal metabolism for one day ($T = 1$). However, 1890 kcal of food energy ingested will not all be available for metabolism. Some will be lost before digestion (as feces), some after digestion in urine, etc. One speaks of metabolizable food energy, the difference between the chemical energy in food and the chemical energy in waste products. This metabolizable energy is the energy available for the building of body substance, milk, or eggs (*anabolism*) and for the production of heat (*katabolism*).

So far, this discussion assumes that the man does no work. When he does work, the source of his work is the chemical energy released when organic compounds are katabolized. The MR can increase dramatically during work and can stay elevated for long periods afterwards. For example, it has been measured at 25% above the basal level 15 hours after work and at 10% above basal level 48 hours after strenuous exercise (Kleiber [22, p. 308]). MR also increases after eating. All of these considerations suggest that the daily caloric requirements for a modestly active man of 81 kg are closer to 3000 kcal than 1890. This result can be thought of as saying that energy requirements are not equal to MR $\times$ T, but proportional to MR $\times$ T, i.e., equal to $k \times$ MR $\times$ T for some appropriate constant k. These energy requirements go up to 4500 kcal if the man is performing heavy physical labor (Brown [7, p. 107]). According to the U.N. Food and Agriculture Organization [42], average caloric intake in most of Central Africa, Pakistan, and India is less than 2000 kcal per day. Brown [7, p. 112] estimates that about 50% of the world population receives less than 2250 kcal per day, barely enough to maintain life.

EXERCISES

1. (a) If $x(t) = kt^n$, k and n constant, find the relative growth rate of x.
   (b) If $x(t) = ae^{bt}$, a and b constant, find the relative growth rate of x.

2. If the relative growth rate of x is constant, find x as a function of time.

3. Suppose x and y are given by

$$x(t) = k_1 t^{n_1}$$

$$y(t) = k_2 t^{n_2},$$

where k_1, k_2, n_1, n_2 are constant. Find the constant c in the allometric law (1).

4. Suppose x and y are given by

$$x(t) = a_1 e^{b_1 t}$$

$$y(t) = a_2 e^{b_2 t},$$

where a_1, a_2, b_1, b_2 are constant. Find the constant c in the allometric law (1).

5. Suppose $x(t)$ is given as in Exercise 3 and $y(t)$ is as in Exercise 4. Could a constant c exist so that the allometric law (1) holds? Why?

6. Derive an allometric law relating surface area (S) to volume (V) for a cube-shaped animal and use it to relate metabolic rate (MR) to weight (W).

7. We shall argue in Section 4.1.1 that weight is proportional to surface area, rather than to volume. If this is true and if the surface law (5) holds, what does this imply about the allometric law (4) for metabolic rate (MR) versus weight (W)?

8. If the surface law (5) holds, graph MR against S in log-log coordinates.

9. (Smith [39]) Laws (6) and (7) can be restated to say that surface area is proportional to the square of some "linear dimension" (such as the radius) and volume is proportional to the cube of this dimension.
   (a) If this dimension doubles, what happens to surface area and to volume?
   (b) Suppose metabolic rate is proportional to the 3/4 power of body weight, as Kleiber argues it is. If body weight is proportional to body volume, then metabolic rate is proportional to some power of the linear dimension. What power?
   (c) The flow of energy into the body is proportional to surface area and hence to the square of the linear dimension. Using your answer to (b), what can you say about the relation between metabolic rate and flow of energy into the body as the animal grows proportionately in size, i.e., as the linear dimension increases? What does this imply about the size of animals of a given shape? Hint: Can the flow of energy into the body be less than MR? (Is there a similar implication if body weight is proportional to surface area rather than to volume?)

10. (Batschelet [3], von Bertalanffy [44])
    (a) If W is the weight of a cell, and weight is proportional to volume, then it follows that surface area is proportional to $W^{2/3}$. Why?
    (b) The growth of a cell depends on the flow of nutrients through the surface. Hence while the cell is growing rapidly,

$$\frac{dW}{dt} = kW^{2/3},$$

some constant k. Solve this equation for W.
    (c) Express surface area S as a function of t.

11. (Kleiber [22]) The rate of weight loss of a starving animal (animal which is not fed) is proportional to its metabolic rate. In particular,

$$\frac{dW}{dt} = -\text{MR}.$$

Suppose

$$\text{MR} = 70W^{3/4}.$$

Find the body weight W of a 25 kg dog t days after it stops eating.

12. (Kleiber [22]) Death from starvation occurs as a rule of thumb when an animal has katabolized (burned up) a certain part of its body substance—50% according to the Law of Chossat. Assuming this 50% law, how long does it take the dog of Exercise 11 to die of starvation?

13. Assuming the Law of Chossat of Exercise 12 and the formulas for dW/dt and MR of Exercise 11, comment on which animal would be expected to have a longer survival time under starvation, a larger animal or a smaller animal.

3. Predators as Efficient Users of Energy

3.1 Definition of Energy Efficiency

Unlike modern man, most predatory creatures spend a large percentage of their time hunting for food. They spend a great deal of energy in trying to obtain the energy value of food. Accordingly, many biologists feel that predators must evolve so as to be efficient in their use of energy. As we pointed out in the Introduction, Hainsworth and Wolf [12] hypothesize that an animal evolves in such a way as to optimize *foraging efficiency*, the energy spent to obtain food relative to the energy value of food. They consider hummingbirds, and argue that optimal body size may be determined by the need to be *energetically efficient*. Schoener [36] argues that for a class of predators which are identical except in size, that sized predator will be optimal (and will evolve) "which is able to obtain enough food to support its requirements in the least amount of feeding time." Emlen [10] assumes that "natural selection will favor the development (by whatever means—innate or learned) of feeding preferences that will, by their direction and intensity, and within the physical and nervous limitations of a species, maximize the net caloric intake per individual of that species per unit time." Thus feeding preferences and habits are dictated (in an unconscious, evolutionary sense) by the need to be energy efficient.

Our basic models will make the hypothesis that predators try to obtain the maximum amount of energy per unit of energy input. That is, they optimize

$$e = \frac{E_O}{E_I}, \tag{12}$$

where E_O is energy "output" or energy obtained from feeding and E_I is energy "input" or energy spent in feeding. (This is the measure of efficiency which was introduced in Section 3.1 of Roberts [33].) In the ecological context, it is sometimes called *energetic efficiency*.

Models which assume optimization of the energetic efficiency omit the role of time. Capturing a large amount of energy per unit of energy expended may take too much time in some cases to be efficient. An alternative model would be that predators optimize the net energy obtained per unit of time spent. The *net energy* obtained is $E_O - E_I$. A measure of net energy obtained per unit time is

$$e' = \frac{E_O - E_I}{T}, \tag{13}$$

where T is the time spent in obtaining E_O. The measure e' might be called the *time-energy efficiency*. In the exercises, we shall consider models of behavior in which e' is optimized. Incidentally, a variant of the measure e is to consider net energy obtained per unit of energy input,

$$e'' = \frac{E_O - E_I}{E_I}.$$

Optimizing e'' reduces to optimizing e, since $e'' = e - 1$.

If a very small food item is taken, then the energy involved in feeding, E_I, might be very small, and so the efficiency e might be very large. Still, an animal might not find it worthwhile to eat such a small source of energy. What defines small? Small is obviously a relative term, relative for example to the predator's food *energy requirements* E_R. (E_R is the total amount of E_O required over a period of time.) It is convenient, therefore, to think in terms of *relative energy output*, E_O/E_R, rather than absolute output E_O, and to think of optimizing the *relative energetic efficiency*

$$e = \frac{E_O/E_R}{E_I}. \tag{14}$$

We shall still use the letter e to represent this efficiency. A similar modification can be made in the measure (13), giving us the *relative time-energy efficiency*,

$$e' = \frac{(E_O - E_I)/E_R}{T}. \tag{15}$$

Here, E_R is the total amount of net energy $E_O - E_I$ required over a period of time. In (14), E_R was the total amount of energy output required. It might be more reasonable to use the total amount of net energy required in (14) as well. However, we shall assume instead that E_R in (14) is calculated in terms of E_O only, but calculated in such a way as to compensate for the "average" energy input expected to be required in obtaining a certain total output. For example, in Section 2.3, we calculated an 81-kg man's net energy requirements per day as 1890 kcal. This assumed no energy used in obtaining food (and no activity, eating, etc.). We compensated for the extra energy use by upping the requirements to 3000 kcal. The latter figure would be used in (14), the former in (15).

Speaking of relative efficiency rather than absolute efficiency is more than just a convenience. The energy output E_O, energy input E_I, and energy requirements E_R can all vary from food item to food item and animal to animal. For example, we shall assume below that both E_I and E_R depend on the animal's body size B, while E_O is independent of B. Then it is possible that for a particular food item,

$$\frac{E_O}{E_I(B)} > \frac{E_O}{E_I(B')}$$

while

$$\frac{E_O/E_R(B)}{E_I(B)} < \frac{E_O/E_R(B')}{E_I(B')}.$$

Hence, for two animals with body sizes B and B', the first animal might be more absolutely efficient in taking the food item than the second animal, but less relatively efficient. An example of this will follow.

3.2 Pure Pursuers and Pure Searchers

Schoener [36] presents several models in which the optimal size of a predator is primarily determined by "trophic-energetic" relationships, the interaction between abundances of food items and the relative amounts of energy obtainable from these by different size predators. These models assume a *solitary predator*, one for which competing species are absent. This allows Schoener to avoid considerations of competition between species for food, which would greatly complicate matters. The models we discuss here are based primarily on Schoener's models for solitary predators. He assumes these predators optimize the relative time-energy efficiency (15). We shall assume that they optimize the relative energetic efficiency (14). (However, we will consider the relative time-energy efficiency in the exercises.) We shall distinguish between two idealized types of solitary predators: pure pursuers and pure searchers. (Schoener calls them Type I and Type II predators, respectively; the terminology pure pursuer is from MacArthur and Levins [25]). The *pure pursuers* expend (little or) no energy in moving about in search of food; they wait at a central location until food is sighted, and then they spend a great deal of energy in pursuing their prey. The pure searchers, on the other hand, spend a great deal of time and energy just searching for food. But when food is sighted, they spend (very little or) none on pursuit. We shall treat pure pursuers and pure searchers in the next two sections. We will find that modeling optimal energy efficient behavior for each of these types of predators will involve considerably different mathematical treatment. In fact, optimally efficient pure pursuers will be modeled deterministically, while optimally efficient pure searchers will be modeled stochastically. For a detailed discussion of the differences between stochastic and deterministic models, see Marcus–Roberts [27].

The models we will consider will look very "quantitative" in the sense that we will have precise formulas for various quantities such as energy used or obtained. However, the predictions we will be able to make from these models will only be "qualitative," for example, that a certain value increases for awhile and then decreases. There are several reasons we will only be able to make such qualitative predictions. First of all, the models will involve a large number of constants whose value is unknown, and indeed vary from predator to predator and prey to prey—these are *parameters* of the models. Second, the level of biological data available is often only useful at the qualitative level, because of the difficulty of measuring, the complications of some of the variables, etc. The reader should not think, however, that modeling which produces only "qualitative" conclusions is not useful, or not mathematical. A qualitative conclusion can be stated in precise mathematical terms, used for predictions, subjected to test, and can lead to understanding of real-world phenomena. Perhaps it will never be possible to produce purely quantitative models of many biological phenomena. We will have to learn to accept such qualitative models.

It should be remarked before we go on that not all animal behavior optimizes. For an example, see the article by Toth [41] on "What the Bees Know and What They Don't Know." Thus the hypothesis that animals optimize energetically is certainly subject to test and refutation.

4. Pure Pursuers

A pure pursuer expends time and energy in pursuing prey, and handling and swallowing prey. However, it is assumed not to spend any time in moving about searching for prey. It locates its prey by monitoring an area until it sees a potential prey. We assume that no energy is used in the monitoring process. Once a pure pursuer locates a potential prey, then it will choose to go after the prey or not, depending on two factors: the size of the prey and the distance of the prey from it. We assume for simplicity that, should the predator choose a given prey, it will succeed in capturing it. Also, we assume that the predator will return to its monitoring point (monitoring locale) after capturing and eating its prey. Although a pure pursuer is an idealization, examples which come close to meeting the description are *Anolis* lizards, kingfishers, many frogs, certain preying mantids, ambush bugs, certain predatory cats, and certain owls (Schoener [36]).

4.1 First Model for Calculation of Energy Inputs and Outputs

Before we can talk about optimizing energetic efficiency, we shall have to develop ways of calculating energy requirements and energy input and output in feeding. The formulas for requirements and input and output will

be developed in steps. Our early models for energy requirements and input
and output will clearly lead to unsatisfactory conclusions.

4.1.1 *Energy Requirements of the Predator.* According to our discussion in
Section 2.3, the energy requirements at rest E_R during a period of time of
length T are given by

$$E_R = MR \times T,$$

where MR is the metabolic rate (at rest). In turn,

$$MR = \alpha W^{3/4},$$

where W is body weight and α is a constant of proportionality. For reasons
of consistency with the literature, in particular with Schoener's models, we
shall use body length or size B of the predator, rather than body weight.
Let $E_R = E_R(B)$ be the energy required during a given period of time—we
shall always think of a day—by a predator of body size B. In order to use
the expression

$$E_R = MR \times T,$$

we shall have to determine the relation between body weight W and body
length B.

In Section 2.2, we observed that, at least for regular geometric figures
such as the sphere or the cube, the surface area S was proportional to the
2/3 power of the volume V. Using the same reasoning, based on (6) and
(7), one can argue that the volume is proportional to the cube of the length
r (or B), and the surface area is proportional to the square of the length.
Now if weight is proportional to volume, as we assumed in the discussion
of Section 2.2, then we should obtain

$$MR = \alpha W^{3/4}$$
$$= \alpha(\beta B^3)^{3/4} = \gamma B^{9/4},$$

where β and γ are constants of proportionality. However, Schoener's experiments suggest that W is proportional to B^2 rather than to B^3, and hence
to surface area rather than volume. Using this fact, one obtains

$$MR = \alpha(\delta B^2)^{3/4} = kB^{3/2},$$

where δ and k are constants of proportionality. In accordance with
Schoener's models, we shall adopt this second condition. Thus we shall
assume that for a given period of one day $(T = 1)$,

$$E_R = MR \times T = MR,$$

or

$$E_R(B) = kB^{1.5},$$

where k is a positive constant. Taking into account increases in metabolic rate during activity, it is perhaps more natural to assume that $E_R(B)$ is proportional to MR $\times$ T, rather than equal to it, and hence to use the equation

$$E_R(B) = k_1 B^{1.5}, \tag{16}$$

where $k_1 > k$. Following Schoener, this is the assumption we shall make rather than calculate $E_R(B)$ in terms of net energy obtained.

4.1.2 *Potential Energy of Food Items.* We shall assume that the (caloric) energy available from a food item is a function of its body size or length i. If a food item has length i, the energy $E(i)$ obtainable from that item can be assumed proportional to the weight of the item, and hence to a power of the body size. (This is again the allometric law.) Schoener assumes that W is proportional to B^2, and hence that

$$E(i) = k_2 i^2, \tag{17}$$

where k_2 is a positive constant. We shall also adopt this assumption.

4.1.3 *Energy Expended in Pursuit.* In pursuing and capturing a food item, a predator uses a certain amount of energy. Presumably, if it will take a large amount of energy to capture an item of food, the item will be pursued only if it contributes a large enough amount of energy. It is natural to assume that the energy used in pursuit depends on the body size of the predator and the time of pursuit TP. In turn, the time of pursuit depends on the distance r that the prey is from the predator. Using an argument similar to that used in deriving (16), Schoener determines the energy used in pursuit EP as proportional to MR times time of pursuit TP, i.e.,

$$EP = k_3 B^{1.5} TP, \tag{18}$$

where k_3 is a positive constant interpreted as the "cost of pursuing." We shall adopt this assumption as well.[6] The value TP depends on the distance r of the prey from the predator, and on the (average) velocity v of the pursuer. For simplicity, we assume that the prey does not try (or is unable) to escape. Then,

$$TP = TP(r) = r/v, \tag{19}$$

and so

$$EP = EP(B, r) = \frac{k_3 B^{1.5} r}{v}. \tag{20}$$

The reader should note that this term is independent of i, the body size of the prey. In the exercises, we shall consider how to modify this formula if the prey should flee.

---

[6] As above, EP is proportional to MR $\times$ TP rather than equal to it because metabolic rate increases over rest rate MR when working.

Before closing this discussion, we must ask how v depends on the other factors, such as B, i, r. Information about the relation of v to B, velocity of a predator to its body size, is not conclusive. Smith [39, pp. 11–12] argues that top speed for animals should be independent of size, at least for sufficiently large animals. Hill [15] also argues that way, at least for "similar" animals of the same taxon. However, other authors (Bonner [6], Hocking [16]) obtain different results. We shall assume that v is a positive constant for all predators under study and independent of B and also of i and r. Exercises 25 and 26 ask the reader to weaken this assumption.

4.1.4 *The Energetic Efficiency.* The basic variables we have used in our model are the body size B of the predator, the body size i of a food item, and the distance r of the food item from the predator. We also have several parameters: k_1, k_2, k_3, and v. Suppose a predator of size B spots a prey of size i at distance r. We shall call such a prey an (i, r) *prey* or (i, r) *food item*. What is the *energetic efficiency* $e(B, i, r)$ for the predator in going after (and capturing) an (i, r) food item? Using our relative energetic efficiency measure (14), we have

$$e(B, i, r) = \frac{E_O/E_R}{E_I} = \frac{E(i)/E_R(B)}{EP(B, r)}, \tag{21}$$

where $E(i)$ is the energy obtained in eating the food item of size i, $E_R(B)$ is the energy requirement for the predator of size B, and $EP(B, r)$ is the energy expended in pursuit. Thus

$$e(B, i, r) = \frac{k_2 i^2/k_1 B^{1.5}}{k_3 B^{1.5} TP(r)} \tag{22}$$

or

$$e(B, i, r) = \frac{k_2 i^2 v}{k_1 k_3 B^3 r}. \tag{23}$$

We are assuming that predators will develop so as to optimize $e(B, i, r)$.

4.1.5 *Predictions from the First Model.* Let us consider the energetic efficiency $e(B, i, r)$ for fixed r and B positive. That is, we let the body size B of the predator be fixed, and we consider prey at a fixed distance r from the predator. Note that by assumption, v is constant. Then we have

$$e(B, i, r) = ai^2, \tag{24}$$

where

$$a = \frac{k_2 v}{k_1 k_3 B^3 r}. \tag{25}$$

If we plot e against i, we obtain a parabola as shown in Figure 11.3, for a is positive since k_1, k_2, k_3, v, r, and B are all positive.

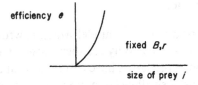

Figure 11.3

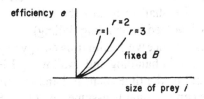

Figure 11.4

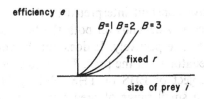

Figure 11.5

Let us ask what happens to e as r increases, i.e., as the prey are at a further distance. We note from (25) that as r increases, a decreases. Hence we obtain a family of parabolas, the wider ones corresponding to larger r, as shown in Figure 11.4. Now e measures the fraction of daily energy requirements obtained per unit of energy used. It is clear from Figure 11.4 that e is higher for fixed i by taking the smallest possible r, i.e., taking prey as close as possible. This is obvious, given our model or given Eq. (23),

Let us consider next a fixed r but a varying body size B. We see again from Equation (25) that a decreases with increasing B. Hence plotting e against i for varying B again gives rise to a family of parabolas, the wider ones corresponding to larger B, much as shown in Figure 11.5. The implication of this result is the following. For any given food size i and any distance r, the predator of smaller body size will obtain a larger fraction of the daily required energy per unit of energy expended than will the predator of larger body size. (This is also clear directly from Eq. (23).) If we take seriously the basic assumption that a predator evolves so as to optimize $e(B, i, r)$, we must predict from our model that all predators will be very tiny. Clearly, this prediction is violated in nature: large predators do exist![7]

---

[7] A similar prediction might be valid if we restrict the range of sizes of a species in advance.

4.2 A Second Model

Faced with a prediction from our model which is wrong, we are forced to inquire about what happened. Why are there large predators in the world? The answer is that large predators have certain advantages over small ones: they can handle (kill) and swallow larger prey. We have omitted in our model any discussion of how much energy is expended in handling (killing) and swallowing the prey, and indeed whether it is possible for a small predator to kill a large prey. We shall disregard the latter problem, and consider here only the energy involved in handling (killing) and swallowing the prey. From our previous experience with estimating energy requirements, we know that the energy required in handling and swallowing EHS will be related to the metabolic rate and to the time spent in handling and swallowing THS, and in particular we can reasonably assume that (as in Equation (18))

$$\text{EHS} = k_4 B^{1.5} \text{THS}, \tag{26}$$

where k_4 is a positive constant interpreted as the "cost of handling and swallowing." THS clearly depends on both the body sizes B and i of the predator and the prey, respectively. It does not, however, depend on the distance r of the predator from the prey. There does not seem to be much literature on the subject of EHS or THS. Holling [17] has found that (for mantids), over a small range of prey sizes, it is suitable to consider eating time as directly proportional to the weight of the food item. Since by our earlier assumptions, weight is proportional to the square of body size, we shall assume that THS is directly proportional to the square of the length i of the food item and that it does not depend on the body weight of the predator. Thus

$$\text{THS} = k_5 i^2, \tag{27}$$

where k_5 is still another positive constant.

Using these assumptions, let us repeat the calculation of the energetic efficiency $e(B, i, r)$. We obtain

$$e(B, i, r) = \frac{E(i)/E_R(B)}{\text{EP} + \text{EHS}}, \tag{28}$$

so

$$e(B, i, r) = \frac{k_2 i^2/k_1 B^{1.5}}{k_3 B^{1.5}\text{TP} + k_4 B^{1.5}\text{THS}}$$

$$= \frac{k_2 i^2}{k_1 k_3 B^3 r/v + k_1 k_4 k_5 B^3 i^2}.$$

For fixed i and r, the function $e(B, i, r)$ still has the problems that our old function $e(B, i, r)$ had: e increases with smaller body size B. Thus, again, if energy use is to be optimized, predators must be tiny.[8]

---

[8] As above, this prediction might be valid if we restrict the range of sizes of a species in advance.

4.3 A Third Model

It should be clear again why this unfortunate prediction has been reached. Our model still shows no advantage to having a larger body. This advantage can arise in the time spent handling and swallowing a prey: larger predators will spend less time disposing of prey they have pursued and caught up to. Thus let us again modify our model by changing our expression for THS. Let us assume for simplicity that THS is not only directly proportional to i^2, but also inversely proportional to some power of B. It should be easy to see that this power of B will have to be relatively large for $e(B, i, r)$ not to have the unfortunate property of increasing with decreasing B. For, suppose

$$\text{THS} = k_5 i^2 B^{-s},$$

where k_5 and s are positive constants. Then, using (28), we have

$$e(B, i, r) = \frac{k_2 i^2 / k_1 B^{1.5}}{k_3 B^{1.5} r / v + k_4 k_5 B^{1.5} i^2 B^{-s}}$$

$$= \frac{k_2 i^2}{k_1 k_3 B^3 r / v + k_1 k_4 k_5 B^{(3-s)} i^2}.$$

We see that s must be greater than 3.[9] We would want to assume this.

With one problem resolved, let us investigate $e(B, i, r)$ further. If r and B are fixed, positive numbers, we obtain

$$e(B, i, r) = \frac{1}{a/i^2 + b}$$

where

$$a = k_1 k_3 B^3 r / k_2 v$$

and

$$b = k_1 k_4 k_5 B^{3-s} / k_2.$$

---

[9] This is the only place in our model where the use of the relative efficiency (14) rather than the (absolute) efficiency (12) makes a difference. If the latter were used, we would have

$$e(B, i, r) = \frac{k_2 i^2}{k_3 B^{1.5} r / v + k_4 k_5 B^{(1.5-s)} i^2}$$

and a choice of $s > 1.5$ would suffice for e to have the desired properties. With $s = 2$ for example, the relative energetic efficiency would be a decreasing function of body size, while the absolute energetic efficiency would not. For some food items, there are two different body sizes B and B' so that a predator of body size B will have greater absolute efficiency in eating the item than a predator of body size B', but would have less relative efficiency! In modeling, therefore, it makes a difference whether we think predators optimize absolute or relative efficiency. (No trouble of this sort will arise if we have a fixed predator and compare his absolute or relative efficiencies for different food items. The absolute efficiency will be larger if and only if the relative efficiency is larger.)

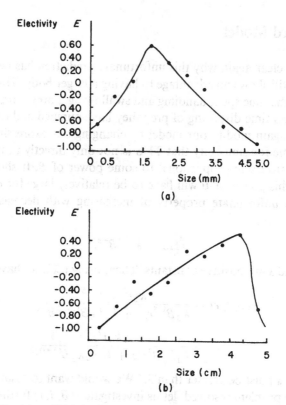

Figure 11.6. Electivity of Fish for Food Items of Various Sizes. (a) Bleak Fed on Water Fleas. (b) Larvae of *Macrodytes circumflexes* Fed on Young Roach. Data Are from Ivlev [19, p. 87]. Reprinted with Permission of Yale University Press.

Since *a* is positive, the function *e* increases as values of *i* get larger. The implication is that, if energy obtained per unit of energy expended is being maximized, then for prey at a fixed distance from a predator, a larger prey will *always* be preferred to a smaller prey. Is that a reasonable prediction? Certain animals eat a variety of sizes of food items. But is that only because of availability? Is it possible that within the range of body sizes of prey which can be reasonably captured, the larger prey will always be preferred?

Ivlev [19] has conducted a variety of studies on fish, in which, among other things, he has measured the fishes' degree of "electivity" (choice) for abundant prey of various sizes. Figure 11.6 shows two typical curves obtained by Ivlev. Ivlev's fish exhibited increasing preferences for increasing size of food items, if the food items were relatively small, but they exhibited decreasing preferences as the sizes got larger. In short, if their preferences do indeed exhibit optimization of energetic efficiency, then $e(B, i, r)$ is not always an increasing function of *i* for fixed *B* and *r*. This prediction leads us again either to question the basic assumption about optimizing energetic efficiency or to modify the model.

4.4 A Fourth Model

4.4.1 *The Model.* The place in our model where we have been the most arbitrary is in the definition of THS. Schoener [36] suggests that time spent handling and swallowing a prey of size i might be more closely related to an exponential function of i than to a power function, in particular, a square.[10] Although substituting another power i^α for i^2 in the formula for THS in our third model might change the unsatisfactory prediction that e increases with increasing i for fixed B and r (Exercise 23), we shall take Schoener's idea as a cue. Continuing to bring in a term inversely proportional to some power of the body size B of the predator, let us investigate the implications of defining THS as

$$\text{THS} = k_5 \exp(k_6 i) B^{-s},$$

where k_5, k_6, and s are positive constants. It will be necessary to choose s larger than 3 in order to avoid the problems with Models 1 and 2. For concreteness, we shall choose s to be 4. (Computations for other values of s are left to the reader.[11]) Thus we are assuming

$$\text{THS} = k_5 \exp(k_6 i) B^{-4}. \tag{29}$$

Using (28), $e(B, i, r)$ becomes

$$e(B, i, r) = \frac{k_2 i^2}{k_1 k_3 B^3 r/v + k_1 k_4 k_5 B^{-1} \exp(k_6 i)}. \tag{30}$$

The assumptions underlying this formula are summarized in Table 1.

4.4.2 *Predictions.* Let us investigate the function $e(B, i, r)$ of (30) for fixed (positive) r and B. We have

$$e(B, i, r) = \frac{ai^2}{b + c \exp(di)} \tag{31}$$

where

$$a = k_2$$
$$b = k_1 k_3 B^3 r/v$$
$$c = k_1 k_4 k_5 B^{-1}$$
$$d = k_6.$$

The function $e(B, i, r)$ will give rise to curves which have the desired property that e is decreasing for increasing i for i sufficiently large, i.e., that de/di (actually $\partial e/\partial i$) is negative for i sufficiently large. To see this, we calculate

---

[10] At least for values of i which are relatively large compared to the size B of the predator.
[11] The reader might wish to decide if other choices of s would change the conclusions *qualitatively.*

Table 1. Assumptions Underlying the Fourth Model

1. Energy Requirements for the Predator per Day $E_R(B) = k_1 B^{1.5}$
2. Potential Energy of Food Items $E(i) = k_2 i^2$
3. Time Expended in Pursuit $TP = r/v$
4. Energy Expended in Pursuit $EP = k_3 B^{1.5} TP$
5. Time Spent Handling and Swallowing $THS = k_5 \exp(k_6 i) B^{-4}$
6. Energy Spent Handling and Swallowing $EHS = k_4 B^{1.5} THS$

Note: B is body size of the predator; i is body size of the prey; r is distance of the the prey from the predator; v is speed of pursuit of the predator, assumed constant independent of B, i, or r; k_1 through k_6 are positive constants.

$$\frac{de}{di} = \frac{[b + c \exp(di)](2ai) - ai^2 cd \exp(di)}{[b + c \exp(di)]^2}.$$

The denominator of de/di is positive for all positive i. The numerator can be rewritten as

$$A(i) = aci \exp(di)[2 - di] + 2abi = ai\{c \exp(di)[2 - di] + 2b\}.$$

Letting

$$x(i) = c \exp(di)[di - 2]$$

we can write

$$A(i) = ai[2b - x(i)].$$

For small positive values of i, $di - 2$ is negative and hence, since c is positive, $x(i)$ is negative. Thus, since a and b are positive, for small positive values of i, $A(i)$ is positive, de/di is positive, and the function e is increasing. For $i > 2/d$, $x(i)$ is positive. For i sufficiently large, $x(i)$ will dominate $2b$, and the function $A(i)$ will be negative. Hence e will be decreasing. Thus e starts out increasing for small positive values of i and decreases after a certain point. In particular, it does have this latter desired property.

To better understand what the graph of e versus i looks like, we need to know what happens to e for "intermediate" values of i. Let us consider dx/di. We have by a simple calculation:

$$\frac{dx}{di} = cd \exp(di)[di - 2] + cd \exp(di)$$

or

$$\frac{dx}{di} = cd \exp(di)[di - 1]. \tag{32}$$

Thus x will be a decreasing function of i for $i < 1/d$ and will increase for $i > 1/d$. Since $x(i)$ starts out less than $2b$ and eventually is larger than $2b$, there must be a first point i_0 where $x(i)$ crosses $2b$. (See Figure 11.7.) Since $x(i)$ is increasing at $i = i_0$, i_0 must be greater than $1/d$. Hence $x(i)$ is increas-

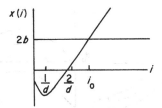

Figure 11.7

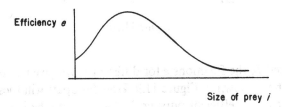

Figure 11.8

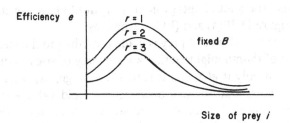

Figure 11.9

ing for $i \geq i_0$, and so $x(i)$ is greater than $2b$ for $i > i_0$. It follows from this discussion that

$$A(i) = ai[2b - x(i)]$$

is positive for $i < i_0$, 0 for $i = i_0$, and negative for $i > i_0$. Hence the curve $e(B, i, r)$ will have a graph which is like the data of Ivlev shown in Figure 11.6, at least to the extent that it is increasing for awhile, has a single peak, and then decreases. At least in a broad qualitative sense, the model does agree with the data.

Let us try to make some additional predictions from our model. First of all, using l'Hospital's rule, we observe that e approaches 0 as i gets large. Thus the line $i = 0$ is an asymptote of the function e. We shall not discuss the concavity of the curves, as that is probably not terribly important for predictive purposes. More or less, the curves e versus i look like the one shown in Figure 11.8.

Let us now consider $e(B, i, r)$ for B and i fixed but r varying. We see clearly from (30) that e decreases as r increases. That is natural: if the sizes of predator and prey are fixed, more energy is used for further pursuit.

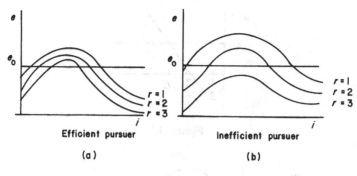

Figure 11.10

Thus, for fixed B, the functions e for different r will give rise to a family of curves like those shown in Figure 11.9. How far apart will these curves be? If a predator is an "efficient pursuer," either because he is fast (v is large) or because his "cost of pursuing" k_3 is small, then we would expect the family of curves to be relatively close together. On the other hand, inefficient pursuers, who lose a lot of energy in pursuit, would have the curves further apart. See Figure 11.10(a) and (b) for examples.

If we assume that choice of prey is made according to the measure e, then a simple rule of thumb might be that a given prey of size i at distance r will be taken if and only if $e(B, i, r)$ is sufficiently large, say larger than some amount e_0. The amount e_0 will be some threshold value and might vary with the abundance of food. We shall show in Section 4.7 that choosing according to some threshold value follows from several additional reasonable assumptions. In terms of our diagram, the prey will be taken if and only if $e(B, i, r)$ lies above a horizontal line at height e_0, as shown in Figure 11.10. Let us look at the different food items taken by the two types of predators. The efficient pursuers (Figure 11.10(a)) will take prey at a larger range of distances (the line $e = e_0$ crosses more r-curves) and a smaller range of prey sizes (the line $e = e_0$ crosses the various r-curves at a smaller range of values of i). The inefficient pursuers will do the opposite.[12] By similar reasoning, the efficient pursuer should have a larger home range,[13] i.e., the maximum distance he travels for food will be larger than that of the inefficient pursuer. However, he will have a smaller *prey-size range*, i.e., the maximum size prey he takes will be smaller. These predictions are made by Schoener [36] and also by MacArthur and Levins [25], MacArthur and Pianka [26], and Rosenzweig [35]. Another way of stating these predictions is that the species with the largest home range will have the smallest prey-size range, and the species with the smallest home range will have the largest prey-size range. Note that these predictions are purely qualitative, in the sense we discussed in Section 3.2. However, they are precise predictions and can be tested by

---

[12] Our reasoning contains a subtle fallacy. We will uncover it later, in Section 4.8.3.
[13] The word "range" is probably not the right word to use for this concept, but we shall use it for conformity with the literature.

looking at data. We shall compare the second prediction to data in the next section.

Before looking at data, let us make one further prediction. As the relative abundance of food increases, the threshold e_0 will increase—the predator can "afford" to take items which are more energetically efficient, since there are more such items available. Hence the home range will decrease, and the prey size range will as well. Since the curves for the efficient pursuers are closer together than the curves for the inefficient pursuers, the *variation* in home range as food abundance changes will be (relatively) greater than the variation for the inefficient pursuers. On the other hand, the variation in the prey size range will be less than the variation in prey size range for the inefficient pursuers. (In terms of the graph, moving the line $e = e_0$ up by a small amount causes a relatively larger variation in maximum size of r traveled for the efficient pursuers than for the inefficient pursuers, and a relatively larger variation in maximum size of i eaten for the inefficient pursuers than for the efficient pursuers.) Put another way, the species with the largest relative variation in home range will have the smallest relative variation in prey-size range, and the species with the smallest relative variation in home range will have the largest relative variation in prey-size range. In the next section, we shall make this prediction more precise, and look at some data.

4.5 Test of the Home Range Predictions

Table 2 gives data on the body weight, home range, and prey-size range for various North American raptors.[14] Unfortunately, the data on size range is in terms of weight, not length, but we shall use it since the length data would be expected to have similar qualitative characteristics, length being an increasing function of weight. The number of observations is shown in the column labeled N, the mean home range and prey-size range are given in the columns marked M. The data in this table is unfortunately incomplete, as some of the prey-size ranges are missing. However, among the birds for which we have both pieces of information, the same raptor, *Falco*, a falcon, does have the largest mean home range (0.78) and the smallest mean prey-size range (84.4). Unfortunately, the raptor with the lowest mean home range, *Buteo*, an owl, does not have the largest mean prey-size range. One reason that these comparisons may not mean too much is that our predictions were derived under the assumption of fixed body size B, and hence fixed body weight, while of the four birds in Table 2 whose home range and prey-size range were measured, none of them have the same body weight. The prediction could have been tested if prey-size range had been obtained for the two *B. jamaicensis*, the Michigan and Wyoming variants, for these had the same weights. This illustrates a common problem in model-building: data is often not in the right form or not available.

[14] Birds of prey with strong notched beaks and strong talons, e.g., falcons, eagles, and owls.

Table 2. Number of Observations (N), Mean (M), Standard Deviation (SD), and Coefficient of Variation (CV = 100SD/M) of Home Range and Prey-Size Range for Some North American Raptors[†]

Species	Body Weight (gm)	Home Range (sq. miles)				Prey-Size Range (gm)			
		N	M	SD	CV	N	M	SD	CV
Buteo lineatus (Michigan)	625	37	0.23	0.13	59	27	759	589	78
B. jamaicensis (Michigan)	1126	5	1.64	0.35	21	...	...	...	...
B. jamaicensis (Wyoming)	1126	8	0.73	0.35	48	7	3025	1786	59
Accipiter cooperi (Michigan)	470	15	0.77	0.64	83	11	1135	142	13
Falco sparverius (Wyoming)	114	11	0.78	0.50	64	8	84.4	63.2	75
B. swainsoni (Wyoming)	988	4	1.12	0.57	51	...	...	...	...

[†] Calculated from data of Craighead and Craighead [9]. Years combined for Michigan raptors. Food-size range data based on records from separate nests. Each nest considered as one observation. Insects not included. Adapted from Schoener [36, p. 290].

Table 3

Mice (oz)	1.7	2.0	2.1	1.9	2.5
Elephants (oz)	320,000	281,600	390,400	281,600	

While we are dealing with this data and recognizing that it is probably not in the right form to test our prediction, let us return to the final prediction made in the previous section, namely, that efficient pursuers will have greater relative variation in home range than inefficient pursuers, but smaller relative variation in prey size range. To test this prediction, we shall have to make more precise what the term "relative variation" means.

Table 2 gives the standard deviation in home range and prey-size range for the different birds in the columns marked SD. The SD alone is not a good measure of variation for comparison purposes if two different variables have quite different means. To give an example, suppose we calculate the weights of mice and elephants as in Table 3. For the mice, the mean weight is 2.04 oz, the standard deviation 0.2966 oz. For the elephants, the mean weight is 318,400 oz, the standard deviation 51,300 oz. Are elephants' weights so much more variable than mice's weights? This question is hard to answer. The standard deviation is larger. Of course, we would get a smaller standard deviation than 51,300 for the elephants' weights if we simply measured their weights in tons. In tons, the mean of their weights is 9.95 and the standard deviation is 1.603. Thus the standard deviation can be large if we simply use large numbers, even though *relative* to the size of the numbers this deviation is small. To compensate for these problems, statisticians calculate the *coefficient of variation* CV, which is a measure of relative dispersion. It is defined as

$$CV = 100 \times \frac{SD}{M}.$$

For the mice, the coefficient of variation is

$$CV = 100 \times \frac{0.2966 \text{ oz}}{2.04 \text{ oz}} = 14.5\%.$$

For the elephants, it is

$$CV = 100 \times \frac{51,300 \text{ oz}}{318,400 \text{ oz}} = 16.1\%.$$

Broadly speaking, the variability of weights of the elephants is comparable to that of the mice. Incidentally, had we found a sample of elephants with mean weight 318,400, but standard deviation 0.2966 oz, the elephants would all have weighed about the same, for all practical purposes. The variability in weight would have been small compared to that of the mice. (The reader should check this.) Also, note that the CV is independent of the units used. For if we use tons for the elephants, we still get a CV of $100 \times (1.603/9.95)$ = 16.1%.

Table 2 gives coefficient of variation for both home range and prey-size range. The species in Table 2 with the greatest CV in home range is also that with the smallest CV in prey-size range. That is the *Accipiter*, a hawk. (Note that *Accipiter* has a higher SD for prey-size range than *Falco*, but it is the CV which is the important measure of variation.) On the other hand, the species with lowest CV home range among those whose prey-size range is known is *B. jamaicensis*, and this does not have the highest CV for prey-size range. Once again, we shall not make much of these observations, because the data does not fit the assumption of equal body size (and hence weight).

Since the Michigan and Wyoming variants of *B. jamaicensis* have the same weight, our predictions for them can be compared. The SD obtained from home range was the same for both species. However, since the means were so different, these represent quite different variations in range. Note that while the Michigan birds have a much greater mean home range, the Wyoming birds have a much higher CV. Our model predicts that for home range, the higher CV and higher M both correspond to greater efficiency of pursuit. This data clearly shows that higher CV does not necessarily correspond to higher M, though we expected it to.[15] We shall return to the relation between M and CV for home-range and prey-size range in Section 4.8.

---

[15] Since we will uncover a subtle fallacy in the reasoning used to obtain this prediction, which seems to be violated here, we will not discard the model.

4.6 Optimal Body Size

Let us continue the analysis of our fourth model and see what it predicts about optimal body size. Suppose first that i and r are fixed, but B is allowed to vary. Then, from (30) we obtain

$$e(B, i, r) = \frac{\alpha}{\beta B^3 + \gamma B^{-1}} = \frac{\alpha B}{\beta B^4 + \gamma},$$

where

$$\alpha = k_2 i^2$$

$$\beta = k_1 k_3 r / v$$

$$\gamma = k_1 k_4 k_5 \exp(k_6 i).$$

Thus

$$\frac{de}{dB} = \frac{(\beta B^4 + \gamma)\alpha - \alpha B(4\beta B^3)}{(\beta B^4 + \gamma)^2}$$

$$= \frac{\alpha\gamma - 3\alpha\beta B^4}{(\beta B^4 + \gamma)^2}.$$

It follows that $de/dB = 0$ when

$$\alpha\gamma - 3\alpha\beta B^4 = 0,$$

or when

$$B = \sqrt[4]{\frac{\alpha\gamma}{3\alpha\beta}},$$

or when

$$B = \sqrt[4]{\frac{k_4 k_5 v \exp(k_6 i)}{3 k_3 r}}. \tag{33}$$

The value of B given by (33) is a maximum point for e, since de/dB is positive for B less than this value and negative afterwards, as can easily be seen from the formula for the derivative. Thus the fraction of required energy provided per unit of energy expended to capture a prey of size i at distance r is maximized by predators of body size given by (33). How does this optimal body size vary with i and r? As r stays fixed and i increases, it is clear from (33) that the optimal B increases. Thus the larger the prey at a fixed distance, the larger the optimal body size. As i stays fixed and r increases, the optimal B decreases. Thus the further the prey of a fixed size, the smaller the optimal body size. (Else, more energy is used in pursuit.) In general, larger B is most efficient if most prey are of large size and are fairly close. It is of interest to consider the sensitivity of optimal body size to some of the other parameters. As "cost of pursuit" k_3 decreases or as speed v increases, an increase occurs in optimal B. Thus "efficient pursuers" can have larger body size. (One reason that this prediction might be a little off is that our model does not compute added energy use by a predator if the speed v is increased. That high speeds and strenuous activity do lead to more energy use would suggest a corresponding mitigation in optimal body size for the speedy pursuers.) Finally, we note that as the "cost of handling and swallowing" k_4 increases, the optimal body size increases.

The authors do not know of precise tests of these various predictions. However, it would be interesting to make such tests. In any case, the model has helped us to carefully think out certain relationships.

All of these predictions treat one factor as varying and hold all of the others fixed. However, at least insofar as i and r are concerned, food items appear in a variety of sizes and at a variety of distances. One body size will be optimal for one i and r and another for different i and r. How can one predict optimal body size if this is the case? To answer this question, we shall have to consider how a predator chooses a diet if faced with a distribution of potential food items of different sizes and at different distances. This we shall do in the next section.

4.7 The Greedy Algorithm

Suppose a predator were completely omniscient about the distribution of potential food items as to size and distance for the coming day. How would he choose food so as to obtain his minimum energy requirements[16] for the day with the least amount of energy used?

Let the food items be listed, together with their (relative) energy outputs E_O/E_R and their energy inputs E_I. Having chosen a set S of these items, the predator could calculate his total relative energetic efficiency for the day as follows:

$$e = \frac{\text{total energy obtained/energy required}}{\text{total energy expended}}$$

or

$$e(S) = \frac{\sum\limits_S E_O/E_R}{\sum\limits_S E_I}, \qquad (34)$$

where the indicator S under the summation sign means that the outputs and inputs are tallied only for items in the set S. The problem of how to choose food items so as to meet the daily requirements and make $e(S)$ of (34) as

---

[16] The reader might wish to consider how the discussion of this section would change if the minimum energy requirements E_R are stated in terms of net energy $E_O - E_I$ rather than energy input E_O.

Table 4

Body Length i (in cm)	Distance r (in m)	Number $N(i, r)$ of (i, r) Food Items	$E_O = E(i)$	$e(B, i, r)$
10	1	12	20	3
10	2	5	20	2
10	3	1	20	1
12	1	2	36	6
12	2	6	36	4
12	3	4	36	2

large as possible was discussed at some length in Section 3.2 of Roberts [33] where it was called a variant of the global optimum efficiency problem or GOE problem (problem (6) of that paper). A natural procedure for optimizing $e(S)$, and one which follows from our assumption that predators choose food items with largest possible relative energetic efficiencies, is for the predator to be greedy. At each stage, he looks at the possible food items that are (still) available and chooses that item which has the maximum relative energetic efficiency

$$e = \frac{E_O/E_R}{E_I}.$$

(If several items have the same maximum value, he chooses any one of them.) He keeps on choosing such items until the daily requirements are met, i.e., until the sum of the E_O/E_R for items chosen just reaches or exceeds 1, or until the sum of the E_O over items chosen just reaches or exceeds E_R.

Let us give a concrete example of how the greedy algorithm would work. Suppose during a 24-hour period, the distribution of food items can be expected to appear (before a predator of given body size B) as in Table 4. Table 4 also lists the amount of energy $E(i)$ attainable from a given item and the relative energetic efficiency $e(B, i, r)$. Suppose the predator's total energy requirement for the 24-hour period is $E_R = E_R(B) = 500$ kcal. The food items with the maximum $e(B, i, r)$ are the $(12, 1)$ items, i.e., items of size 12 cm and at distance 1 m. There are two such items, which should be eaten first, supplying a total of $2 \times 36/500 = 72/500$ kcal of food energy per kcal of energy required. The next most efficient food item is the $(12, 2)$ item. Six of these are available, supplying $6 \times 36/500$ kcal per kcal required, making a total of $288/500$ so far. The next most efficient source of food is the $(10, 1)$ item. Twelve of these exist, to supply a total of $12 \times 20/500 = 240/500$ kcal per kcal required. However, $288/500 + 240/500 = 528/500$, which is larger than 1. Eating 11 of the 12 $(10, 1)$ items will supply just enough energy to meet the requirements, since

$$11 \times \frac{20}{500} = \frac{220}{500},$$

and

$$\frac{288}{500} + \frac{220}{500} = \frac{508}{500},$$

while

$$10 \times \frac{20}{500} = \frac{200}{500},$$

and

$$\frac{288}{500} + \frac{200}{500} = \frac{488}{500}.$$

Thus the greedy strategy for the predator omiscient about the distribution of food will be to eat two of the (12, 1) items, six of the (12, 2) items, 11 of the (10, 1) items, and none of the other items.

Not all of the items will be present at one time. However, knowing ahead of time how many items of each kind can be expected, the predator can calculate the number $m(i, r)$ of (i, r) items to be eaten in his greedy solution. Then he can use these numbers to calculate a threshold value e_0, which is the minimum $e(B, i, r)$ over all (i, r) for which $m(i, r) \neq 0$. If an item of type (i, r) appears, he can choose to pursue it if $e(B, i, r)$ is above threshold value and if he has not yet eaten $m(i, r)$ such items. Schoener [36] speaks of the predator as somehow being "programmed" to choose its prey according to this procedure. As the food supply fluctuates, the distribution of food items will change. According to Schoener, "hunger" functions to change the program, "telling" the predator to change its threshold e_0 and its numbers $m(i, r)$. This assumption seems to be satisfied by data. Holling [17] has shown that mantids will travel greater distances to capture prey when hungry than when near satiation.

Does the greedy strategy or greedy algorithm necessarily lead to the optimal selection of food items, or is there a selection of food items which would lead to a higher $e(S)$? In [33, section 3.2] we showed that the latter could be the case. For example, suppose Table 5 gives the information about the available food items and suppose that $E_R = 760$. Then the greedy algorithm would say to choose first the (12, 2) item and then the (11, 3) item. However, choosing the (12, 2) item and (10, 4) item would also just meet daily requirements $E_R = 760$. We shall see that the latter would be a

Table 5

Body Length i	Distance r	$N(i, r)$	$E_O = E(i)$	$e(B, i, r)$
12	2	1	750	7.5
11	3	1	250	5.0
10	4	1	10	1.0

better solution. Now, by definition,

$$\frac{E_O/E_R}{E_I} = e(B, i, r),$$

so

$$E_I = \frac{E_O/E_R}{e(B, i, r)}.$$

Thus the energy inputs for the items in Table 5 are as follows.

Item	E_I
(12, 2)	0.132
(11, 3)	0.066
(10, 4)	0.013

Thus the greedy solution $S = \{(12, 2), (11, 3)\}$ has

$$e(S) = \frac{750/760 + 250/760}{0.132 + 0.066} \approx 6.6,$$

while the solution $T = \{(12, 2), (10, 4)\}$ has

$$e(S) = \frac{750/760 + 10/760}{0.132 + 0.013} \approx 6.9.$$

(This example is obtained from one given in Roberts [33, table 4]).

Roberts [33, section 3.2] showed that this greedy algorithm sometimes leads to an optimal solution to the (variant of the) GOE problem, i.e., a selection of items which maximizes $e(S)$ of (34), and sometimes it does not. However, he argued that it was a natural procedure to use and that we probably use variants of it in our daily decisions about investments. Thus, although it might not be the best procedure to use, in building a *descriptive* model of behavior it is not unreasonable to assume that the animal whose behavior is being described does indeed use this procedure. (If we were building a *prescriptive* model, i.e., one which tried to show how the animal should behave, we would have to worry about the procedure.) Thus we shall assume that our pure pursuer uses the greedy algorithm.

Let us remark before leaving this section that we are making several assumptions which are reasonable alone but which in combination might appear peculiar. We are assuming that the predator somehow "knows" the forthcoming food distribution but that he will not know enough to stay away from a procedure which will not always get him an optimal total energetic efficiency. Rather, he finds the greedy procedure easier in practice. Perhaps the explanation is that he does not actually "know" the distribution but "learns" by experience which levels e_0 and $m(i, r)$ to use to be as efficient as possible given that he will use the greedy procedure.

4.8 Using the Greedy Algorithm for Further Predictions: Computer Simulation and Assumptions about Food Distribution

When a model is as complicated as the one we have presented, its ramifications can sometimes be better understood by using computer simulation. In particular, various predictions of our energetic efficiency model can be highlighted using this procedure, and new predictions can be derived. The procedure is the following. For a given choice of parameters k_1 to k_6, and v, and of variable B, one can calculate values of $E(i)$, $E_R(B)$, and $e(B, i, r)$. Using the greedy algorithm, one can calculate the number of prey $m(i, r)$ of each type (i, r) taken from a given population. Using the numbers $m(i, r)$, one can calculate such quantities as the mean and maximum r for food items taken, the mean and maximum i, the coefficient of variation of the r, or the coefficient of variation of the i. In the example given in the previous section,

$$m(12, 1) = 2$$

$$m(12, 2) = 6$$

$$m(10, 1) = 11$$

$$m(i, r) = 0, \quad \text{otherwise.}$$

Thus the mean distance of prey taken is

$$\frac{2 \times 1 + 6 \times 2 + 11 \times 1}{19} = 25/19 \approx 1.3,$$

the standard deviation of the distance is

$$\sqrt{\frac{(2 \times 1^2 + 6 \times 2^2 + 11 \times 1^2) - 19 \times (25/19)^2}{19 - 1}} \approx 0.48$$

and the coefficient of variation of the distance is

$$100 \times \frac{0.48}{1.3} \approx 37\%.$$

Having such statistics, one can get a better feel for various predictions about the relation of these statistics to the parameters or variables, for example, the prediction that as a pursuer becomes more efficient, i.e., as k_3 decreases or v increases, the maximum r (home range) will increase and the maximum i (prey-size range) will decrease. This is one prediction about efficient versus inefficient pursuers we studied in Section 4.5. Also, the predictions can be used, with data, to help estimate the parameters of the model.

What is needed to perform a computer simulation is to have examples like that of the previous section, namely sample populations or numbers $N(i, r)$ giving the number of (i, r) food items of each type. In this section we shall discuss how to generate such populations for use in computer

Figure 11.11

simulations. Then we shall give an example of such a population and carry out several calculations with it. Our discussion of generation of the populations follows closely that of Schoener [36].

4.8.1 *Abundance of Food at a Given Distance.* It is natural to assume, as a start, that the appearance of food items over a large time period such as a day is uniform over the area in question. For the purposes of computer simulations we will want a discrete selection of distances, say only integer values. Such a selection can be obtained as follows. Suppose D is the density of food items, i.e., the total number of items appearing per unit area during the day. The number of such items appearing in a circle of radius ρ is $\pi\rho^2 D$. Let us consider all points at distances between $r - 1$ and r from the center of the area considered (the predator's perch, or monitoring point). These points fall in an annulus bounded by the circles of radius $r - 1$ and r. (See Figure 11.11.) The number of food items appearing in the annulus is given by

$$N(r) = \pi r^2 D - \pi(r - 1)^2 D$$

or

$$N(r) = \pi D(2r - 1). \tag{35}$$

This number can be used as an estimate of the number of food items at distance r. One normally performs the calculation for a "reasonable" number of integer values of r, for example $r = 1, 2, \cdots, 10$. Or one uses the formula (35) in the calculation of optimal solutions using the greedy algorithm.

The discussion of food abundance at the end of Section 4.4 can now be made more precise. If D increases (food becomes more abundant), e_0 (the threshold of energetic efficiency of food items eaten) should increase. Then the home range and prey-size range should decrease.

Remark.[17] We might be a little more precise in the determination of the number of food items occurring at distance r if we used the annulus between $r - 1/2$ and $r + 1/2$. To see this, we will show that for $d \geq 1$, the mean distance from the origin of all items occurring between distances $d - 1$ and d is between $d - 1/2$ and $d - 1/3$ and approaches $d - 1/2$ as d increases. Hence the mean distance from the origin of items in an annulus of width 1 is close to the midpoint of the distances from the origin of items in the annulus. It follows that the number of food items at distance r, at least

---

[17] This remark may be omitted, and if it is, the reader should turn immediately to Section 4.8.2. To appreciate the proof, a student should be familiar with continuous probability density functions.

for reasonably large r, can be estimated by using the annulus between $r - 1/2$ and $r + 1/2$, and counting the number of items in here, namely (by Eq. (35))

$$\pi D[2(r + 1/2) - 1] = 2\pi Dr.$$

This is a better estimate of the number of food items at distance r than (35).

To verify our claim about mean distance, suppose all food items are contained in a circle of radius Δ. Then the probability that a given item is found in a circle of radius d is given by

$$F(d) = \frac{\pi d^2 D}{\pi \Delta^2 D} = \frac{d^2}{\Delta^2}.$$

The probability density function corresponding to this cumulative distribution function is given by

$$f(d) = F'(d) = 2d/\Delta^2.$$

Now the expected distance e_d of a food item from the origin given that the food item is in the interval between $d - 1$ and d is given by

$$e_d = \frac{1}{p_d} \int_{d-1}^{d} sf(s)ds,$$

where p_d is the probability that the food item is in the interval between $d - 1$ and d. By earlier calculation, the number of items in this interval is $\pi D(2d - 1)$, so

$$p_d = \frac{\pi D(2d - 1)}{\pi \Delta^2 D} = \frac{2d - 1}{\Delta^2}.$$

Hence

$$e_d = \frac{\Delta^2}{2d - 1} \int_{d-1}^{d} s \frac{2s}{\Delta^2} ds$$

$$= \frac{\Delta^2}{2d - 1} \int_{d-1}^{d} \frac{2s^2}{\Delta^2} ds$$

$$= \frac{2}{3} \frac{1}{2d - 1} [s^3]_{d-1}^{d}$$

$$= \frac{2}{3} \frac{1}{2d - 1} [3d^2 - 3d + 1]$$

$$= \frac{1}{3} \frac{1}{d - 1/2} [3d^2 - 3d + 1]$$

$$= \frac{1}{d - 1/2} [d^2 - d + 1/3]$$

$$= \frac{1}{d - 1/2} \left[(d - 1/2)^2 + \frac{1}{12} \right]$$

$$= d - 1/2 + \frac{1}{12d - 6}.$$

Since $d \geq 1$, the term $1/(12d - 6)$ is between 0 and $1/6$, and so e_d is between $d - 1/2$ and $d - 1/3$. As d gets large,

$$e_d - (d - 1/2) = \frac{1}{12d - 6} \to 0,$$

which is what we wanted to show.

4.8.2 *Distribution of Food Sizes.* Food items are not uniformly distributed as to size. Data of Schoener and Janzen [37] suggest that food sizes have a log-normal distribution. A variable i is distributed *log-normally*, with mean μ and standard deviation σ, if $\ln i$ is distributed normally with mean $\ln \mu$ and standard deviation σ. For the purposes of computer simulation, we will want a discrete selection of food sizes, say only integer values. We shall see how to obtain such a distribution of food sizes using a log-normal distribution.

First, we shall fix the parameters, mean μ and standard deviation σ, needed to define a log-normal. Schoener and Janzen give values of these parameters obtained from distributions of real food items. Suppose we have calculated the number $N(r)$ of food items at distance r, for example, by the procedures of the previous subsection. The fraction of these food items which are between sizes $i - 1/2$ and $i + 1/2$ can be used for the fraction at size i in a computer simulation. This fraction p_i can be calculated by using a normal table and calculating the probability that a normally distributed random variable with mean $\ln \mu$ and standard deviation σ will lie between $\ln (i - 1/2)$ and $\ln (i + 1/2)$. Specifically, one would look in a table of the standard normal distribution (mean 0, standard deviation 1) for the probability that a standard normal lies between

$$\frac{\ln (i - 1/2) - \ln \mu}{\sigma} \quad \text{and} \quad \frac{\ln (i + 1/2) - \ln \mu}{\sigma}.$$

This fraction of the items of size i would be multiplied by the number of food items at distance r to obtain the number $N(i, r)$ of (i, r) food items. In sum,

$$N(i, r) = p_i N(r).$$

The number $N(i, r)$ would be rounded to the nearest integer. (This procedure assumes that the distribution of food sizes at a given distance is independent of the distance, a not unreasonable assumption.)

To give an example, suppose $D = 1$, $\mu = 10$, and $\sigma = 0.5$. Then by Equation (35), the number of food items at distance $r = 10$ is given by

$$N(10) = \pi D(2r - 1) = 19\pi \approx 59.7.$$

The fraction p_i of these items which have size $i = 2$ is given as follows: find the probability that a standard normal is between

$$\frac{\ln(2 - 1/2) - \ln 10}{0.5} \quad \text{and} \quad \frac{\ln(2 + 1/2) - \ln 10}{0.5}$$

or between

$$-3.79 \text{ and } -2.77.$$

This probability is given by $p_i = 0.003$, and so the number of $(i, r) = (2, 10)$ items is

$$N(2, 10) = p_2 N(10) = 0.003 \times 59.7 = 0.18,$$

i.e., 0 rounded to the nearest integer.

It is interesting to calculate what range of values of i we will need to consider. We will want i's so that $N(i, r)$ comes out to be at least 0.5, since we are rounding off to the nearest integer. Thus we want

$$p_i \times \pi D(2r - 1) \geq 0.5.$$

If $r = R$ is the maximum value of r considered, we want

$$p_i \geq \frac{0.5}{\pi D(2R - 1)} = \lambda.$$

We will certainly obtain all such i's if we eliminate i's beyond which the two tails of the log-normal are both less than λ. That is, suppose we pick an integer i_L so that if

$$\frac{\ln(i_L - 1/2) - \ln \mu}{\sigma} = k,$$

then the probability that a standard normal is below k is less than λ. Then any integer $i < i_L$ will certainly have $p_i < \lambda$. Similarly, if integer i_U is chosen so that if

$$\frac{\ln(i_U + 1/2) - \ln \mu}{\sigma} = l,$$

then the probability that a standard normal is above l is less than λ, then for $i > i_U$, p_i is certainly less than λ.

From the above equations, we have

$$i_L = 1/2 + \exp[\sigma k + \ln \mu]$$
$$i_U = -1/2 + \exp[\sigma l + \ln \mu].$$

In our example, $\mu = 10$, $\sigma = 0.5$, and $D = 1$. Suppose $R = 10$. Then

$$\lambda = \frac{0.5}{19\pi} = 0.008.$$

Thus

$$k = -2.41$$
$$l = 2.41,$$

and so

$$i_L = 3.50, \text{ which must be treated as 3}$$

$$i_U = 32.87, \text{ which must be treated as 33.}$$

Thus values of i between 3 and 33 will capture all of the cases needed. (This explains why we obtained such a low probability of 0.003 in our calculations with $i = 2$ above.)

4.8.3 *A Sample Simulation.* In this section, we shall perform a sample simulation. We shall want to check some of the home range predictions of Section 4.4. In particular, let us check how changes in food density D affect the distances traveled and sizes of food items eaten, and let us see how changes in velocity v of the predator affect these values. We shall start with a predator of fixed size $B = 1$. For the sake of discussion, we choose the following values of the parameters k_i:

$$k_1 = 500, \quad k_2 = 1, \quad k_3 = 1/500, \quad k_4 = 1/500, \quad k_5 = 0.01, \quad k_6 = 1.$$

We shall consider, for comparison, two values of v, $v = 1$ and $v = 2$.

Table 6. Probability p_i that a Log-Normal Random Variable with $\mu = 5$ and $\sigma = 0.5$ Lies between $i - 1/2$ and $i + 1/2$.

i	p_i
<1	0
1	0.0080
2	0.0743
3	0.1566
4	0.1779
5	0.1585
6	0.1232
7	0.0925
8	0.0644
9	0.0443
10	0.0309
11	0.0219
12	0.0139
13	0.0103
14	0.0067
15	0.0047
16	0.0035
17	0.0024
>17	0.0060

Table 7. Number $N(i, r)$ of Prey of Type (i, r) if Food Density $D = 1$ and Log-Normal Distribution Has Parameters $\mu = 5$ and $\sigma = 0.5$[†]

i \ r	1	2	3	4	5	6	7	8	9	10
<1	0	0	0	0	0	0	0	0	0	0
1	0.03	0.08	0.13	0.18	0.23	0.28	0.33	0.38	0.43	0.48
2	0.23	0.70	1.17	1.63	2.10	2.57	3.03	3.50	3.97	4.43
3	0.49	1.48	2.46	3.44	4.43	5.41	6.40	7.38	8.36	9.35
4	0.56	1.68	2.80	3.91	5.03	6.15	7.27	8.38	9.50	10.62
5	0.498[a]	1.49	2.49	3.49	4.48	5.48	6.47	7.47	8.47	9.46
6	0.39	1.16	1.94	2.71	3.48	4.26	5.03	5.81	6.58	7.35
7	0.29	0.87	1.45	2.03	2.62	3.20	3.78	4.36	4.94	5.52
8	0.20	0.61	1.01	1.42	1.82	2.23	2.63	3.03	3.44	3.84
9	0.14	0.42	0.70	0.97	1.25	1.53	1.81	2.09	2.37	2.64
10	0.10	0.29	0.49	0.68	0.87	1.07	1.26	1.46	1.65	1.84
11	0.07	0.21	0.34	0.48	0.62	0.76	0.89	1.03	1.17	1.31
12	0.04	0.13	0.22	0.31	0.39	0.48	0.57	0.66	0.74	0.83
13	0.03	0.10	0.16	0.23	0.29	0.36	0.42	0.49	0.55	0.61
14	0.02	0.06	0.11	0.15	0.19	0.23	0.27	0.32	0.36	0.40
15	0.01	0.04	0.07	0.10	0.13	0.16	0.19	0.22	0.25	0.28
16	0.01	0.03	0.05	0.08	0.10	0.12	0.14	0.16	0.19	0.21
17	0.01	0.02	0.04	0.05	0.07	0.08	0.10	0.11	0.13	0.14
>17	0.02	0.06	0.09	0.13	0.17	0.21	0.25	0.28	0.32	0.36

[†] $N(i, r)$ must be rounded to nearest integer. If $D = d$, multiply these numbers by d and then round.

[a] Three digits are included because writing this as 0.50 would round to 1 prey, whereas 0.498 rounds to 0 prey.

We start by considering prey at distances $r = 1, 2, \cdots, 10$, and setting $D = 1$. We also choose $\mu = 5$ and $\sigma = 0.5$. With these values, we calculate $i_L = 1$ and $i_U = 17$, using the method of the end of the previous section. It will turn out that with the rest of the parameters chosen, we shall never have to consider i's at the ends of these ranges, or r's at the higher end of the range.

With all of the parameters chosen, we now compute p_i in Table 6, $N(i, r)$ in Table 7, and $e(B, i, r)$ in Table 8. The reader might wish to check some of the calculations. If v is changed from 1 to 2, the values of $e(B, i, r)$ change. The new values are shown in Table 9. Values of D can also be changed. Multiplying D by d will simply multiply all values of $N(i, r)$ by d. We will consider the cases $D = 2$ and $D = 4$ as well as $D = 1$. (Of course, for larger D, it might be necessary to consider larger ranges of i. It turns out that with the other parameters as chosen, i's other than those represented in the computations displayed are not needed.)

Since $k_1 = 500$ and $B = 1$,

$$e_R(B) = k_1 B^{1.5} = 500.$$

A greedy algorithm with this value of $e_R(B)$ is carried out for each choice of D and v. The results of this algorithm for each case are shown in Table 10,

Table 8. Values of $e(B, i, r)$ if $B = 1$, $k_1 = 500$, $k_2 = 1$, $k_3 = 1/500$, $k_4 = 1/500$, $k_5 = 0.01$, $k_6 = 1$, and $v = 1$.

i \ r	1	2	3	4	5	6	7	8	9	10
1	0.97	0.49	0.33	0.25	0.20	0.17	0.14	0.12	0.11	0.10
2	3.72	1.93	1.30	0.98	0.79	0.66	0.57	0.50	0.44	0.40
3	7.49	4.09	2.81	2.14	1.73	1.45	1.25	1.10	0.98	0.88
4	10.35	6.28	4.51	3.52	2.88	2.44	2.12	1.87	1.68	1.52
5	10.06	7.18	5.58	4.56	3.86	3.34	2.95	2.64	2.38	2.18
6	7.15	5.97	5.12	4.48	3.98	3.59	3.26	2.99	2.76	2.57
7	4.09	3.78	3.51	3.27	3.07	2.89	2.73	2.58	2.45	2.34
8	2.08	2.01	1.95	1.89	1.84	1.79	1.74	1.69	1.65	1.61
9	0.99	0.98	0.96	0.95	0.94	0.93	0.92	0.91	0.90	0.89
10	0.45	0.45	0.45	0.45	0.44	0.44	0.44	0.44	0.44	0.43
11	0.20	0.20	0.20	0.20	0.20	0.20	0.20	0.20	0.20	0.20
12	0.09	0.09	0.09	0.09	0.09	0.09	0.09	0.09	0.09	0.09
13	0.04	0.04	0.04	0.04	0.04	0.04	0.04	0.04	0.04	0.04
14	0.02	0.02	0.02	0.02	0.02	0.02	0.02	0.02	0.02	0.02
15	0.01	0.01	0.01	0.01	0.01	0.01	0.01	0.01	0.01	0.01
16	0	0	0	0	0	0	0	0	0	0
17	0	0	0	0	0	0	0	0	0	0

Table 9. Values of $e(B, i, r)$ Modified from Those of Table 8 if $v = 2$.

i \ r	1	2	3	4	5	6	7	8	9	10
1	1.90	0.97	0.65	0.49	0.40	0.33	0.28	0.25	0.22	0.20
2	6.97	3.72	2.54	1.93	1.55	1.30	1.12	0.98	0.87	0.79
3	12.84	7.49	5.29	4.09	3.33	2.81	2.43	2.14	1.91	1.73
4	15.30	10.35	7.82	6.28	5.25	4.51	3.95	3.52	3.17	2.88
5	12.60	10.06	8.38	7.18	6.27	5.58	5.02	4.56	4.18	3.86
6	7.94	7.15	6.50	5.97	5.51	5.12	4.78	4.48	4.22	3.98
7	4.27	4.09	3.93	3.78	3.64	3.51	3.39	3.27	3.17	3.07
8	2.11	2.08	2.04	2.01	1.98	1.95	1.92	1.89	1.87	1.84
9	0.99	0.99	0.98	0.98	0.97	0.96	0.96	0.95	0.95	0.94
10	0.45	0.45	0.45	0.45	0.45	0.45	0.45	0.45	0.44	0.44
11	0.20	0.20	0.20	0.20	0.20	0.20	0.20	0.20	0.20	0.20
12	0.09	0.09	0.09	0.09	0.09	0.09	0.09	0.09	0.09	0.09
13	0.04	0.04	0.04	0.04	0.04	0.04	0.04	0.04	0.04	0.04
14	0.02	0.02	0.02	0.02	0.02	0.02	0.02	0.02	0.02	0.02
15	0.01	0.01	0.01	0.01	0.01	0.01	0.01	0.01	0.01	0.01
16	0	0	0	0	0	0	0	0	0	0
17	0	0	0	0	0	0	0	0	0	0

Table 10. Results of Greedy Algorithm—Items and Numbers Chosen (in the Order Chosen) until $e_R(B) = 500$ Is Reached, for Different Values of D and v.

$D = 1, v = 1$

Item											
(i, r)	(4, 1)	(5, 2)[a]	(4, 2)	(6, 2)	(5, 3)	(6, 3)	(5, 4)	(4, 3)	(6, 4)	(3, 2)	(6, 5)[b]
Number											
$m(i, r)$	1	1	2	1	2	2	3	3	3	1	1

$D = 2, v = 1$

(i, r)	(4, 1)	(5, 1)	(3, 1)	(5, 2)	(6, 1)	(4, 2)	(6, 2)	(5, 3)	(6, 3)
$m(i, r)$	1	1	1	3	1	3	2	5	3

$D = 4, v = 1$

(i, r)	(4, 1)	(5, 1)	(3, 1)	(5, 2)	(6, 1)	(4, 2)	(6, 2)
$m(i, r)$	2	2	2	6	2	7	2

$D = 1, v = 2$

(i, r)	(4, 1)	(4, 2)	(5, 2)	(5, 3)	(4, 3)	(3, 2)	(5, 4)	(6, 2)	(6, 3)	(4, 4)	(5, 5)
$m(i, r)$	1	2	1	2	3	1	3	1	2	4	3

$D = 2, v = 2$

(i, r)	(4, 1)	(3, 1)	(5, 1)	(4, 2)	(5, 2)	(5, 3)	(6, 1)	(4, 3)	(3, 2)	(5, 4)
$m(i, r)$	1	1	1	3	3	5	1	6	3	2

$D = 4, v = 2$

(i, r)	(4, 1)	(3, 1)	(5, 1)	(4, 2)	(5, 2)	(5, 3)
$m(i, r)$	2	2	2	7	6	6

---

[a] This is second because, by Table 7, no (5, 1) items or (3, 1) items occur.
[b] The total energy output here is $\Sigma E(i^2) = 1(4^2) + 1(5^2) + 2(4^2) + \cdots = 507$.

where the items chosen up until $e_R(B)$ is reached are shown in the order in which they are chosen. Some summary data is included in Table 11. The reader will notice that, as predicted, if v is fixed, then both home range R_r and prey-size range R_i are decreasing (nonincreasing) with increasing D. For example, with $v = 1$, the home range (largest distance travelled) decreases from 5 with $D = 1$ to 3 with $D = 2$ to 2 with $D = 4$. Similarly, for fixed D, the prediction was that as the efficiency of a pursuer increased (v increased), then the home range would increase (not decrease) and the prey-size range would decrease (not increase). The results in Table 11 uphold this prediction as well.

Let us suppose that a predator of given speed v is observed on three different days. On each day, the food sizes are distributed log-normally with mean 5 and standard deviation 0.5. On one day, the density D is 1, on a second day D is 2, and on a third day D is 4. One can calculate the home range R_r and prey-size range R_i on each day, and then calculate the mean, standard deviation, and coefficient of variation of the home range and prey-

Table 11. Summary Data from Results of Greedy Algorithms.[†]

	$D = 1$	$D = 2$	$D = 4$
$v = 1$			
M_i	4.950	5.000	4.609
SD_i	0.9445	0.8584	0.8913
CV_i	19.08%	17.17%	19.34%
R_i	6	6	6
Range i	$[3, 6]$	$[3, 6]$	$[3, 6]$
M_r	3.050	2.200	1.652
SD_r	0.9987	0.7678	0.4870
CV_r	32.74%	34.90%	29.48%
R_r	5	3	2
Range r	$[1, 5]$	$[1, 3]$	$[1, 2]$
$v = 2$			
M_i	4.609	4.346	4.480
SD_i	0.7827	0.7971	0.6532
CV_i	16.98%	18.34%	14.58%
R_i	6	6	5
Range i	$[3, 6]$	$[3, 6]$	$[3, 5]$
M_r	3.261	2.423	2.000
SD_r	1.0962	0.8566	0.7071
CV_r	33.62%	35.35%	35.36%
R_r	5	4	3
Range r	$[1, 5]$	$[1, 4]$	$[1, 3]$

[†] M_i, SD_i, and CV_i give the mean, standard deviation, and coefficient of variation of the size of food items taken, R_i is the maximum value of i, and Range i gives the range of sizes of items taken. M_r, SD_r, CV_r, R_r, and Range r give similar data for the distance traveled.

Table 12. Mean M, Standard Deviation SD and Coefficient of Variation CV of Home Range and Prey-Size Range with R_i and R_r from Table 11 Taken as Particular Observations.

	Home Range			Prey-Size Range		
	M	SD	CV	M	SD	CV
$v = 1$						
	3.33	1.5275	45.8%	6	0	0%
$v = 2$						
	4	1	25%	5.67	0.5774	10.2%

Table 13. Threshold Values e_0
Resulting from the Greedy
Algorithm.

D	1	2	4	1	2	4
v	1	1	1	2	2	2
e_0	3.98	5.12	5.97	6.27	7.18	8.38

size range over the different observations.[18] We show the results of such a computation for $v = 1$ and $v = 2$ in Table 12. For example, for home range with $v = 2$, the observations are $R_r = 5$ with $D = 1$, 4 with $D = 2$, and 3 with $D = 4$. Hence the mean home range is $(5 + 4 + 3)/3 = 4$. It was predicted in Section 4.4 (the prediction was made more precise in Section 4.5) that as v increased, the coefficient of variation of home range would increase while the coefficient of variation of prey-size range would decrease. However, Table 12 shows just the opposite: the coefficient of variation of home range decreased from 45.8% to 25%, while the coefficient of variation of prey-size range increased from 0% to 10.2%.

This violation of the prediction is a little strange. After all, it was not arrived at with "real" data but with data simulated using the assumptions of the model. It can only follow that our model does not make the prediction we thought it made. Let us see why this is so.

In the case $D = 1$, $v = 1$, the last food items taken are the (6, 5) items. The corresponding $e(B, i, r)$ is 3.98. Thus e_0, the threshold value, is 3.98. Other threshold values are shown in Table 13. The reader will notice that for fixed v, e_0 increases with increasing D, as expected. However, for fixed D, e_0 can be different for different v. If the reader will look back to the discussion in Section 4.4, he will notice that in our suggestive diagram of Figure 11.10, we had the e_0 lines at the same horizontal level for both the efficient and inefficient pursuers. We implicitly assumed, in deriving our prediction about coefficients of variation of home range and prey-size range, that a similar change in food abundance would result in a similar change in e_0 for both an efficient and an inefficient pursuer. This clearly is not the case. This fallacy in our reasoning also makes us suspect most of the predictions made in Section 4.4. For example, if the lines $e = e_0$ are at different levels in the two parts of Figure 11.10, then it may not necessarily be the case that efficient pursuers have a higher home range and a lower prey-size range. The prediction that home range and prey-size range will both decrease with increasing D for a fixed level of efficiency *still holds*: it uses only one part of Figure 11.10 at a time. It is interesting that it took a computer simulation to show us our mistake. Sometimes with a very complicated model, one only learns to understand its implications by doing exactly what we have done. It is a good check on our reasoning power.

---

[18] Of course, three observations would not be nearly enough in practice, but we are merely illustrating a procedure.

Using the results of this simulation, specifically those in Table 11, we do learn several things about our models. In particular, the reader will notice that for fixed v and varying D, the mean distance traveled to eat decreases with increasing D. There is no similar pattern to mean size of food items as D increases. With fixed D and variable v, the mean prey size decreases and the mean distance travelled increases with increasing v. No similar pattern occurs for coefficients of variation. The reader is left to think about whether our observations about means are "reasonable" results for a pure pursuer, and whether they can be derived mathematically from our model.

EXERCISES

14. Assume that $v = k_1 = k_2 = k_3 = k_4 = k_5 = k_6 = 1$, and $s = 4$. Let $B = 2$, $i = 2$, and $r = 2$.
    (a) Calculate $E_R(B)$ under all four models.
    (b) Calculate $E(i)$ under all four models.
    (c) Calculate TP and EP under all four models.
    (d) Calculate THS and EHS under all four models.

15. Adopt the assumptions of our fourth model (Table 1). Suppose $v = k_1 = k_2 = k_3 = k_4 = k_5 = k_6 = 1$.
    (a) If $B = 1$, calculate $e(B, i, r)$ for all combinations of $i = 1, 2, 3$ and $r = 1, 2$. Plot the curves of e versus i for each r on the same set of axes.
    (b) Do the same if $B = 2$.
    (c) For $r = 1$, plot the curves of e versus i for $B = 1$ and e versus i for $B = 2$ on the same set of axes.
    (d) Do the same for $r = 2$.

16. Repeat Exercise 15 if v is changed to 10.

17. In our discussion of Section 2.3, we calculated $E_R(B)$ for an 81 kg man doing moderate activity as 3000 kcal per day. What value of k_1 were we using?

18. Suppose $N(i, r)$, $E(i)$, $e(B, i, r)$ are as in Table 14, and $E_R(B) = 200$.
    (a) Calculate the numbers $m(i, r)$ for the greedy solution.
    (b) Calculate e_0.
    (c) Calculate M_i, SD_i, CV_i, R_i, range i, M_r, SD_r, CV_r, R_r, and range r as defined in Table 11.

Table 14

i	r	$N(i, r)$	$E(i) = i^2$	$e(B, i, r)$
2	5	2	4	0.79
3	6	5	9	1.45
4	5	5	16	2.88
7	4	2	49	3.27
9	3	1	81	0.96
2	8	4	4	0.50

Table 15

i	r	$N(i, r)$	$E(i) = i^2$	$e(B, i, r)$
8	5	2	64	1.84
7	4	2	49	3.27
8	6	2	64	1.79
3	4	3	9	2.14
4	3	3	16	4.51
6	6	4	36	3.59
10	4	1	100	0.44

19. Repeat Exercise 18 for the data of Table 15 with $E_R(B) = 300$.

20. Calculate $N(r)$, p_i, and $N(i, r)$ if
    (a) $\mu = 2$, $\sigma = 0.1$, and $D = 1$,
    (b) $\mu = 10$, $\sigma = 1$, $D = 1$,
    (c) $\mu = 2$, $\sigma = 0.5$, $D = 10$.

21. How do your answers to Exercise 20(a) change if D is changed to 100?

22. Calculate i_L and i_U for each of the cases of Exercise 20.

23. Investigate the third model with i^2 in THS replaced by i^α, some $\alpha > 0$. Show that for some α, e is not an increasing function of i for fixed r and B.

24. Suppose W is proportional to B^3 rather than to B^2, as we have assumed in all of our models. This changes MR to $\gamma B^{9/4}$, as we indicated in Section 4.1.1.
    (a) How does this change $E_R(B)$?
    (b) How does it change $E(i)$?
    (c) How does it change EP?
    (d) How does it change EHS if THS is known?
    (e) Discuss the effect on the predictions of Model 1.
    (f) Discuss the effect on the predictions of Model 2.
    (g) Discuss the effect on the predictions of Model 3.
    (h) Discuss the effect on the predictions of Model 4.

25. Suppose that instead of being constant, v depends on B. For example, let $v = kB^\gamma$, for some constants k and γ.
    (a) How does this change the predictions of Model 1? Does your answer depend on γ?
    (b) How does it change the predictions of Model 2?
    (c) How does it change the predictions of Model 3?
    (d) How does it change the predictions of Model 4?

26. Project: Consider the effect of letting v depend not only on B, but also on r. (Is it reasonable to make it depend on i?)

27. Consider the following statement of Schoener [36, p. 290]. "Only relatively large prey are taken at great distances, though the largest prey taken at a given distance will not be as large as the largest taken at smaller distances."
    (a) Does this statement follow from the curves for e vs. i for different r derived from our fourth model, and from the use of the thresholds $e = e_0$?
    (b) Is this statement upheld by the data of Tables 10 or 11?

28. Suppose the prey does not sit still, waiting for capture, but heads directly away from the predator at a speed $w < v$.
   (a) How long will it take the predator to pursue the prey and catch up if both continue to go in a straight line?
   (b) How does this modify TP and EP in our models?
   (c) If w is independent of i, B, and r, how does this modify $e(B, i, r)$ in our first model? Is the unsatisfactory prediction still made?
   (d) What happens to the fourth model?
   (e) How would you calculate TP if the prey started out on a straight line in a certain direction and the predator had to choose in what direction to head in order to "intercept" the prey? (This problem arises in calculating rendezvous points at sea. See Baker [2] for a discussion).

29. In our models, we have assumed that THS depends on the size of the prey eaten. However, for prey which are relatively small in comparison to the predators, the prey might be swallowed without much fuss and the eating time might be constant (Watt [45]). This suggests that there is a cutoff value i_B, depending on body size B of the prey, so that THS is a constant if $i \leq i_B$ but increases with $i - i_B$ if $i > i_B$. Thus Schoener [36] assumes that

$$\text{THS} = \begin{cases} k_7, & \text{if } i \leq i_B \\ k_7 + k_8 \exp(i - i_B), & \text{if } i > i_B, \end{cases} \qquad (36)$$

where k_7 and k_8 are positive constants. (Schoener also considers replacing the exponential $\exp(i - i_B)$ by a power function $\alpha(i - i_B)^\beta$, which might be equally plausible, but then decides not to do so.). For many cases, B/i_B is on the order of 7. It should be pointed out that if THS is defined by (36), then THS is not a continuous function of i. There is a jump discontinuity at $i = i_B$. The reader should check this by plotting THS against i.

30. If THS is discontinuous, then so is $e(B, i, r)$, which does not seem reasonable. Apparently, Schoener did not intend either THS or $e(B, i, r)$ to be discontinuous. One can avoid the problem by using the following formula for THS:

$$\text{THS} = \begin{cases} k_7, & \text{if } i \leq i_B \\ k_7 \exp[k_8(i - i_B)], & \text{if } i > i_B. \end{cases} \qquad (37)$$

The reader is urged to modify the fourth model with this definition of THS and try to make some predictions about $e(B, i, r)$.

31. The student with access to a computer (or a hand calculator) might wish to continue the analysis of Section 4.8.3 by taking two more values of D, e.g., 0.5 and 10, and perhaps two more values of v, e.g., 4 and 10.

4.9 Variations on the Model: Time-Energy Efficiency

The model we have considered so far is based on the assumption that an animal optimizes by maximizing the fraction of daily energy required per unit of energy expended, the relative energetic efficiency. As we have pointed out before, Schoener [36] considers a somewhat different idea: an animal optimizes by maximizing the net fraction of daily energy requirement obtained per unit time expended. This measure would be calculated using what we called in Section 3 the relative time-energy efficiency:

$$e' = \frac{(E_O - E_I)/E_R}{T}.^{[19]}$$

The following exercises develop Schoener's model. Underlying all of them are the assumptions given in lines 1–4 and line 6 of Table 1. These are the assumptions common to all four of the models we considered above.

EXERCISES

32. In a model analogous to our first model,

$$e'(B, i, r) = \frac{[E(i) - EP]/E_R(B)}{TP}.$$

   Calculate $e'(B, i, r)$ and discuss it as we discussed $e(B, i, r)$ in Section 4.1.5.

33. Introduce THS as in the second model (Section 4.2, equation (27)), and calculate $e'(B, i, r)$ as

$$e'(B, i, r) = \frac{[E(i) - EP - EHS]/E_R(B)}{(TP + THS)}.$$

   Discuss $e'(B, i, r)$ as we discussed $e(B, i, r)$ in Section 4.2.

34. Modify THS as in the third model, i.e., take

$$THS = k_s i^2 B^{-s}.$$

   Use the formula for $e'(B, i, r)$ of the previous exercise, and discuss this function as we did in Section 4.3.

35. Modify THS as in Table 1 (the fourth model), calculate $e'(B, i, r)$ as in Exercise 33, and discuss $e'(B, i, r)$.

36. Modify THS by using (37) of Exercise 30 of the previous section, and use this to calculate $e'(B, i, r)$ of Exercise 33 above. Discuss the properties of $e'(B, i, r)$.

37. Discuss a possible greedy algorithm for the minimization of relative time-energy efficiency. Note that it is $\Sigma(E_O - E_I)$ which must reach E_R.

38. Do some computer simulations, using the function $e'(B, i, r)$ of Exercise 36 and food distributions generated using the procedures of Section 4.8.

5. Pure Searchers

Many predators are quite different from the "pure pursuers" we have been studying. Indeed, many predators spend a great deal of time moving around, searching for food, and expending energy *in the search*. As a second idealized

---

[19] The major difference is that E_R will be thought of as a requirement for the sum of the net energy $E_O - E_I$, and hence the constant k_1 of Eq. (16) will change.

type of predator, we consider a "pure searcher," a predator which, when it finds a prey, needs to spend no time on pursuit. It simply has to decide whether or not to expend the time and energy required to handle and swallow the prey, or whether it can expect to do better by continuing its search. According to Schoener [36], examples of such predators are such birds as warblers, kinglets, and titmice, some lizards, and many skinks.

Models of pure searchers will be quite different in character from models of pure pursuers. The key element will be an element of *uncertainty*: what is the *probability* of finding a better food item soon enough to make the extra energy and time used in the search worthwhile? While the pure pursuer can rest or perform other activities while waiting for the "right" prey to come along, the pure searcher is wasting energy on his search. He must take chances to conserve energy. Thus, in contrast to the deterministic models of behavior of the previous section, the models of behavior in this section will involve a chancy or stochastic element.

5.1 Two Food Types

Perhaps the simplest model of a pure searcher is that of Emlen [10]. We shall present a model which has as its source some of the ideas of Emlen but which is quite different from his model. In contrast to the complexity of the models we have been considering, Emlen's models assume, for the sake of discussion, just two types (sizes) of food; we shall call them types 1 and 2. Our basic assumption continues as before: feeding preferences or physical characteristics will develop so as to maximize the (relative) energy intake per unit of energy expended.

We imagine the pure searcher moving over an essentially linear strip. When he comes upon a given food item, he can either accept it or reject it. We shall want to trace him from food item to food item.

Our notation will be the same as in Section 4. Thus let B be the body size of the pure searcher. Let $E_R(B)$ be his daily energy requirements. Let $E(i)$ be the caloric value to the predator of an item of food i. We do not need a term EP, energy spent in pursuit. However, we will need EHS and THS, energy and time spent handling and swallowing. We shall want to emphasize the dependence of these terms on food type i, and so subscript them as $(EHS)_i$ and $(THS)_i$. In this elementary model, we shall not need to make assumptions about the specific ways of determining E_R, $E(i)$, EHS, and THS. However, in Section 5.2 and in some of the exercises following this section, we shall adopt the assumptions of Table 1.

To complete our model of the pure searcher, we shall have to introduce a term describing the *energy used in searching*, ES, which of course is related to the *time spent searching*, TS. At first, we will not have to specify how ES is related to TS. However, one natural assumption is that $ES = kB^{1.5}TS$, for k a positive constant. To calculate TS, let us assume that the searcher travels over his territory at a constant speed v'. This will certainly be different from the speed of pursuit v, discussed in Section 4. Before we can calculate TS, we shall have to make some assumptions about the distribution of food items in the predator's territory. The simplest assumption is that the items are uniformly distributed in the territory, which we are thinking of as a linear strip. Suppose the items are distributed in this strip with a mean distance between them of δ. The predator searches the strip, heading always in the same direction, say left to right. If he encounters a food item, the expected distance to the next food item is δ. The time to reach the next item, TS, is estimated by calculating its expected value. We estimate

$$\text{TS} = \frac{\delta}{v'}. \tag{38}$$

Finally, we shall have to make an assumption about the distribution of different food items. Let us assume that the proportion of i items in the population is μ_i, $i = 1, 2$. We assume the items are independently distributed, so that if the predator has just found an item of type i, the probability that the next item he finds is of type j is μ_j, independent of i and j. (Here, j can equal i.) Of course $\mu_1 + \mu_2 = 1$.

Since there are only two different food items, calculation of the number of items of each kind eaten (what we called $m(i, r)$ in Section 4.7) reduces to the calculation of ρ_i, the proportion of each type i of food eaten. We shall want to relate ρ_i to μ_i.

5.1.1 *The Patient Strategy: Waiting for the Right Type of Food.* If a pure searcher, without spending time searching, finds a food item of type i, his relative[20] energetic efficiency (14) or fraction of his daily energy requirements obtained per unit of energy input is given by

$$\frac{E(i)/E_R}{(\text{EHS})_i}.$$

Let us assume that

$$\frac{E(1)/E_R}{(\text{EHS})_1} < \frac{E(2)/E_R}{(\text{EHS})_2}.$$

We shall say that type 2 foods are more energetically efficient. Thus, if a predator finds an item of type 2 food, he will certainly eat it. He can only lose energy by waiting for a type 1 food to be found. Suppose the predator comes upon an item of type 1. Should he eat it or continue the search? To continue the search is worth his while if he expects to achieve a higher relative energy accumulation per unit of energy spent. Suppose the predator did not spend the energy in eating the item he just found, but instead he continued looking.

---

[20] In all of Section 5.1, where we just consider a fixed predator and will compare his energetic efficiencies for different food items, we could just as well use his absolute energetic efficiency (12). For the sake of consistency, however, we will continue to use the relative efficiency.

His time of search TS before finding the next food item is estimated by (38) and his energy use in searching is determined by TS. If the next food item is again an item of type 1 and he eats that item, he will have a relative energy output of $E(1)/E_R$. He will have used $(EHS)_1$ units of energy in handling and swallowing the item, and ES units of energy in the search. Thus his relative energetic efficiency would be

$$A = \frac{E(1)/E_R}{(EHS)_1 + ES},\qquad(39)$$

which is less than

$$B = \frac{E(1)/E_R}{(EHS)_1},\qquad(40)$$

if we assume that ES is positive when TS is positive. Indeed, should the predator ever give in and eat an item of type 1, after spending some time searching for it, his relative energetic efficiency would be clearly less than it would have been had he eaten the original type 1 food encountered. Thus, suppose he adopts the patient strategy of waiting until he first meets a type 2 item. Let us suppose for the sake of argument that TS now denotes the length of time the predator can expect to wait before he encounters a type 2 item. We shall see below how he might calculate TS. The energy spent in searching is given by ES, which is related to TS.

In general, by waiting until he finds the type 2 item, the predator obtains $E(2)$ units of energy. He uses $(EHS)_2$ units of energy in handling and swallowing plus the energy used in the search, ES, which is calculated from TS. His relative energetic efficiency can be estimated by

$$C = \frac{E(2)/E_R}{(EHS)_2 + ES}.\qquad(41)$$

This should be compared to his relative energetic efficiency if he ate the original type 1 item; this efficiency is given by B of (40). If the predator is energetically efficient, then he eats a type 1 item whenever he encounters it if and only if his relative energetic efficiency by eating the type 1 item (B of Equation (40)) is at least as large as his estimated relative energetic efficiency of waiting until he finds a type 2 item (C of Equation (41)), i.e., if and only if $B \geq C$. He always eats a type 2 item when he encounters it, since we assumed that type 2 foods were more energetically efficient. Thus, if $B < C$, he eats only type 2 items. If $B \geq C$, he eats items whenever he encounters them. (The proportion ρ_i of type i items he eats is therefore comparable to the proportion μ_i of type i items in the population.) Is this a reasonable prediction? The answer is no. Predators certainly have preferred foods, pass some foods up for others, and yet have a mixed diet. (We will mention data to this effect below.) Thus we will want to modify our model.

Before doing so, let us for completeness go back to the missing point, namely an indication of how the predator with the patient strategy can estimate the time of search until he finds a type 2 prey. How long can he expect to wait? Let us first ask how many food items he can expect to encounter having just passed up a type 1 item until he encounters a type 2 item for the first time. The probability of finding a type 2 item as the first item is μ_2. The probability of first finding a type 1 item and then a type 2 item is $\mu_1\mu_2$. In general, the probability that he first finds a type 2 item as the kth item encountered after passing up $k-1$ type 1 items is $\mu_1^{k-1}\mu_2$. Thus the expected number of encounters until finding a type 2 item is given by the expression

$$1\mu_2 + 2\mu_1\mu_2 + 3\mu_1^2\mu_2 + \cdots = \sum_{k=1}^{\infty} k\mu_1^{k-1}\mu_2$$

$$= \mu_2 \sum_{k=1}^{\infty} k\mu_1^{k-1}$$

$$= \frac{\mu_2}{(1-\mu_1)^2}$$

$$= \frac{1}{\mu_2},$$

since $\mu_2 = 1 - \mu_1$. We have used the well-known identity

$$\sum_{k=1}^{\infty} kx^{k-1} = \frac{1}{(1-x)^2}.$$

The amount of time spent searching until a type 2 item is encountered can now be estimated by

$$\text{TS} = \frac{\delta}{v'\mu_2}. \tag{42}$$

If μ_2 is small, this is large, and the predator is probably better off eating item 1. That is, scarcity of the preferred food leads to the strategy of eating whatever comes along.

5.1.2 *The Impatient Strategy.* How can we modify our model to obtain a prediction of a mix of food items eaten, without getting the prediction that the predator will eat every food item offered? One natural thing to do is to ask if a predator who has adopted a "wait until type 2" strategy will be patient enough to carry this out. If after a certain number of sightings he still fails to encounter a type 2 food item, he might lose patience or get hungry and decide to take the next food item sighted, regardless of its type. To consider the impact of this type of impatience, let us consider the most extreme case: if the predator passes up a type 1 food item, he will take the next food item regardless of its type. Assuming this type of strategy, when is it in his interest to pass up a type 1 item? What can happen if he does pass up a type 1 item? He can encounter either a type 1 item on the next sighting, which happens with probability μ_1, or a type 2 item, which happens with probability μ_2. If he next encounters a type 1 item and eats it, his relative energetic efficiency is given by A of (39). Similarly, if he next encounters a type 2 item and eats it, his relative energetic efficiency is given by C of Equation (41). Observe that the term ES in both of these equations is now the same, and it depends on the time of search TS, which is the time to find the next item, estimated by (38). Thus his relative energetic efficiency if he passes up a type 1 item and eats the next item which comes along can be estimated by

$$D = \mu_1 A + \mu_2 C. \tag{43}$$

To decide whether or not to pass up the original type 1 item, the predator must compare his relative energetic efficiency of eating that item, which is given by B of (40), with his estimate of his relative energetic efficiency of waiting, which is given by D of (43). Under the assumption of optimizing energetic efficiency, the predator will pass up the type 1 item and wait for the next item if and only if $D > B$. Thus, if $B \geq D$, he will always eat any item encountered, and his proportion ρ_i of type i items eaten is comparable to μ_i, the proportion of type i items in the population. However, if $D > B$, the proportion ρ_i is different from μ_i. What is the value of ρ_i? Having just eaten, what is the probability that the predator next eats an item of type 1? He does so if and only if the next two items he encounters are type 1's, and this occurs with probability $\mu_1 \mu_1 = \mu_1^2$. Thus the proportion of type 1 items eaten is given by

$$\rho_1 = \mu_1^2,$$

the proportion of type 2 items eaten by

$$\rho_2 = 1 - \mu_1^2 = 1 - (1 - \mu_2)^2.$$

(Note that our model assumes that the predator just keeps on eating: there is no discussion of meeting daily energy requirements here.)

Suppose we plot the observed frequency ρ_i of eating an item i against μ_i. Our model predicts that one of the curves in Figure 11.12 will be obtained. (The first curve is the graph $y = x$; the second the graph $y = x^2$, and the

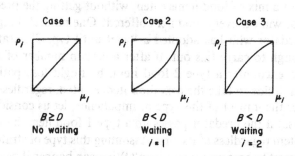

Figure 11.12

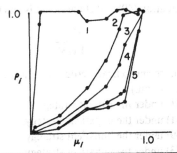

Predator	i	Foods Available
1) *Thais emarginata*	*Balanus glandula*	*B. glandula, B. cariosus*
2) Carp	Chironomid larvae	Chironomid larvae, amphipods, fresh water isopods, mollusks
3) Carp	Amphipods	
4) Carp	Fresh water isopods	
5) Carp	Mollusks	

Figure 11.13. Relation between the Frequency ρ_i of Food i in the Diet and the Frequency μ_i of Food i in the Environment. From Emlen [10]. Reprinted with Permission of the University of Chicago Press and of the Author.

third the graph $y = 1 - (1 - x)^2$; the latter is the graph of the parabola $y = -x^2$ shifted up by one unit and to the right by one unit.)

Figure 11.13, using data obtained in experiments by Ivlev [19] and Emlen (unpublished), shows curves which are qualitatively very much like those of cases 2 and 3.

Before closing this section, we might ask when we would expect cases 2 or 3 to hold, and when we would expect case 1 to hold. One answer is that D of Equation (43) decreases if δ increases. This is because both A and C decrease when ES increases, since it is natural to assume that ES increases when TS increases, and since TS increases when δ increases. The number δ measures the mean distance between food items, and so is a measure of food abundance. As food abundance decreases, i.e., as food becomes scarce, δ increases and D decreases. Then eventually B becomes bigger than D, and case 1 is obtained: the predator is no longer selective but eats any food item he finds. It would be interesting to test this prediction more precisely by investigating what values of δ result in a change of behavior.

EXERCISES

39. Suppose i represents size, and $E(i)$, E_R, EHS, and THS are given by our fourth model for pure pursuers (Table 1). Suppose $\mu_1 = \mu_2 = 1/2$, $v' = 1$, $\delta = 1$, $B = 1$, and $k_1 = k_2 = k_3 = k_4 = k_5 = k_6 = 1$. Suppose analogously to our fourth model,

$$ES = k_9 B^{1.5} TS,$$

and assume $k_9 = 1$.

(a) Calculate B of Equation (40) and show that it is less than

$$\frac{E(2)/E_R}{(EHS)_2}.$$

(Thus food 2 is more energetically efficient than food 1, as is assumed in our discussion of this section.)

(b) Calculate C of (41) under the patient strategy.

(c) Calculate C of (41) under the impatient strategy.

(d) Calculate A of (39) under the impatient strategy.

(e) Calculate D of (43) under the impatient strategy.

(f) Determine ρ_1 and ρ_2 under the patient strategy.

(g) Estimate ρ_1 and ρ_2 under the impatient strategy.

40. (a) Redo Exercise 39 if $\delta = 0.1$.

(b) Redo Exercise 39 if $\delta = 10$.

(c) What is the effect of changing δ?

41. (a) Redo Exercise 39 if $\mu_1 = 0.9$.

(b) What will be the effect in general of increasing μ_1?

42. What will be the effect in general of increasing v'?

43. Suppose there are three food types, 1, 2, and 3. Consider what happens if relative energetic efficiency is maximized, and

$$\frac{E(3)/E_R}{(EHS)_3} > \frac{E(2)/E_R}{(EHS)_2} > \frac{E(1)/E_R}{(EHS)_1}.$$

(a) What are the predictions if the predator adopts the strategy which gives him the following choice: either eat an item of food encountered or search until a type 3 item comes along?

(b) What if the predator either eats an item encountered or searches until some better one comes along?

(c) What if the predator either eats an item encountered or decides to eat the next item he encounters?

44. In the two-item situation, what happens if the predator either eats an item encountered, or waits no more than m encounters before eating the next item encountered?

45. Consider what happens in the two-item situation if instead of the relative energetic efficiency the time-energy efficiency (15) is used.

46. Project: Consider what happens in the two-item situation if the probability of encountering next an item of type j just after encountering an item of type i is p_{ij}, dependent possibly on both i and j. Perhaps you can extend your results to more than two items.

5.2 Many Food Types

Let us now assume that there are many food types. Let the type i correspond to the length of the food item, as in our models of Section 4. We shall continue to use the notation of the previous section, but our analysis will be somewhat different, following Schoener's model [36] of what he calls Type II predators. We shall assume that the expressions $E_R(B)$, $E(i)$, THS, and EHS take on the values in our fourth model, as given in Table 1. We shall also assume that

$$ES = k_9 B^{1.5}TS, \qquad (44)$$

in analogy with the expressions for EP and EHS used in our models in Section 4. (The reader might wish to reread the derivation of these expressions to remember the rationale used.)

One factor neglected in the previous section was a pure searcher's need to meet its daily energy requirements. We envisaged such a pure searcher eating so as to be energetically efficient, without paying heed to meeting his daily requirements. We also did not consider that the searcher might stop eating once he had met those requirements, though that is easily assumed with little change in our previous discussion. If we disregard search time, the relative energetic efficiency of eating an item of size i is given by

$$e(B, i) = \frac{E(i)/E_R(B)}{(EHS)_i}. \qquad (45)$$

This corresponds to the function we call $e(B, i, r)$ in Section 4. Under the assumptions of Table 1, the properties of the function $e(B, i)$ are similar to those of $e(B, i, r)$ as described in Section 4.4. In particular, for fixed B, $e(B, i)$ will have a graph like that shown in Figure 11.14.

Suppose we limit our predator to the following types of strategies: find a set Δ of food sizes which are acceptable, and take a food item if and only if its size is in the set Δ. Suppose moreover that the predator takes a given food item of size i if and only if $e(B, i)$ is at least as large as a threshold level e_0. The threshold level, as we saw in Section 4.4, will correspond to a line parallel to the i axis, and this line in turn corresponds to an interval $[i_1, i_2]$ of acceptable i values, as shown in Figure 11.15. Thus the sets Δ for us to consider are intervals of numbers.

In the case of a pure pursuer, we could choose the threshold e_0 for a known distribution of food items, so that choosing only items above threshold would lead to just meeting the daily requirements and using the food items with highest possible energetic efficiencies or measures of energy spent in obtaining daily energy requirements. In the case of a pure searcher, the choice is made differently. Even for fixed food distributions, different choices of threshold or of sets Δ will, in our model, still lead to obtaining

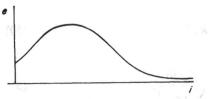

Figure 11.14

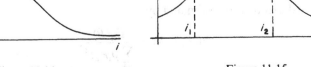

Figure 11.15

the daily requirements. However, these different choices will lead to different expectations about energy spent in obtaining daily requirements. We will want the expected energy to be spent minimized or, equivalently, the (global) energetic efficiency maximized. We are led naturally to this goal, while we were not in the case of the pure pursuer, where we showed that his strategy might not maximize global energetic efficiency.

How will we measure the energetic efficiency of the strategy corresponding to the interval $\Delta = [i_1, i_2]$? The efficiency will depend on the body size B of the predator and on the distribution of food sizes—we shall use the letter f to stand for this distribution. Based on B, f, and Δ, we shall determine the expected amount of time $TS(B, f, \Delta)$ spent in searching for food items before meeting the daily requirements, the expected amount of time $THS(B, f, \Delta)$ spent handling and swallowing the food items eaten, and the expected energy value $E(B, f, \Delta)$ obtained from these items. Then the energetic efficiency corresponding to B, f, Δ is given by

$$e(B, f, \Delta) = \frac{E(B, f, \Delta)/E_R(B)}{EHS(B, f, \Delta) + ES(B, f, \Delta)}, \tag{46}$$

where $EHS(B, f, \Delta)$ and $ES(B, f, \Delta)$ are the energy inputs corresponding to $THS(B, f, \Delta)$ and $TS(B, f, \Delta)$, respectively, and are given by

$$EHS(B, f, \Delta) = k_4 B^{1.5} THS(B, f, \Delta) \tag{47}$$

and

$$ES(B, f, \Delta) = k_9 B^{1.5} TS(B, f, \Delta). \tag{48}$$

How would we determine the required numbers $E(B, f, \Delta)$, $TS(B, f, \Delta)$, and $THS(B, f, \Delta)$? Suppose we assume that i takes on only integer values, that the fraction of food items of size i in the population is μ_i, that food items are uniformly distributed along the strip the predator is searching, with mean distance apart δ, and that the distribution is independent in the sense that if the searcher has just found a food item of size i, the probability of finding a food item of size j next is μ_j, independent of i and j. This information defines the distribution we have called f. Then we can calculate the expected energy obtained from a given food item by

$$E^\circ(B, f, \Delta) = \sum_{i \in \Delta} \mu_i k_2 i^2, \tag{49}$$

since $E(i) = k_2 i^2$ is the energy obtainable from a food item of size i which is eaten and 0 is the food energy obtainable from a food item which is not eaten. The expected number of trials (number of encounters) before the energy requirements

$$E_R(B) = k_1 B^{1.5} \tag{50}$$

are reached can then be estimated by

$$n(B, f, \Delta) = \frac{E_R(B)}{\sum_{i \in \Delta} \mu_i k_2 i^2}. \tag{51}$$

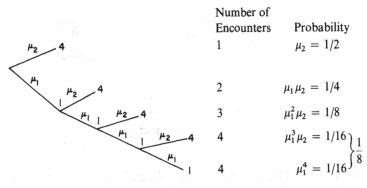

Figure 11.16

This is only a crude estimate. Let us see why. Suppose $E_R(B) = 4, \Delta = [1, 2]$, $k_2 = 1$, and $\mu_1 = \mu_2 = 1/2$, $\mu_j = 0$, otherwise. Then the tree diagram of Figure 11.16 indicates how we might reach the required amount of energy. The expected number of trials to reach E_R is

$$\tfrac{1}{2} \times 1 + \tfrac{1}{4} \times 2 + \tfrac{1}{8} \times 3 + \tfrac{1}{8} \times 4 = 15/8.$$

The estimate (51) is

$$n(B, f, \Delta) = \frac{4}{(\tfrac{1}{2} \times 1) + (\tfrac{1}{2} \times 4)} = 8/5.$$

To obtain an actual calculation in general of the expected number of trials is a hard problem and so we shall be content with this crude estimate (51). This in turn gives an estimate for $E(B, f, \Delta)$ of $E_R(B)$, for $E(B, f, \Delta)$ would be estimated as

$$E(B, f, \Delta) = n(B, f, \Delta)E^\circ(B, f, \Delta) = E_R(B), \qquad (52)$$

with $n(B, f, \Delta)$ as in (51) and $E^\circ(B, f, \Delta)$ as in (49).

The time spent searching depends on the speed of search, which we have assumed is a constant v'. Thus the time spent searching for the *next* food item is expected to be δ/v', and the time spent searching for enough food to meet the daily energy requirements can be estimated as

$$TS(B, f, \Delta) = n(B, f, \Delta)\delta/v'. \qquad (53)$$

The time spent handling and swallowing the ith item is estimated to be

$$THS(B, f, \Delta) = \sum_{i \in \Delta} \mu_i(THS)_i, \qquad (54)$$

since $(THS)_i$ is the time spent handling and swallowing item i if it is handled and swallowed and 0 is the time spent otherwise. From equations (46) through (53) we obtain

$$e(B, f, \Delta) = \frac{E_R(B)/E_R(B)}{k_4 B^{1.5} \sum_{i \in \Delta} \mu_i(THS)_i + k_9 B^{1.5} n(B, f, \Delta)\dfrac{\delta}{v'}}$$

or

$$e(B, f, \Delta) = \cfrac{1}{k_4 B^{1.5} \displaystyle\sum_{i \in \Delta} \mu_i (THS)_i + k_9 B^{1.5} \cfrac{k_1 B^{1.5}}{\displaystyle\sum_{i \in \Delta} \mu_i k_2 i^2} \cfrac{\delta}{v'}}$$

or

$$e(B, f, \Delta) = \cfrac{1}{k_4 k_5 B^{-2.5} \displaystyle\sum_{i \in \Delta} \mu_i \exp(k_6 i) + \cfrac{k_1 k_9 B^3 \delta}{v' \displaystyle\sum_{i \in \Delta} \mu_i k_2 i^2}} , \qquad (55)$$

using the value of THS given in Table 1. As awful as expression (55) looks, it is possible to obtain some predictions from it. For example, since $\exp(k_6 i)$ gets large much faster than $k_2 i^2$, it follows from (55) that for i sufficiently large, adding i to Δ will decrease $e(B, f, \Delta)$. Thus an upper bound will exist beyond which it is not reasonable to eat food items.

Expression (55) can also be used to estimate by computer which value Δ_M of Δ will maximize $e(B, f, \Delta)$, under different assumptions about B, f (and hence δ and the μ_i's), and about the constants k_1, k_2, k_4, k_5, k_6, k_9, and v'. This can be done if we limit i_2 in $\Delta = [i_1, i_2]$ to a reasonable size, which can be accomplished, for example, by limiting it to a multiple of B such as $(3/2)B$, or by using a log-normal distribution as in Section 4.8.2. If a predator is assumed to choose the optimal Δ_M strategy, then the optimal

Table 16. Values of $e(B, f, \Delta)$ of (55) if $B = 4$ cm, Food Items of Sizes 1 through 5 Are Equally Likely, $\delta = 1$, $v' = 1$, and All Parameters k_i are 1. The Column Labeled $e'(B, f, \Delta)$ Shows $e(B, f, \Delta)$ if k_4 Is Changed to 50.

Δ	$e(B, f, \Delta)$	$e'(B, f, \Delta)$
{1}	0.003	0.003
[1, 2]	0.016	0.015
[1, 3]	0.043	0.031
[1, 4]	0.089	0.027
[1, 5]	0.137	0.013
{2}	0.012	0.012
[2, 3]	0.040	0.030
[2, 4]	0.087	0.027
[2, 5]	0.136	0.013
{3}	0.028	0.024
[3, 4]	0.075	0.028
[3, 5]	0.128	0.013
{4}	0.049	0.027
[4, 5]	0.110	0.014
{5}	0.073	0.017

Δ_M will give an estimate of the sizes of prey fed on by the predator as a function of the body size and the food distribution. These predictions can be compared to data.

Table 16 illustrates the procedure. We assume B is 4 cm, and take integer values of i from 1 up to 5. (5 is less than $(3/2)B = 6$, but will be useful to compare with real data.) We assume an equal distribution of food items among the possible sizes 1–5. We also choose $\delta = 1$, $v' = 1$, and all parameters k_i to be 1. In Table 16, the column labeled Δ gives a possible interval of food items, and the column labeled $e(B, f, \Delta)$ gives the estimated relative energetic efficiency corresponding to Equation (55). Note that the highest $e(B, f, \Delta)$ is 0.137, which corresponds to $\Delta = [1, 5]$. The optimal energetically efficient strategy for this predator is to prey on items of all food sizes from 1 cm to 5 cm. This seems a bit peculiar: such a predator will eat some food items larger than himself. To compare this prediction to data, we note that Ivlev [19] (pp. 82–90, especially p. 87, fig. 21d), which we reprinted as Figure 11.6), discovers that fish (larvae of *Macrodytes circumflexus*) of about 4.2 cm exposed to a uniform distribution of prey sizes (prey was young roach) from 0 to about 5 cm will prey on *all* sizes. This behavior is similar to what we have predicted.

What our prediction does not do is say anything about the frequency p_i with which a predator will eat food items of a given size in its "acceptable" set Δ. It simply predicts what sets $\Delta = \Delta_M$ will be chosen. Perhaps the numbers $e_i = e(B, f, \{i\})$ can be used to give estimates of p_i. In particular, we would use

$$p_i = \begin{cases} 0, & \text{if } i \notin \Delta_M \\ \dfrac{e_i}{\sum\limits_{i \in \Delta} e_i}, & \text{if } i \in \Delta_M. \end{cases} \tag{56}$$

In our example, we obtain the values shown in Table 17. These values are plotted in Figure 11.17. The reader will notice that p_i increases with i. In Ivlev's data, the frequency with which food items are "elected" increases until about 4 cm (the maximum), and then decreases sharply. Thus our simulation has not predicted the curves that Ivlev obtained (Figure 11.6).

Table 17. Values
of p_i of (56)
Estimated from
Data of Table 16.

$p_1 = 0.018$
$p_2 = 0.073$
$p_3 = 0.170$
$p_4 = 0.297$
$p_5 = 0.442$

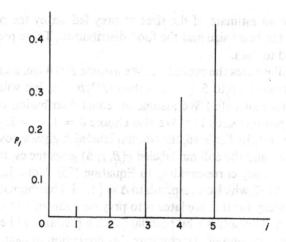

Figure 11.17. Plot of ρ_i from Table 17.

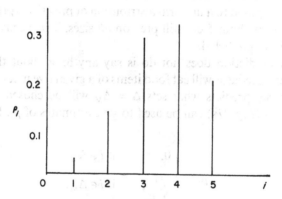

Figure 11.18. Plot of ρ_i from First Column of Table 18.

However, modifying the parameters can lead to predictions closer to Ivlev's. For example, our current choice of parameters may give too much advantage to a predator of large body size in overcoming large prey. Increasing the "penalty" for large body size—for example, the coefficient k_4 in EHS—should change the results. Changing k_4 to 50 gives rise to the numbers $e'(B, f, \Delta)$ shown in the last column of Table 16, and the numbers e_i and ρ_i shown in Table 18. Notice that now, with $\Delta = [1, 5]$, ρ_i increases until $i = 4$, and then decreases. (See Figure 11.18) Unfortunately, the interval Δ with the highest $e'(B, f, \Delta)$ is now a relatively small interval $[1, 3]$. Thus the prediction is that only the items of sizes 1, 2 or 3 will be eaten. Hence, using the numbers e_i of Table 18, we predict that items of size 3 will be eaten about 61.5% of the time, items of size 2 about 30.8% of the time, and items of size 1 the rest of the time. The reader with access to a computer or a calculator might wish to see if, by adjusting some of the other parameters of this model, he can obtain the prediction that the Δ with highest $e(B, f, \Delta)$

Table 18. Values of $e_i = e'(B, f, \{i\})$
and ρ_i of (56) Estimated from Data of
Table 16, Third Column.

		If $\Delta_M = [2, 3]$
	If $\Delta_M = [1, 5]$	(which it is)
$e_1 = 0.003$	$\rho_1 = 0.036$	$\rho_1 = 0.077$
$e_2 = 0.012$	$\rho_2 = 0.145$	$\rho_2 = 0.308$
$e_3 = 0.024$	$\rho_3 = 0.289$	$\rho_3 = 0.615$
$e_4 = 0.027$	$\rho_4 = 0.325$	$\rho_4 = 0$
$e_5 = 0.017$	$\rho_5 = 0.205$	$\rho_5 = 0$

is $[1, 5]$, while e_i's increase from 1 up through 4 and then decreased. Our model has so many parameters that we can use observed data to determine reasonable values for some of these parameters. Once these parameter values are determined, we will want to use them to make additional predictions. This is a common exercise in modeling.

EXERCISES

47. Suppose $\mu_1 = \mu_3 = 1/2$, and $\mu_j = 0$ otherwise. Suppose $E_R(B) = 13$, and all parameters k_i, δ, and v' are 1.
    (a) If $\Delta = [1, 3]$, find $E^\circ(B, f, \Delta)$.
    (b) If $\Delta = [1, 3]$, find $n(B, f, \Delta)$ and compare to the expected number of trials to reach $E_R(B)$.
    (c) Calculate $e(B, f, \Delta)$ as estimated in (55) as a function of B and Δ.

48. Repeat Exercise 47 if $\mu_1 = \mu_2 = \mu_3 = 1/3$, $\mu_j = 0$ otherwise, $E_R(B) = 13$, and all parameters k_i, δ, and v' are 1.

49. (a) Calculate $e(B, f, \Delta)$ of (55) in the case where just two types of food items are available, sizes 1 and 2, and $\mu_1 = \mu_2 = 1/2$, and all parameters k_i, δ, and v' are 1.
    (b) Calculate Δ_M if $B = 1$
    (c) Calculate the corresponding ρ_i.
    (d) Show that Δ_M can change if B changes.

50. Discuss how changes in the various parameters affect $e(B, f, \Delta)$ of (55).

51. The maximum element of Δ_M defines the prey-size range R_i. Suppose for fixed B and f, we vary v'. Would you expect this to affect the prey-size range? Why?

52. Suppose for fixed B and v', we keep the μ_i fixed and vary δ. For different δ, Δ_M will change and so will the prey-size range R_i.
    (a) Taking $\mu_1 = \mu_2 = \mu_3 = 1/3$, $\mu_j = 0$ otherwise, and $B = v' = 1$, find Δ_M and R_i for $\delta = 1$, 10, and 100.
    (b) Find mean, standard deviation, and coefficient of variation of R_i.

53. The number $e(B, f, \{l\})$ gives the relative energetic efficiency of the strategy of eating only food item l.

(a) If we could calculate $e(B, f, \{l\})$ exactly (by the method of (46)), would we discover the following:

$$e(B, i) > e(B, j) \text{ iff } e(B, f, \{i\}) > e(B, f, \{j\}), \tag{57}$$

for all i, j and "distributions" f.

(b) Is (57) still the case if we *estimate* $e(B, f, \{l\})$ using (55)?

54. The function $e(B, f, \Delta)$ of (46) or (55) may not have the property that Δ must be an interval to maximize $e(B, f, \Delta)$. For example, using the data in the last column of Table 16, show that for the function of (55),

$$e(B, f, \{3, 5\}) > e(B, f, [3, 5]).$$

55. Explore the implications of this section if the relative time-energy efficiency replaces the relative energetic efficiency.

6. Discussion

We have presented several mathematical models of the energy efficient predator. For a summary of related work, see the bibliographies in the papers by Belovsky [4] and Belovsky and Jordan [5]. In discussing what our models have accomplished, we shall paraphrase Schoener [36]. Models which are both hypothetical and complex such as those presented depend on a variety of unsubstantiated assumptions and involve a great many difficult-to-measure parameters. Some of these parameters can be estimated by trying to fit the models to data, and these parameters in turn can be used in making predictions. Since we are mostly interested in making qualitative predictions, it should not be overly surprising that many different types of qualitative behavior can be predicted. What is interesting to see is how difficult capturing the right qualitative behavior can be, even with such flexibility. Attempts to define the various functions needed to build our models, functions such as THS, point to important gaps in ecological knowledge. Finally, the models suggest interesting and nonobvious new ecological hypotheses, which in turn can give direction to future empirical research in ecology.

References

[1] H. L. Alder and E. B. Roessler, *Introduction to Probability and Statistics*. San Francisco, CA: W. H. Freeman, 1968.

[2] R. Baker, "Five nautical models," this series, volume III, 1982.

[3] E. Batschelet, *Introduction to Mathematics for Life Scientists*. New York: Springer-Verlag, 1971.

[4] G. E. Belovsky, "Diet optimization in a generalist herbivore: The moose," *Theoretical Population Biology*, vol. 14, pp. 105–134, 1978.

[5] G. E. Belovsky and P. A. Jordan, "The time-energy budget of a moose," *Theoretical Population Biology*, vol. 14, pp. 76–104, 1978.

[6] J. T. Bonner, *Size and Cycle*. Princeton, NJ: Princeton Univ. Press, 1965.

[7] H. Brown, *The Challenge of Man's Future*, New York: Viking, 1958.

[8] P. A. Colinvaux, *Introduction to Ecology*. New York: Wiley, 1973.

[9] J. J. Craighead and F. C. Craighead, *Hawks, Owls, and Wildlife*. Harrisburg, PA: Stackpole, 1956.

[10] J. M. Emlen, "The role of time and energy in food preference," *Amer. Natur.*, vol. 100, pp. 611–617, 1966.

[11] F. Grande and H. L. Taylor, "Adaptive changes in the heart, vessels, and patterns of control under chronically high loads," in *Handbook of Physiology*, J. Field, Ed., vol. 3. Washington, D. C.: Amer. Physiol. Soc., 1965, section 2, pp. 2615–2677.

[12] F. R. Hainsworth and L. L. Wolf, "Power for hovering flight in relation to body size in hummingbirds," *Amer. Natur*, vol. 106, pp. 589–596, 1972.

[13] A. M. Hemmingsen, "The relation of standard (basal) energy metabolism to total fresh weight of living organisms," *Rept. Steno Hosp.* (Copenhagen), vol. 4, pp. 7–58, 1950.

[14] ——, "Energy metabolism as related to body size and respiratory surfaces, and its evolution," *Rept. Steno Hosp.*, vol. 9, pp. 7–110, 1960.

[15] A. V. Hill, "The dimensions of animals and their muscular dynamics," *Sci. Progress*, vol. 150, pp. 209–230, 1950.

[16] B. Hocking, "The intrinsic range and speed of flight of insects," *Roy. Entomol. Soc. London Trans.*, vol. 104, pp. 223–345, 1953.

[17] C. S. Holling, "The functional response of invertebrate predators to prey density," *Entomol. Soc. Can. Mem.*, vol. 48, pp. 1–86, 1966.

[18] J. S. Huxley, *Problems of Relative Growth*. London: Methuen, 1932.

[19] V. S. Ivlev, *Experimental Ecology of the Feeding of Fishes*. New Haven, CT: Yale Univ. Press, 1961.

[20] M. Kleiber, "Body size and metabolism," *Hilgardia*, vol. 6, pp. 315–353, 1932.

[21] ——, "Dietary deficiencies and energy metabolism," *Nutrition Abstracts and Reviews*, vol. 15, pp. 207–222, 1945–1946.

[22] ——, *The Fire of Life (An Introduction to Animal Energetics)*. New York: Wiley, 1961.

[23] R. C. Lasiewski and W. R. Dawson, "A re-examination of the relation between standard metabolic rate and body weight in birds," *Condor*, vol. 69, pp. 13–23, 1967.

[24] A. L. Lehninger, *Bioenergetics*. Menlo Park, CA: W. A. Benjamin, 1973.

[25] R. H. MacArthur and R. Levins, "Competition, habitat selection, and character displacement in a patchy environment," *Nat. Acad. Sci. Proc.*, vol. 51, pp. 1207–1210, 1964.

[26] R. H. MacArthur and E. Pianka, "On optimal use of a patchy environment," *Amer. Natur.*, vol. 100, pp. 603–609, 1966.

[27] H. Marcus-Roberts, "A comparison of some deterministic and stochastic models of population," this volume, chapter 3.

[28] G. T. Miller, *Energetics, Kinetics, and Life: An Ecological Approach*. Belmont, CA: Wadsworth, 1971.

[29] E. P. Odum, *Ecology*. New York: Holt, Rinehart and Winston, 1966.

[30] J. Phillipson, *Ecological Energetics*. New York: St. Martin's, 1966.

[31] K. Reid, *Nature's Network*. London: Aldus Books, 1969.

[32] R. E. Ricklefs, *Ecology*. Newton, MA: Chiron Press, 1973.

[33] F. S. Roberts, "Efficiency of energy use in obtaining food, I: Humans," this volume, chapter 10.

[34] R. Rosen, *Optimality Principles in Biology*. London: Butterworths, 1967.

[35] M. I. Rosenzweig, "Community structure in sympatric carnivora," *J. Mammal.*, vol. 47, pp. 602–612, 1966.

[36] T. W. Schoener, "Models of optimal size for solitary predators," *Amer. Natur.*, vol. 103, pp. 277–313, 1969.

[37] T. W. Schoener and D. H. Janzen, "Some notes on tropical versus temperate insect size patterns," *Amer. Natur.*, vol. 101, pp. 207–224, 1968.

[38] G. G. Simpson, A. Roe, and R. C. Lewontin, *Quantitative Zoology*, rev. ed. New York: Harcourt, Brace, 1960.

[39] J. M. Smith, *Mathematical Ideas in Biology*. New York: Cambridge Univ. Press, 1968.

[40] G. Teissier, "Relative growth," in *The Physiology of Crustacea*, T. H. Waterman, Ed., vol. 1. New York: Academic Press, 1960, ch. 16.

[41] F. Toth, "What the bees know and what they don't know," *Bull. Amer. Math. Soc.*, vol. 17, 1964.

[42] U. N. Food and Agriculture Organization, *Provisional Indicative World Plan for Agricultural Development*. Rome: U. N. Food and Agriculture Organization, 1970.

[43] E. Voit, "Über die Grösse des Energiebedarfs der Tiere in Hungerzustande." *Ztschr. Biol.*, vol. 41, pp. 113–154, 1901.

[44] L. von Bertalanffy, *Theoretische Biologie*, vol. 2, *Stoffwechsel, Wachstum*, 2nd ed. Bern: Francke 1951.

[45] K. E. F. Watt, *Ecology and Resource Management*. New York: McGraw-Hill, 1968.

[46] J. P. Wesley, *Ecophysics: The Application of Physics to Ecology*. Springfield, IL: Charles C. Thomas, 1974.

[47] K. M. Wilbur and G. Owen, "Growth," in *Physiology of Mollusca*, K. M. Wilbur and C. M. Yonge, Eds., vol. 1. New York: Academic Press, 1964, ch. 7.

[48] E. Zeuther, "Oxygen uptake as related to body size in organisms," *Quart. Rev. Biol.*, vol. 28, pp. 1–12, 1953.

Notes for the Instructor

Objectives. This is the second of a series of two chapters on efficiency of energy use in obtaining food. The first chapter deals with human behavior. The two chapters are essentially independent, except that the second chapter depends in places on a few parts of Sections 2 and 3 of the first one.

Prerequisites. Differential and integral calculus are used here, primarily differential calculus as an aid in curve plotting and identifying maxima and minima. Probability theory is also used, but not until Section 4.8, and a few places use techniques from statistics such as mean, SD, and normal distribution. *Most of the chapter can be understood with just the calculus as prerequisite.*

Time. It will probably take several weeks to do this in detail. However, pieces of it, such as the discussion of the allometric law, can be worked into existing courses in less than an hour.

Remarks. The first chapter could be used in a finite math course, a linear programming course, or an introductory O.R. course. Parts of this second chapter might be appropriate in a calculus course, in particular the models of the pure pursuer and the treatment of the allometric law. The two modules taken together, or either chapter alone, would be suitable for a modeling course with the appropriate prerequisites. An attempt is made, especially in this second chapter, to show the development of a mathematical model through several iterations, with predictions from earlier versions tested against information about behavior. Each of the chapters is prepared with possible "open-ended" use in mind. Namely, students could be involved in extending the models presented, investigating alternative approaches, and the like.

If these chapters are used in modeling courses, attention should be drawn to the following:

(1) the difference between the normative or prescriptive approach to human energy use and descriptive approach to animal energy use;

(2) the difference between the deterministic models of the pure pursuer and the stochastic models of the pure searcher;

(3) the large number of different mathematical techniques which are brought to bear on one problem;

(4) the constant attempt, at least in the descriptive models, to test predictions of the models, and to modify them if the predictions do not measure up.

CHAPTER 12

The Spatial Distribution of Cabbage Butterfly Eggs

Daniel L. Solomon*

1. Purpose

The intent of this chapter is to demonstrate, in a realistic biological setting, the usefulness of some of the basic tools of probability theory. It also points out an important feature of mathematical models of biological (or other) phenomena, namely, that several different sets of underlying biological assumptions can lead to the same mathematical model. Thus even if a model is consistent with observation, we cannot conclude that the assumed biological mechanisms on which the model is based are realistic.

2. The Biology

We seek a probability model for the number of eggs of the common cabbage butterfly *Pieris rapae crucivora* found on individual cabbage plants. Experimental evidence (Harcourt [4] and Kobayashi [5]) indicates that this number is well described by the negative binomial distribution. That is, the probability function of the number of eggs, H, per plant is

$$P(H = h) = \binom{h + k - 1}{h} p^k (1 - p)^h, \qquad h = 0, 1, 2, \cdots$$

where $k > 0$ and $0 < p < 1$ are parameters. We do not require k to be an integer and have taken liberty with notation in writing the binomial coefficient with noninteger entries. We mean

* Department of Statistics, North Carolina State University, Raleigh, NC 27650.

$$\binom{h + k - 1}{h} \equiv \frac{(h + k - 1)!}{h!(k - 1)!} \equiv \frac{\Gamma(h + k)}{h!\Gamma(k)}$$

where $\Gamma(\alpha) = \int_0^\infty z^{\alpha-1} e^{-z} dz$ is the gamma function, defined for all $\alpha > 0$. It can be shown using integration by parts that for any $\alpha > 0$, $\Gamma(\alpha + 1) = \alpha\Gamma(\alpha)$. Thus if α is a positive integer, repeated application of this result gives $\Gamma(\alpha + 1) = \alpha!$. In this sense, the gamma function is a generalization of the factorial to nonintegers. Readers unfamiliar with the gamma function will lose little by restricting the parameter k to being a positive integer.

EXERCISE

1. Bliss and Fisher [2] report the following data collected by Dr. Philip Garman of the Connecticut Agricultural Experiment Station. On July 18, 1951, 150 leaves on McIntosh apple trees were selected at random and the number of adult female European red mites on each leaf counted. The 150 leaves were categorized according to the number of mites present and the results are presented in Table 1.

   The negative binomial distribution was postulated as an appropriate model and the parameters of the distribution estimated by $k = 1.0$ and $p = 0.47$. Calculate the negative binomial probabilities, $P(H = h)$ for $h = 0, 1, 2, \cdots, 7$ and $P(H \geq 8)$ for these values of k and p. Multiply each by 150 and compare these frequencies predicted by the negative binomial model with those actually observed. Would you say that the model provides an adequate fit to the data? Hint: Show that $P[H = 0] = p^k$ and that $P[H = h] = [(h + k - 1)/h](1 - p) P[H = h - 1]$ for $h = 1, 2, \cdots$. Use these facts to calculate the required probabilities recursively.

Returning to the cabbage butterfly, we describe a different sort of evidence for the adequacy of the negative binomial model. We note that for the negative binomial distribution, the variance (denoted by σ^2) and mean (denoted by μ) are related by $\sigma^2 = \mu + \mu^2/k$ (see Exercise 2). Thus in *samples* of cabbages, this relationship should be mimicked by the sample

Table 1

Number of Mites per Leaf h	Number of Leaves with h Mites
0	70
1	38
2	17
3	10
4	9
5	3
6	2
7	1
8+	0
Total	150

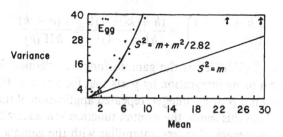

Figure 12.1. Variance-mean Relationships for Counts of Eggs of the Imported Cabbage-worm on Cabbage. Each Point Plotted Is Based on a Sample of 64 to 96 Plants.

variance (S^2) and sample mean (m). Figure 12.1 (after Harcourt [4]) demonstrates that this indeed occurs in data collected during 1957–1960 at Merivale, Ontario. For those data, the parameter k was estimated to be 2.82.

The line denoted $S^2 = m$ represents the Poisson probability law which has variance equal to mean ($\sigma^2 = \mu$) and is often used to describe spatial randomness. Clearly, the negative binomial provides a better fit to these data. Formal statistical tests confirm these graphical results. We now propose two different sets of biological mechanisms, each consistent with a negative binomial model.

3. Biological Assumptions I

Adult female butterflies visit individual plants "at random," laying clusters of eggs. The environment is homogeneous in that all plants are equally attractive to the females. We also suppose that the number of eggs in a cluster follows the same probability distribution for each cluster, and that the number of eggs in a given cluster is independent of the number in any other and of the number of clusters. Thus the females are assumed, in particular, not to become depleted or be influenced by the number of clusters that they see already deposited.

Mathematical Model I

We interpret "at random" to mean that the number of egg clusters N found per cabbage plant can be adequately described by a Poisson distribution. That this is a reasonable choice may be argued as follows. The plant can be viewed as a collection of a large number of potential cluster sites. Suppose each site receives or fails to receive a cluster independently of all other sites. Suppose further that the probability that a site does receive a cluster is small and the same for all sites. Then the number of clusters on the plant has the binomial distribution. Thus decisions to fill or not fill each site with a cluster could be achieved by a mechanism equivalent to flipping a biased coin, and so the term "at random." Now it can be shown (most easily using probability generating functions) that the binomial distribution with large number of "trials" (sites) each with small probability of "success" (containing a cluster) can be well approximated by a Poisson distribution.

The homogeneity of plants is taken to mean that the parameter $\lambda > 0$ of this Poisson distribution is the same for each plant. Symbolically,

$$P[N = n] = \frac{e^{-\lambda}\lambda^n}{n!}, \qquad n = 0, 1, 2, \cdots.$$

If we assume that the probability distribution for the number X of eggs per cluster, is the logarithmic, then X has probability function

$$P[X = x] = -\frac{1}{\ln p}\frac{(1-p)^x}{x}, \qquad x = 1, 2, \cdots,$$

where p is a parameter $0 < p < 1$. Note that a cluster must contain at least one egg. Some motivation for this choice of distribution is given in Fisher et al. [3].

If now we let H denote the number of eggs per cabbage plant, then the independence assumptions imply that H is the sum of a random number N of independent random variables, i.e., $H = X_1 + X_2 + \cdots + X_N$, where $X_1, X_2, \cdots$ is a sequence of independent random variables, each with the logarithmic distribution and each independent of the random variable N.

We will demonstrate that H has the negative binomial distribution by calculating its probability generating function (PGF). Recall that the PGF of a discrete random variable H taking values 0, 1, 2, $\cdots$ is defined for $|t| \leq 1$, by

$$\phi_H(t) \equiv E(t^H).$$

Here $H = X_1 + X_2 + \cdots + X_N$ and using properties of PGF's and conditional expectation, it can be shown that

$$\phi_H(t) = \phi_N(\phi_X(t)).$$

To apply this result here, we first derive the PGF ϕ_X of the logarithmic distribution.

$$\phi_X(t) \equiv E(t^X) = \sum_{x=1}^{\infty} t^x P[X = x]$$

$$= -\frac{1}{\ln p}\sum_{x=1}^{\infty} t^x \frac{(1-p)^x}{x}$$

$$= -\frac{1}{\ln p}\sum_{x=1}^{\infty} \frac{[t(1-p)]^x}{x}$$

$$= \frac{1}{\ln p}\ln[1 - t(1-p)], \qquad \text{for } |t(1-p)| < 1,$$

where the last equality follows from the series expansion of the natural logarithm. Also, since N has the Poisson distribution with parameter λ, its PGF is (for all real numbers s),

$$\phi_N(s) = e^{\lambda(s-1)}.$$

Thus

$$\phi_H(t) = \phi_N(\phi_X(t)) = e^{\lambda(\phi_X(t)-1)}$$

$$= \exp\left\{\lambda\left[\frac{\ln\left[1 - t(1 - p)\right]}{\ln p} - 1\right]\right\}, \quad \text{for } |t(1 - p)| < 1.$$

If we now substitute $k = -\lambda/\ln p \ (>0)$, we have

$$\phi_H(t) = \exp\left\{-k \ln\left[1 - t(1 - p)\right] + k \ln p\right\}$$

$$= \exp\left\{\ln\left[1 - t(1 - p)\right]^{-k}\right\} \cdot \exp\left\{\ln p^k\right\}$$

$$= \left[1 - t(1 - p)\right]^{-k} p^k$$

$$= \left[\frac{p}{1 - t(1 - p)}\right]^k, \quad \text{for } |t(1 - p)| < 1.$$

However, this is the PGF of a random variable with the negative binomial distribution with parameters k and p. By the uniqueness theorem for PGF's, H must have probability function

$$P[H = h] = \binom{h + k - 1}{h} p^k(1 - p)^h, \quad h = 0, 1, 2, \cdots.$$

EXERCISE

2. Use the probability generating function to calculate the mean (μ) and variance (σ^2) of H and confirm that the relationship $\sigma^2 = \mu + \mu^2/k$ asserted earlier indeed holds.

We now describe a different and contradictory set of biological assumptions which we will show lead to the same distribution for H.

4. Biological Assumptions II

Contrary to the assumptions in the first model, eggs are not laid in clusters but are spatially distributed at random on the cabbage plants. Furthermore, unlike the first model, individual heads are not equally attractive to the female butterflies, differing in size, condition, and location (e.g., border versus interior of the plot or orientation with respect to the sun), and so the mean number of eggs varies from head to head according to some probability law.

Mathematical Model II

We interpret the assumptions to mean that for a given plant, the number of eggs H has a conditional Poisson distribution with mean λ, characteristic of the plant. The Poisson assumption is motivated as in the first model but here applied to individual eggs rather than clusters. Values of λ vary across the population of plants, and we suppose that its probability law can be adequately represented by a gamma distribution. Thus the conditional probability function of H for given λ is

$$P[H = h|\lambda] = \frac{e^{-\lambda}\lambda^h}{h!}, \qquad h = 0, 1, 2, \cdots, \lambda > 0,$$

and we have taken the probability density function for λ to be

$$f(\lambda) = \frac{\mu^k}{\Gamma(k)}\lambda^{k-1}e^{-\lambda\mu}, \qquad \lambda > 0$$

where $\mu > 0$ and $k > 0$ are parameters. We argue that by varying μ and k we can generate a rich class of distributions among which we should be able to find one to adequately describe the variability of λ across the population of plants. Notice that H is a discrete random variable but that λ is continuous. We seek the marginal probability function of H which for $h = 0, 1, 2, \cdots$ is

$$P[H = h] = \int_0^\infty P[H = h|\lambda] f(\lambda)d\lambda$$

$$= \int_0^\infty \frac{e^{-\lambda}\lambda^h}{h!} \frac{\mu^k}{\Gamma(k)}\lambda^{k-1}e^{-\lambda\mu}d\lambda$$

$$= \frac{\mu^k}{h!\Gamma(k)} \int_0^\infty \lambda^{h+k-1}e^{-\lambda(\mu+1)}d\lambda.$$

EXERCISE

3. Verify the next equality.

$$= \frac{\mu^k}{h!\Gamma(k)} \frac{\Gamma(h + k)}{(\mu + 1)^{h+k}}$$

$$= \frac{\mu^k}{h!(k - 1)!} \frac{(h + k - 1)!}{(\mu + 1)^{h+k}}.$$

We have again taken liberty with notation in writing $\Gamma(k) = (k - 1)!$ even for non-integral k.

$$= \binom{h + k - 1}{h} \left(\frac{\mu}{\mu + 1}\right)^k \left(1 - \frac{\mu}{\mu + 1}\right)^h$$

$$= \binom{h + k - 1}{h} p^k(1 - p)^h$$

where we have written $0 < p \equiv \mu/(\mu + 1) < 1$.

Thus as in model I, H has the negative binomial distribution with parameters k and p. Of course, the interpretation of the parameters is different under the two models. We conclude that even though the observed number of eggs per plant is well fit by the negative binomial distribution, more information is required to decide between the two possible mechanisms (neither of which need, of course, be correct). We emphasize that the biological assumptions on which the two models are based are not only different but are in fact *contradictory*. In the absence of additional information we might, nevertheless, make predictions about, say, the mean number of eggs per plant $(E(H) = k(1 - p)/p)$ and thus about future butterfly population sizes. Such predictions could have implications for control decisions with important economic consequences.

For the curious reader, we remark that, for this particular population, experiments have been performed in a net house to observe the detailed behavior of the female cabbage butterfly. Peripheral plants and those nearer the light source were favored, but under uniform light conditions, the butterflies visited interior plants at random (Poisson). The independence assumption made in model I was also tested and found tenable. Model I is thus currently held as the most appropriate description of the biological mechanism. Details are available in Kobayashi [5].

There are numerous other sets of plausible biological assumptions which might be proposed, several of which lead to the negative binomial distribution. We briefly describe one more here, leaving the mathematical details to the reader.

5. Biological Assumptions III

Each cabbage plant has k "sites" upon which eggs can be laid. There are enough female butterflies so that every site on every cabbage will be visited, and some number (perhaps 0) of eggs will be laid on each site. Each site is visited exactly once.

The reproductive mechanism is such that occasionally a "defective" egg is produced. This happens with probability p independently of the number of eggs previously produced. Eggs are laid by a given female on a given site, one at a time, until the first defective egg is deposited. Then she stops.

Mathematical Model III

Denote by Y_i, the number of nondefective eggs laid on the ith site. Then Y_1, $Y_2, \cdots, Y_k$ are independent random variables with the same probability function, and the total number of nondefective eggs per cabbage is $H = Y_1 + Y_2 + \cdots + Y_k$.

4. Deduce the common probability function of $Y_1, Y_2, \cdots, Y_k$ and its probability generating function. Use this to deduce the probability generating function of H and thus its probability function. Compare your results with models I and II.

6. Suggestions for Further Study

There are several other ways to construct a mathematical model for biological population sizes which lead to the negative binomial distribution. The models we have considered are spatial, i.e., describe the number of individuals per unit area (e.g., per cabbage plant). Other models are temporal, allowing for features like birth, death and immigration and describing the number of individuals present at a given time after the inception of the process. The mathematical techniques required are slightly more advanced than those used here, and the interested reader is referred in this regard to Bailey [1] for an introduction to this field of probability known as stochastic processes. We note that although not easily applicable to the cabbage butterfly biology, at least three processes lead to the negative binomial distribution for $H(t)$, the number of individuals present at time t.

1. The "pure birth process" (Bailey [1, pp. 84–87]). Suppose $H(t)$ is the number of offspring at time t of k independently reproducing individuals, each of whom gives birth to a single offspring (or divides into two new individuals) in the small time interval $(t, t + \Delta t)$ with probability approximately $\lambda \Delta t$. If also, new offspring follow the same reproductive behavior, then $H(t)$ has the negative binomial distribution with parameters k and $p \equiv p(t) = e^{-\lambda t}$.

2. The "Polya process" (Bailey [1, pp. 107–110]). If we allow both random immigration and birth with probabilities specified as follows, then the resulting process is known as the Polya process. In particular, if an immigrant arrives in a short interval $(t, t + \Delta t)$ with probability approximately $\lambda(1 + \lambda \mu t)^{-1} \Delta t$ and if an existing individual gives birth in such an interval with probability $\lambda \mu (1 + \lambda \mu t)^{-1} \Delta t$ and if births and immigrations are all independent, then $H(t)$, the number of individuals present at time t has the negative binomial distribution with parameters $k = 1/\mu$ and $p \equiv p(t) = (1 + \lambda \mu t)^{-1}$. Note that we start with no individuals and that the environment is assumed to be degraded in such a way that the immigration and birth probabilities decrease with time.

3. The "linear birth, death, and immigration process" (Bailey [1, pp. 99–101]). Suppose that the population begins with zero individuals and that in a short time interval $(t, t + \Delta t)$, an immigrant arrives, an existing individual gives birth to a single offspring, or an existing individual dies, with respective probabilities approximately $v\Delta t$, $\lambda \Delta t$, or $\mu \Delta t$. Then $H(t)$, the number of individuals present at time t follows the negative binomial distribution with parameters $k = v/\lambda$ and $p \equiv p(t) = (\lambda - \mu)/(\lambda e^{(\lambda - \mu)t} - \mu)$.

Appendix: Probability Generating Functions

We assume that the reader is already familiar with the basic properties of discrete and continuous random variables, their joint, marginal, and conditional probability (density) functions and expectations. The notation should be self-explanatory. We will introduce a set of tools which are useful both for calculating moments of distributions and for finding distributions of certain functions of random variables.

Definition. Let X be a *discrete* random variable taking values 0, 1, 2, 3, $\cdots$ and with probability function $f_X(x) = P[X = x]$. For real numbers t let

$$\phi_X(t) = Et^X.$$

Then (provided that the expectation exists for $|t| \leq 1$) ϕ_X is called the *probability generating function* (PGF) of X. It is also referred to as the *factorial moment generating function* of X.

Note: A corresponding theory, that of moment generating functions, applies to both discrete and continuous random variables. Most probability textbooks at this level treat that theory.

By writing

$$\phi_X(t) = Et^X = \sum_{x=0}^{\infty} t^x f_X(x)$$

$$= f_X(0) + t f_X(1) + t^2 f_X(2) + \cdots + t^k f_X(k) + \cdots$$

we observe that $\phi_X(0) = f_X(0) = P[X = 0]$ and $\phi_X(1) = 1$. Now

$$\frac{\partial}{\partial t} \phi_X(t) \equiv \phi_X'(t) = f_X(1) + 2t f_X(2) + 3t^2 f_X(3) + \cdots + k t^{k-1} f_X(k) + \cdots$$

so that $\phi_X'(0) = f_X(1) = P[X = 1]$ and

$$\phi_X'(1) = 1 f_X(1) + 2 f_X(2) + 3 f_X(3) + \cdots + k f_X(k) + \cdots$$

$$= \sum_{x=0}^{\infty} x f_X(x) = EX.$$

Similarly,

$$\phi_X''(t) = 2 \cdot 1 f_X(2) + 3 \cdot 2t f_X(3) + 4 \cdot 3t^2 f_X(4) + \cdots$$

$$+ k(k - 1)t^{k-2} f_X(k) + \cdots$$

so that $\phi_X''(0) = 2 f_X(2) = 2P[X = 2]$ and $\phi_X''(1) = EX(X - 1)$. By repeatedly differentiating we see that for $k = 1, 2, \cdots$, the kth derivative of $\phi_X(t)$ with respect to t has the following properties:

Theorem A1. *If X is a discrete random variable with probability generating function $\phi_X(t)$, then for $k = 1, 2, \cdots$*

$$\left.\frac{\phi_X^{(k)}(t)}{k!}\right|_{t=0} = P[X = k]$$

and

$$\phi_X^{(k)}(t)|_{t=1} = E[X(X - 1)(X - 2) \cdots (X - k + 1)].$$

Thus ϕ_X generates probabilities and factorial moments. $(E[X(X - 1)(X - 2) \cdots (X - k + 1)]$ is called the kth factorial moment of X.)

EXAMPLE A1. Suppose that X has the distribution binomial (n, p). Then the PGF of X is

$$\phi_X(t) = Et^X = \sum_{x=0}^{n} t^x \binom{n}{x} p^x(1 - p)^{n-x}$$

$$= \sum_{x=0}^{n} \binom{n}{x} (tp)^x(1 - p)^{n-x}$$

$$= (1 - p + tp)^n \qquad \text{by the binomial theorem.}$$

Now $\phi_X(0) = (1 - p)^n = P[X = 0]$ and

$$\phi_X(1) = (1 - p + p)^n = 1.$$

Also $\phi_X'(t) = np(1 - p + pt)^{n-1}$ so that

$$\phi_X'(0) = np(1 - p)^{n-1} = P[X = 1]$$

and

$$\phi_X'(1) = np = EX.$$

Finally, $\phi_X''(t) = n(n - 1)p^2(1 - p + pt)^{n-2}$ and so

$$\phi_X''(0) = n(n - 1)p^2(1 - p)^{n-2} = 2!P[X = 2]$$

$$\phi_X''(1) = n(n - 1)p^2 = EX(X - 1).$$

Thus

$$\begin{aligned}
\text{var}(X) &= E(X^2) - (EX)^2 \\
&= EX(X - 1) + EX - (EX)^2 \\
&= n(n - 1)p^2 + np - (np)^2 \\
&= np(1 - p).
\end{aligned}$$

By similar calculations, we can show that

$$\phi_X^{(k)}(0) = k!\binom{n}{k} p^k(1 - p)^{n-k}$$

$$\phi_X^{(k)}(1) = k!\binom{n}{k} p^k, \qquad \text{for } k = 1, 2, \cdots, n.$$

EXERCISE

A1. Find the probability generating function for a random variable Y with the Poisson distribution with parameter λ. Use theorem A1 to find the kth factorial moment of Y.

Theorem A2. *If X is a random variable with PGF ϕ_X, if a and b are real numbers, and if we define a random variable $Y = aX + b$, then the PGF of Y is $\phi_Y(t) = t^b \phi_X(t^a)$.*

PROOF. $\phi_Y(t) = E(t^{aX+b}) = E(t^{aX} t^b) = t^b E\left[(t^a)^X\right] = t^b \phi_X(t^a).$ $\qquad\square$

Theorem A3. *If X and Y are independent random variables with PGF's ϕ_X and ϕ_Y respectively, then the PGF of their sum is $\phi_{X+Y}(t) = \phi_X(t)\phi_Y(t)$.*

EXERCISE

A2. Prove theorem A3.

Corollary. *If $X_1, X_2, \cdots, X_n$ are independent random variables with PGF's $\phi_1, \phi_2, \cdots, \phi_n$ respectively, then the PGF of the sum $S = X_1 + X_2 + \cdots + X_n$ is $\phi_S(t) = \prod_{i=1}^{n} \phi_i(t)$.*

EXAMPLE A2. Suppose $X_1, X_2, \cdots, X_k$ are independent random variables, each with the geometric distribution with common probability function $f_X(x) = P(X = x) = p(1 - p)^x; x = 0, 1, 2, \cdots, \quad 0 < p < 1.$

EXERCISE

A3. Show that the common PGF of the X_i is $\phi(t) = \dfrac{p}{1 - t(1 - p)}$ for $|t(1 - p)| < 1$.

Now letting $Z = X_1 + X_2 + \cdots + X_k$, the PGF of Z is

$$\phi_Z(t) = \prod_{i=1}^{k} \phi_{X_i}(t) = [\phi(t)]^k = \left[\frac{p}{1 - t(1 - p)}\right]^k.$$

From a table of PGF's or by direct calculation, we could show that this is the PGF of a random variable with the negative binomial distribution with parameters k and p. Can we conclude that Z has this distribution? Yes, but to do so we need a "uniqueness theorem" which asserts that there is a one-to-one correspondence between PGF's and probability functions. The following is such a theorem.

Theorem A4. *If X and Y are random variables taking values $0, 1, 2, \cdots$ with PGF's ϕ_X and ϕ_Y, respectively, and if $\phi_X(t) = \phi_Y(t)$ for all $|t| \leq 1$, then the corresponding probability functions are equal, i.e., $P[X = k] = P[Y = k]$, $k = 0, 1, 2, \cdots$.*

PROOF. The proof requires familiarity with power series expansions and follows directly from a uniqueness theorem for such series.   □

Theorem A5. *Suppose $X_1, X_2, \cdots$ is a sequence of discrete random variables, independent and identically distributed with common PGF $\phi_X(t)$. Suppose that N is a positive integer valued random variable independent of the X_i and with PGF $\phi_N(t)$. Then the random sum $Z = X_1 + X_2 + \cdots + X_N$ has PGF $\phi_Z(t) = \phi_N(\phi_X(t))$.*

PROOF. $\phi_Z(t) = Et^Z = E[E\{t^{X_1 + X_2 + \cdots + X_N} | N\}]$.

by the properties of conditional expectation;

$$= E[E(t^{X_1}|N)E(t^{X_2}|N) \cdots E(t^{X_N}|N)]$$
$$= E[E(t^{X_1})E(t^{X_2}) \cdots E(t^{X_N})]$$

by the independence of N from the X_i;

$$= E[\phi_X(t) \cdot \phi_X(t) \cdots \phi_X(t)]$$

since the X_i are identically distributed with PGF ϕ_X;

$$= E[\phi_X(t)]^N$$
$$= \phi_N(\phi_X(t))$$

by the definition of the PGF of N, when evaluated at $\phi_X(t)$.   □

EXERCISE

A4. Suppose that the number N of fish eggs laid on a unit area of stream bottom has the Poisson distribution with parameter λ. Suppose that laid eggs hatch independently with probability p. Define a sequence of independent and identically distributed random variables $X_1, X_2, \cdots$ where $P(X_i = 1) = 1 - P(X_i = 0) = p$. Then the total number of hatchlings found per unit area of stream bottom is the random sum $Z = X_1 + X_2 + \cdots + X_N$. Use theorems A5 and A4 to deduce the PGF and then the probability function of Z.

We state a final theorem without proof and then provide an example of its applicability.

Theorem A6. (Continuity Theorem). *Suppose that $X_1, X_2, \cdots$ is a sequence of random variables taking values $0, 1, 2, \cdots$ with PGF's $\phi_{X_1}, \phi_{X_2}, \cdots$ and probability functions $f_{X_1}, f_{X_2}, \cdots$ respectively. Let X be a random variable with PGF ϕ_X and probability function f_X. Then $\lim_{n \to \infty} f_{X_n}(x) = f_X(x)$ for all $x = 0, 1, 2, \cdots$, if and only if*

$$\lim_{n \to \infty} \phi_{X_n}(t) = \phi_X(t), \quad \text{for all } |t| \le 1.$$

EXAMPLE A3. For each positive integer $n = 1, 2, \cdots$, suppose that X_n has the binomial distribution with parameters n and p. Then from example A1, the PGF of X_n is $\phi_{X_n}(t) = (q + pt)^n$ where $q \equiv 1 - p$. We write $\lambda = EX_n = np$ and ask about the limiting distribution of X_n as $n \to \infty$ and $p \to 0$ in such a way that λ remains constant. Thus

$$\phi_{X_n}(t) = (q + pt)^n = \left(1 - \frac{\lambda}{n} + \frac{\lambda}{n}t\right)^n = \left(1 + \frac{\lambda(t - 1)}{n}\right)^n \text{ and so}$$

$$\lim_{n \to \infty} \phi_{X_n}(t) = \lim_{n \to \infty} \left(1 + \frac{\lambda(t - 1)}{n}\right)^n = e^{\lambda(t-1)}.$$

This is the PGF of a random variable with the Poisson distribution with parameter λ and so from the continuity theorem we conclude that for all $x = 0, 1, 2, \cdots$,

$$\lim_{n \to \infty} \binom{n}{x} p^x q^{n-x} = \frac{e^{-\lambda} \lambda^x}{x!},$$

where the limit is taken with $\lambda = np$ fixed. Thus for large n and small p, we may *approximate*

$$\binom{n}{x} p^x (1 - p)^{n-x} \quad \text{by} \quad \frac{e^{-np}(np)^x}{x!}.$$

EXERCISE

A5. Find a large k, small $q = 1 - p$ approximation to the negative binomial distribution. That is, suppose that X_k has the negative binomial distribution with PGF $\phi_{X_k}(t) = [p/(1 - qt)]^k$. Write $\lambda = kq$ and substitute for p and q in terms of λ in $\phi_X(t)$. Then take the limit as $k \to \infty$ and appeal to the continuity theorem as in example A3.

Solutions to the Exercises

1. $P(H = h) = \dfrac{\Gamma(h + k)}{h!\Gamma(k)} p^k (1 - p)^h, \qquad h = 0, 1, 2, \cdots$

   $= \dfrac{(h + k - 1)\Gamma(h + k - 1)}{h(h - 1)!\Gamma(k)} p^k (1 - p)^{h-1}(1 - p), \qquad h = 1, 2, \cdots$

   $= \dfrac{(h + k - 1)}{h}(1 - p)\dfrac{\Gamma(h - 1 + k)}{(h - 1)!\Gamma(k)} p^k (1 - p)^{h-1}$

   $= \dfrac{(h + k - 1)}{h}(1 - p)P(H = h - 1).$

Also $P[H = 0] = p^k$. Thus the probabilities can be computed recursively. For $p = 0.47, k = 1, P(H = 0) = 0.47$ and so $150P(H = 0) = 70.50$. Also for $h = 1, 2, \cdots$, $P(H = h) = [(h + 1 - 1)/h] (1 - 0.47) P(H = h - 1) = 0.53P(H =$

$h - 1$). That is, $P(H = 1) = 0.53P(H = 0) = (0.53)(0.47)$, $P(H = 2) = (0.53)^2$ (0.47), and so on. Multiplying each probability by 150 gives the predicted frequencies tabulated below. The fit to the observed data is clearly quite good. The fit can even be slightly improved using other estimators for k and p.

h	Observed Frequency	Predicted Frequency
0	70	70.50
1	38	37.37
2	17	19.80
3	10	10.50
4	9	5.56
5	3	2.95
6	2	1.56
7	1	0.83
8+	0	0.93
Total	150	150.00

2. $\phi_H(t) = \left[\dfrac{p}{1 - t(1 - p)}\right]^k$.

$\phi_H'(t) = k\left[\dfrac{p}{1 - t(1 - p)}\right]^{k-1} \dfrac{p(1 - p)}{[1 - t(1 - p)]^2} = \dfrac{k(1 - p)}{p}\left[\dfrac{p}{1 - t(1 - p)}\right]^{k+1}$.

$\mu \equiv EH = \phi_H'(1) = \dfrac{k(1 - p)}{p}$.

$\phi_H''(t) = \dfrac{k(1 - p)(k + 1)}{p}\left[\dfrac{p}{1 - t(1 - p)}\right]^k \dfrac{p(1 - p)}{[1 - t(1 - p)]^2}$

$= \dfrac{k(k + 1)(1 - p)^2}{p^2}\left[\dfrac{p}{1 - t(1 - p)}\right]^{k+2}$.

$EH^2 - EH = EH(H - 1) = \phi_H''(1) = \dfrac{k(k + 1)(1 - p)^2}{p^2}$.

$\sigma^2 \equiv \operatorname{var} H = EH^2 - (EH)^2 = EH(H - 1) + EH - (EH)^2$

$= \dfrac{k(k + 1)(1 - p)^2}{p^2} + \dfrac{k(1 - p)}{p} - \left[\dfrac{k(1 - p)}{p}\right]^2$

$= \dfrac{k(1 - p)^2}{p^2} + \dfrac{k(1 - p)}{p}$

$= \mu^2/k + \mu$.

3. $\int_0^\infty \lambda^{h+k-1} e^{-\lambda(\mu+1)}\, d\lambda$ can be evaluated at least two ways. The integral is (up to a constant) the density of the gamma distribution with parameters $\mu + 1$ and $h + k$. The constant required to make it a probability density with integral 1 is $(\mu + 1)^{h+k}/\Gamma(h + k)$ and so its reciprocal is the value of the required integral. An alternative derivation follows by the change of variable $z = \lambda(\mu + 1)$ and $d\lambda = dz/(\mu + 1)$.

4. The biological assumptions imply that egg laying proceeds as a sequence of independent (Bernoulli) trials with probability $p(0 < p < 1)$ of a defective egg ("success") being produced on each trial. Thus if Y is the number of nondefective eggs laid on a particular site,

$$P[Y = y] = P[y \text{ nondefective eggs produced followed by a defective one}]$$

$$= (1 - p)^y \cdot p, \quad \text{for } y = 0, 1, 2, \cdots.$$

The probability generating function for Y is thus

$$\phi_Y(t) = Et^Y = \sum_{y=0}^{\infty} t^y (1 - p)^y p = p \sum_{y=0}^{\infty} [t(1 - p)]^y$$

$$= \frac{p}{1 - t(1 - p)}, \quad \text{for } |t(1 - p)| < 1$$

from the geometric series. Now $H = Y_1 + Y_2 + \cdots + Y_k$ and $Y_1, Y_2, \cdots, Y_k$ are independent and identically distributed so that

$$\phi_H(t) = Et^H = E(t^{Y_1 + Y_2 + \cdots + Y_k})$$

$$= (Et^{Y_1})(Et^{Y_2}) \cdots (Et^{Y_k})$$

$$= [\phi_Y(t)]^k$$

$$= \left[\frac{p}{1 - t(1 - p)} \right]^k$$

which is the PGF for the negative binomial distribution with parameters k and p.

This is the same result as in models I and II, so that we have established yet another mechanism consistent with experimental evidence.

A1. $\phi_Y(t) = Et^Y = \sum_{y=0}^{\infty} t^y \frac{e^{-\lambda} \lambda^y}{y!}$

$$= e^{-\lambda} \sum_{y=0}^{\infty} (\lambda t)^y / y!$$

$$= e^{-\lambda} e^{\lambda t}$$

$$= e^{\lambda(t-1)}.$$

$\phi_Y^{(k)}(t) = \lambda^k e^{\lambda(t-1)}$ so that the kth factorial moment is $EY(Y - 1) \cdots (Y - k + 1)$
$= \phi_Y^{(k)}(1) = \lambda^k$.

A2. $\phi_{X+Y}(t) = E(t^{X+Y})$

$$= E(t^X t^Y)$$

$$= (Et^X)(Et^Y),$$

by independence;

$$= \phi_X(t) \phi_Y(t).$$

A3. $\phi(t) = Et^X = \sum_{x=0}^{\infty} t^x p(1 - p)^x$

$$= p \sum_{x=0}^{\infty} [t(1-p)]^x$$

$$= p \frac{1}{1 - t(1-p)}, \quad \text{if } |t(1-p)| < 1 \text{ by the geometric series.}$$

A4. $\phi_Z(t) = \phi_N(\phi_X(t))$ where $\phi_N(t) = e^{\lambda(t-1)}$ and $\phi_X(t) = \Sigma_{x=0}^1 t^x P(X = x) = P(X = 0) + tP(X = 1) = q + pt$ where $q = 1 - p$. Thus

$$\phi_Z(t) = e^{\lambda[(q+pt)-1]} = e^{\lambda[1-p+pt-1]} = e^{\lambda p(t-1)}.$$

Thus Z has the Poisson distribution with parameter λp.

A5.
$$\phi_{X_k}(t) = \left(\frac{p}{1 - qt} \right)^k = \frac{(1 - \lambda/k)^k}{(1 - \frac{\lambda}{k}t)^k}.$$

So

$$\lim_{\substack{k \to \infty \\ q \to 0}} \phi_{X_k}(t) = \frac{e^{-\lambda}}{e^{-\lambda t}} = e^{\lambda(t-1)}.$$

$$\lambda = kq \text{ fixed.}$$

Thus for large k and small q (large p) we can approximate the negative binomial probability function with parameters k and p by the Poisson with parameter $\lambda = k(1 - p)$.

References

[1] N. T. J. Bailey, *The Elements of Stochastic Processes with Applications to the Natural Sciences.* New York: Wiley, 1964.
[2] C. I. Bliss and R. A. Fisher, "Fitting the negative binomial distribution to biological data," *Biometrics*, vol. 9, pp. 176–200, 1953.
[3] R. A. Fisher, A. S. Corbett, and C. B. Williams, "The relation between the number of species and the number of individuals in a random sample of an animal population," *J. Animal Ecol.*, vol. 12, pp. 42–58, 1943.
[4] D. G. Harcourt, "Spatial pattern of the imported cabbageworm, *Pieris rapae* (L.) (Lepidoptera: Pieridae), on cultivated cruciferae," *Can. Ent.*, vol. 93, pp. 945–52, 1961.
[5] S. Kobayashi, "Influence of parental density on the distribution pattern of eggs in the common cabbage butterfly, *Pieris rapae crucivora*," *Res. Popul. Ecol.*, vol. 7, pp. 109–17, 1965.
[6] ——, "Process generating the distribution pattern of eggs of the common cabbage butterfly, *Pieris rapae crucivora*," *Res. Popul. Ecol.*, vol. 8, pp. 51–61, 1966.

Notes for the Instructor

Objectives. To be used in a first course in post-calculus probability. The intent is to provide applications of conditional expectation, probability generating functions, and other basic tools in a realistic biological setting and to emphasize the inductive component of mathematical modelling.

Prerequisites. One year of calculus and the basic notions of random variables, probability distributions, and expectations.

Time. If used as lecture material, the application can be covered in one to two hours. The required probability theory, provided as an appendix, can be treated in one to two further hours assuming that the basic properties of discrete and continuous random variables, their joint, conditional and marginal distributions and expectations have been previously studied. Exercises are distributed throughout the text, and solutions are provided separately.

Remarks. This chapter is intended to be used in connection with an introductory probability course with one year of calculus as prerequisite. The chapter has two components, both of which can be given to the student for self study. Solutions to the homework problems appearing within the text are provided separately.

One component is an appendix which serves as a compendium of the standard results concerning probability generating functions. It includes examples and exercises and can be used either to supplement class lectures or form a basis for them.

The other component is a biological application which assumes knowledge of the technical material in the appendix but does not refer to the appendix explicitly. Thus if the appendix material has been previously covered, the application can be distributed separately. The intent of the application is several-fold. It demonstrates the use of some basic tools of probability theory, it provides a realistic biological setting to illustrate the usefulness of the mathematics, and it makes an important point about mathematical modelling, namely, that goodness of fit of a mathematical model to an observable phenomenon does not guarantee that the biological (or other) premises of the model are correct.